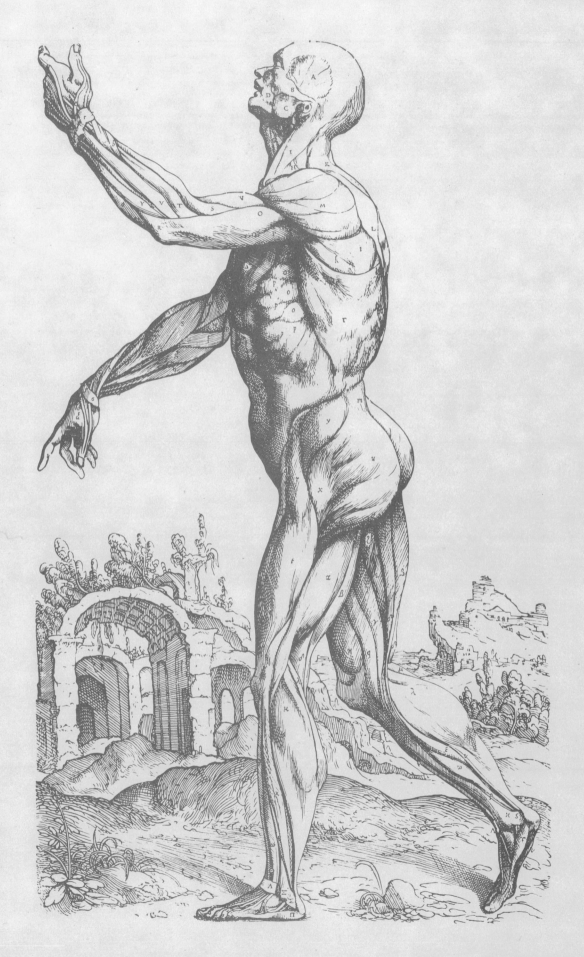

ANATOMY

ANATOMY

A Regional Atlas of the Human Body

CARMINE D. CLEMENTE PH.D.

Professor of Anatomy,

*University of California
at Los Angeles School of Medicine;*

Professor of Surgery (Anatomy),

Charles R. Drew

*Postgraduate Medical School,
Los Angeles, California*

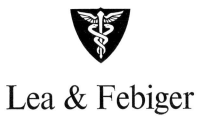

Lea & Febiger

Philadelphia · 1975

The pictures on the end leaves of the present volume show reproductions of the work of "Andreas Vesalii de corporis humani fabrica libri septem", which appeared in Basel in 1542. Andreas Vesalius (* Brussels 1514, † 1564) urged and practiced the dissection of human bodies and may be considered to be the founder of Modern Anatomy.

Editor's address:

Carmine D. Clemente, Ph. D., Professor of Anatomy, Department of Anatomy, UCLA School of Medicine, Los Angeles, California 90024/USA

The illustrations of this atlas were originally published in
    Sobotta/Becher, Atlas der Anatomie des Menschen, edited by H. Ferner and J. Staubesand,
    Urban & Schwarzenberg, München–Berlin–Wien
with the exception of figures 216, 229, 231, 257, 276, 282, 284, 363, 374, 435, 442, 443, 454, 458, 460 – 462, 540, 546, 549, 577, 579, 585, 594 (from Benninghoff/Goerttler, Lehrbuch der Anatomie des Menschen, edited by H. Ferner and J. Staubesand, Urban & Schwarzenberg, München–Berlin–Wien).
Figures 13, 14, 88, 156, 162, 359, 361 have been drawn for this atlas by Jill Penkhus.

This edition may only be distributed in the United States of America, Canada and Latin America.

Library of Congress Cataloging in Publication Data

Clemente, Carmine D.   Anatomy.

1. Anatomy, Human-Atlases.   I. Title.
[DNLM: 1. Anatomy, Regional-Atlases.   QS17 C626c   1974]
QM25.C56   611'.0022'2   73-23046

ISBN 0-8121-0496-X

Printed in Germany by Kastner & Callwey, Buch- und Offsetdruckerei, München. 041179

ISBN 0-8121-0496-X

PREFACE

Twenty-five years ago, while a student at the University of Pennsylvania, I marvelled at the clarity, completeness, and boldness of the anatomical illustrations of the original German editions of Professor Johannes Sobotta's Atlas and their excellent three-volume, English counterparts, the recent editions of which were authored by the late Professor Frank H. J. Figge. It is a matter of record that before World War II these atlases were the most popular ones consulted by American medical students. In the United States, with the advent of other anatomical atlases, the shortening of courses of anatomy in the medical schools, and the increase in publishing costs, the excellent but larger editions of the Sobotta atlases have become virtually unknown to a full generation of students. During the past twenty years of teaching Gross Anatomy at the University of California at Los Angeles I have found only a handful of students who are familiar with the beautiful and still unexcelled Sobotta illustrations.

With this background I enthusiastically accepted the proposal of creating a single-volume atlas from the Sobotta plates and those subsequently drawn by Professor Erich Lepier of Vienna, with the objective of making this teaching resource material once again available to American students, this time at a relatively low cost.

This volume introduces several departures from the former Sobotta atlases. It is the first English edition that presents the Sobotta plates in a regional sequence—the pectoral region and upper extremity, the thorax, the abdomen, the pelvis and perineum, the lower extremity, the back, vertebral column and spinal cord, and finally the neck and head. This sequence is consistent with that followed in many courses presented in the United States and Canada and one which should be useful to students in other countries.

English instead of Latin labels have been used in all the figures. In most instances the terminology of the labels represents the English translation of the Nomina Anatomica designations. In rare instances in which the problem and discrepancies in nomenclature found among modern anatomical texts could not be resolved by consulting the Nomina Anatomica, I have elected to be consistent with the terminology presented in the Twenty-ninth American Edition of Gray's Anatomy. The text consists simply of notes intended to amplify the illustrations but not to exclude the need for an anatomy textbook. The index provides cross-references to the Twenty-ninth American Edition of Gray's Anatomy, making it possible for the student to obtain quickly further information on any structure or subject mentioned in the Atlas.

Several illustrations never before published are presented in this Atlas. These have been drawn by Jill Penkhus, who for a number of years has been the resident medical artist in the Anatomy Department 'at the UCLA School of Medicine.

Many have contributed to bringing this Atlas to fruition. I wish to thank Dr. David S. Maxwell, Professor and Vice Chairman for Gross Anatomy and my colleague at UCLA, for his encouragement and suggestions. I also wish to express my appreciation to my friends Mr. John Febiger Spahr and Mr. George Mundorff, of Lea & Febiger in Philadelphia, and Mr. Michael Urban, of Urban and Schwarzenberg in Munich, for proposing this work and for assistance in seeing it to completion. I am indebted to Klaus Gullath, and Sabine Rheineck, of Urban and Schwarzenberg, who have contributed much to the editing and format of this Atlas, and to Caroline Mitchell and Louise Campbell, who spent many hours proofreading and typing the original text. I especially wish to thank Mary Mansor, of Lea & Febiger, for constructing the index . . . a most laborious task. I am grateful to Barbara Robins for her assistance in typing some of the early parts of the manuscript, and, above all, her sister Julie, who is my wife and who makes all of my efforts worthwhile through her encouragement and devotion.

Los Angeles, California   CARMINE D. CLEMENTE

VI

CONTENTS

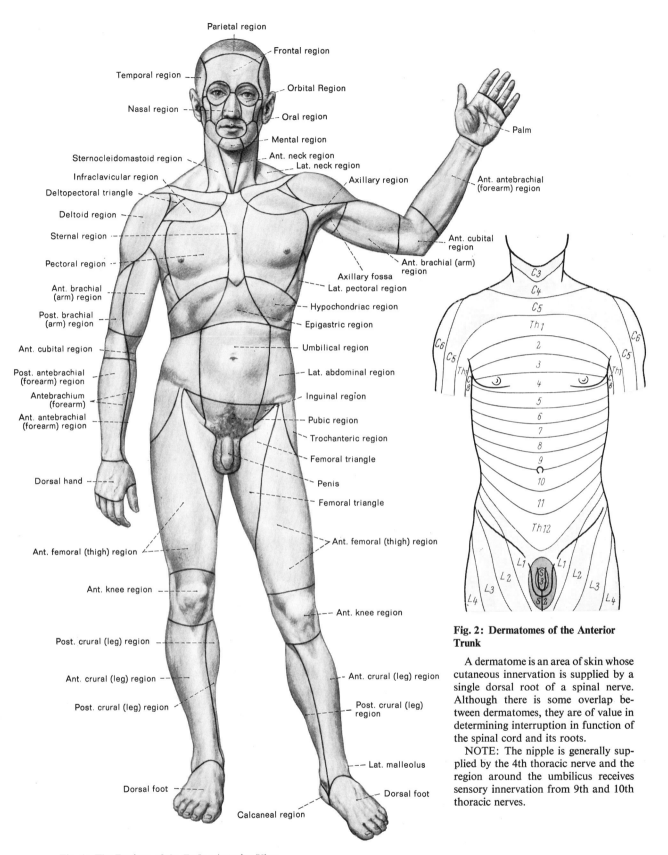

Fig. 2: Dermatomes of the Anterior Trunk

A dermatome is an area of skin whose cutaneous innervation is supplied by a single dorsal root of a spinal nerve. Although there is some overlap between dermatomes, they are of value in determining interruption in function of the spinal cord and its roots.

NOTE: The nipple is generally supplied by the 4th thoracic nerve and the region around the umbilicus receives sensory innervation from 9th and 10th thoracic nerves.

Fig. 1: The Regions of the Body: Anterior View

Become familiar with the names of the various regions of the body in order to describe more precisely the location of anatomical structures.

NOTE: Some regions are named after underlying or adjacent bones (sternal, parietal, frontal, temporal, infraclavicular, femoral) while other regions are named for underlying muscles (sternocleidomastoid, deltoid, pectoral). Still other regions are named after specialized anatomical structures (umbilical, oral, nasal).

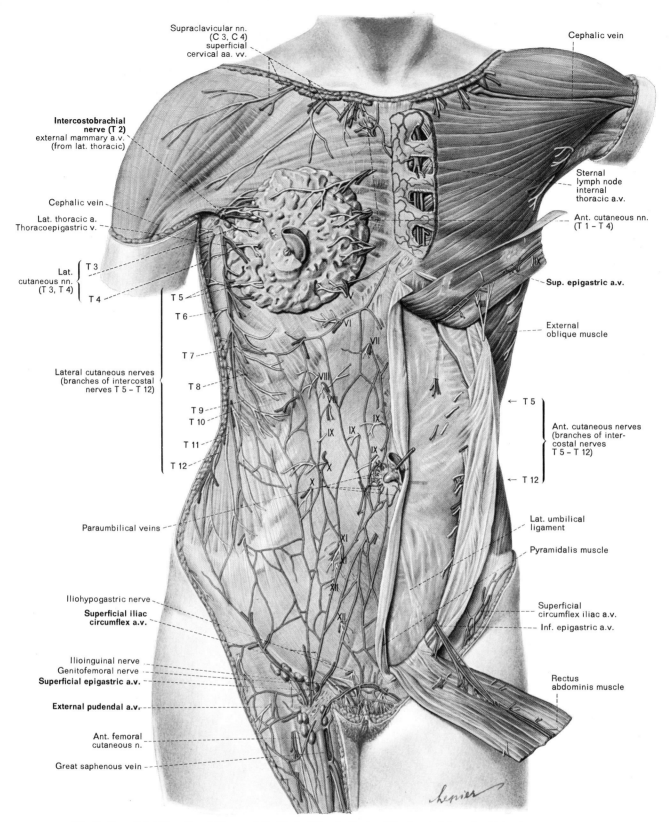

Fig. 3: Superficial Vessels and Nerves of the Ventral Trunk: Pectoral Region and Anterior Abdominal Wall

OBSERVE: 1) the cutaneous innervation of the anterior trunk which is derived from a) the supraclavicular nerves (C_3, C_4); b) the intercostal nerves (anterior cutaneous T 1 – T 12; lateral cutaneous T 2 – T 12); c) iliohypogastric and ilioinguinal nerves (L 1).

2) the thoracoepigastric venous anastomosis between the thoracoepigastric and lateral thoracic veins superiorly and the superficial circumflex iliac and superficial epigastric veins inferiorly.

3) the mammary gland: its innervation (T 2 – T 6) and its blood supply (branches of internal thoracic artery, lateral thoracic artery). Additionally the mammary gland may receive small branches from the intercostal arteries which may enter the deep surface of the gland.

4) the nipple at the level of T 4 and the umbilicus at the level of T 10.

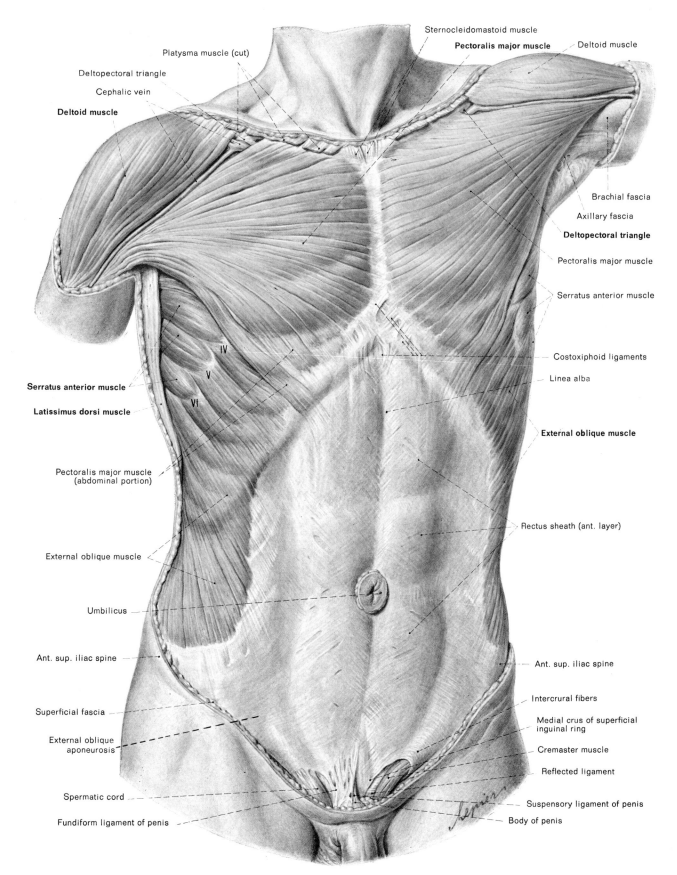

Sternocleidomastoid muscle
Platysma muscle (cut)
Deltopectoral triangle
Cephalic vein
Deltoid muscle
Pectoralis major muscle
Deltoid muscle

Brachial fascia
Axillary fascia
Deltopectoral triangle
Pectoralis major muscle
Serratus anterior muscle
Costoxiphoid ligaments
Linea alba
External oblique muscle

IV
V
VI

Serratus anterior muscle
Latissimus dorsi muscle

Pectoralis major muscle
(abdominal portion)

Rectus sheath (ant. layer)

External oblique muscle

Umbilicus

Ant. sup. iliac spine

Ant. sup. iliac spine

Intercrural fibers

Medial crus of superficial
inguinal ring

Superficial fascia

Cremaster muscle

External oblique
aponeurosis

Reflected ligament

Spermatic cord

Suspensory ligament of penis

Fundiform ligament of penis

Body of penis

Fig. 4: The Superficial Thoracic and Abdominal Muscles

Observe that the pectoralis major arises from the medial half of the clavicle, the costal margin of the sternum, the 2nd to 6th ribs and the upper part of the aponeurosis of the external oblique. Also note the deltopectoral triangle and the course of the cephalic vein as it empties into the axillary vein.

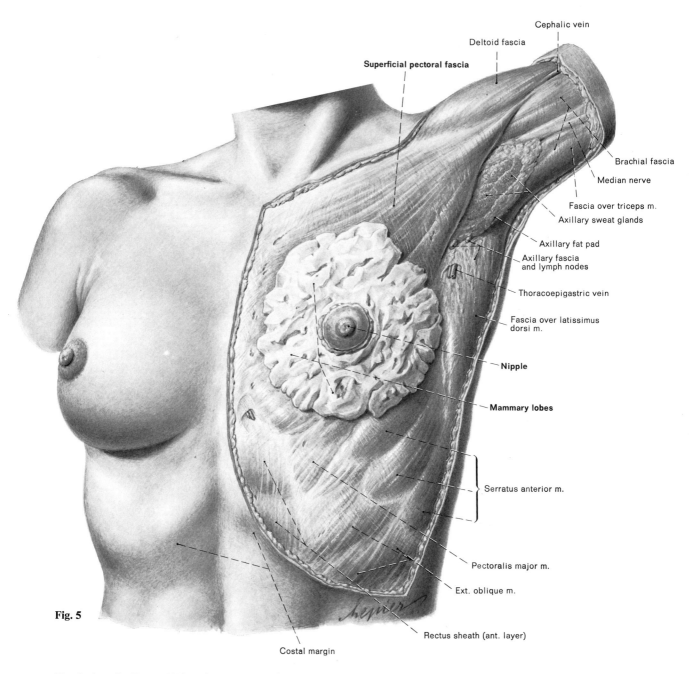

Cephalic vein
Deltoid fascia
Superficial pectoral fascia
Brachial fascia
Median nerve
Fascia over triceps m.
Axillary sweat glands
Axillary fat pad
Axillary fascia and lymph nodes
Thoracoepigastric vein
Fascia over latissimus dorsi m.
Nipple
Mammary lobes
Serratus anterior m.
Pectoralis major m.
Ext. oblique m.
Rectus sheath (ant. layer)
Costal margin

Fig. 5

Fig. 5: Anterior Pectoral Dissection (Adult Female)

NOTE: 1) the lobular nature of the mammary gland extending toward the axilla and its location anterior to the pectoralis major muscle.

2) the superficial axillary lymph and sudoriferous (sweat) glands.

Fig. 6: Sagittal Section through Mammary Gland of Gravid Female

NOTE: 1) the radial arrangement of the lobes of glandular tissue. These lobes are comprised of smaller lobules and are ▶ separated from one another by fat and the supporting connective tissue.

2) the lactiferous duct system. Each of the 15 to 20 lobes has its own duct which opens by means of a small orifice onto the nipple.

3) that the mammary gland is separated from the pectoralis major muscle by the pectoral fascia and that connective tissue strands (suspensory ligaments of Cooper) within the gland extend toward this fascia.

Fig. 7: Right Mammary Gland: Dissection of the Nipple

A circular piece of skin has been removed in this dissection. With the incised margin of the skin around the nipple retracted, the lactiferous ducts can be observed perforating onto the surface and arranged circumferentially around the nipple.

Fig. 8: Two Typical Spinal Nerves: Their Origin, Branches and Connections to the Sympathetic Trunk

NOTE: 1) each spinal nerve attaches to the spinal cord by two roots: an afferent or sensory dorsal root and an efferent or motor ventral root. Each dorsal root contains a spinal ganglion comprised of afferent neuron cell bodies.

2) the two spinal roots join to form the spinal nerve which in turn divides into a dorsal ramus coursing posteriorly and a ventral ramus coursing anteriorly. During their course, these rami divide further to innervate the body segment with both sensory and motor fibers.

3) the spinal nerve communicates with the sympathetic trunk carrying preganglionic sympathetic fibers to the trunk (white ramus) and postganglionic fibers from the trunk (gray ramus).

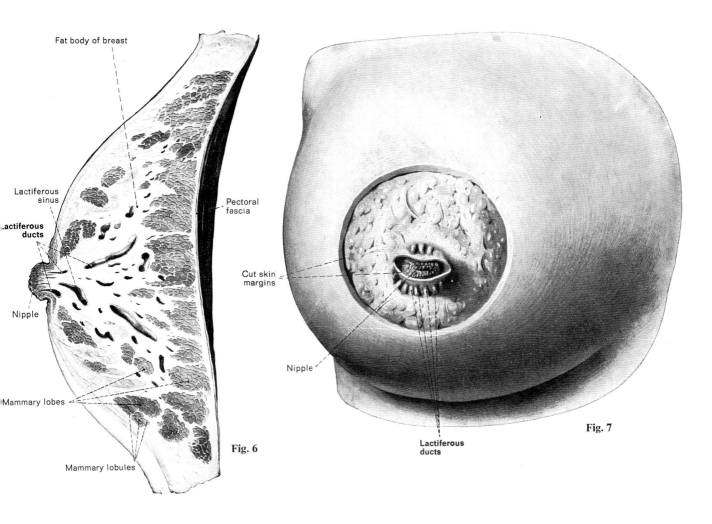

Fat body of breast

Lactiferous sinus

actiferous ducts

Nipple

Mammary lobes

Mammary lobules

Pectoral fascia

Fig. 6

Cut skin margins

Nipple

Lactiferous ducts

Fig. 7

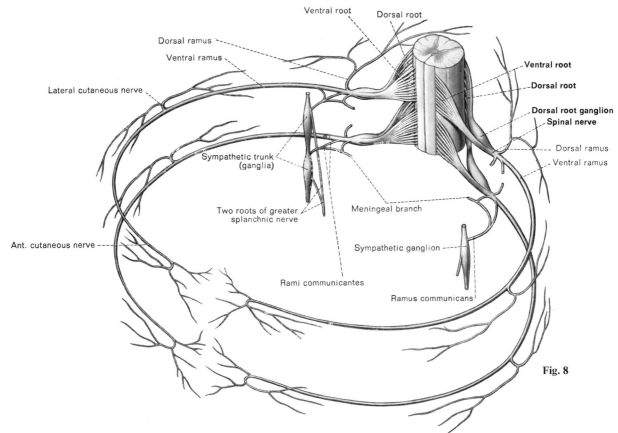

Ventral root

Dorsal root

Dorsal ramus

Ventral ramus

Lateral cutaneous nerve

Ventral root

Dorsal root

Dorsal root ganglion
Spinal nerve

Dorsal ramus

Ventral ramus

Sympathetic trunk (ganglia)

Meningeal branch

Two roots of greater splanchnic nerve

Ant. cutaneous nerve

Sympathetic ganglion

Rami communicantes

Ramus communicans

Fig. 8

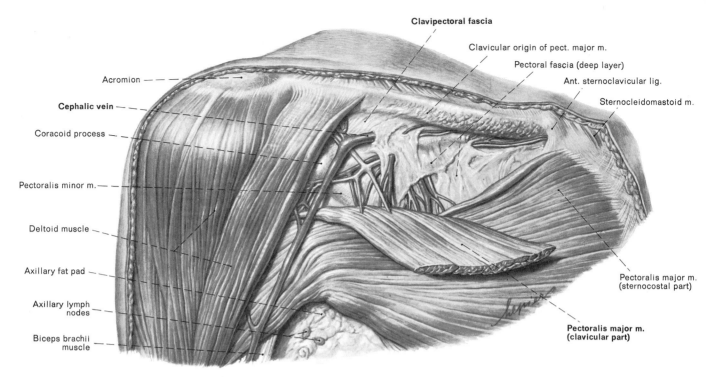

Clavipectoral fascia

Clavicular origin of pect. major m.

Pectoral fascia (deep layer)

Ant. sternoclavicular lig.

Sternocleidomastoid m.

Acromion

Cephalic vein

Coracoid process

Pectoralis minor m.

Deltoid muscle

Axillary fat pad

Axillary lymph nodes

Biceps brachii muscle

Pectoralis major m. (sternocostal part)

Pectoralis major m. (clavicular part)

Fig. 9: The Deltopectoral Triangle

With the clavicular head of the pectoralis major muscle severed,
OBSERVE: 1) the internal investing layer of fascia deep to the pectoralis major;
2) the clavipectoral fascia which lies between the pectoralis major and the thoracic wall;
3) the course of the cephalic vein as it pierces the clavipectoral fascia to join the axillary vein.

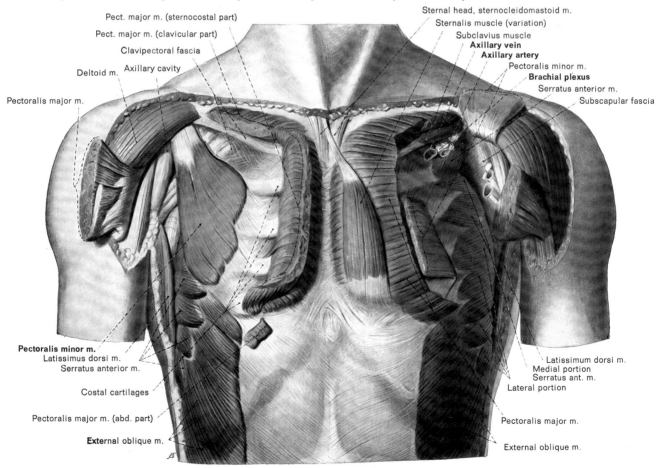

Pect. major m. (sternocostal part)

Pect. major m. (clavicular part)

Clavipectoral fascia

Deltoid m.   Axillary cavity

Pectoralis major m.

Sternal head, sternocleidomastoid m.

Sternalis muscle (variation)

Subclavius muscle

Axillary vein

Axillary artery

Pectoralis minor m.

Brachial plexus

Serratus anterior m.

Subscapular fascia

Pectoralis minor m.
Latissimus dorsi m.
Serratus anterior m.

Costal cartilages

Pectoralis major m. (abd. part)

External oblique m.

Latissimum dorsi m.
Medial portion
Serratus ant. m.
Lateral portion

Pectoralis major m.

External oblique m.

Fig. 10: The Pectoralis Minor and Anterior Axillary Structures

With the pectoralis major muscle reflected,
OBSERVE the relationship of the pectoralis minor muscle to the axillary vessels and nerves.

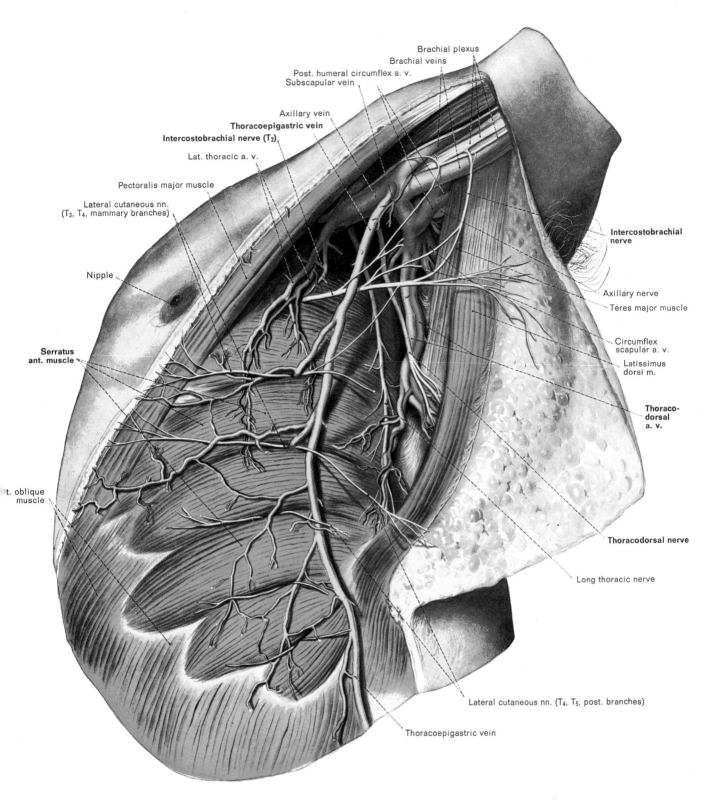

Brachial plexus
Brachial veins
Post. humeral circumflex a. v.
Subscapular vein
Axillary vein
Thoracoepigastric vein
Intercostobrachial nerve (T₂)
Lat. thoracic a. v.
Pectoralis major muscle
Lateral cutaneous nn.
(T₃, T₄, mammary branches)
Nipple
Serratus
ant. muscle
t. oblique
muscle

Intercostobrachial
nerve
Axillary nerve
Teres major muscle
Circumflex
scapular a. v.
Latissimus
dorsi m.
Thoraco-
dorsal
a. v.
Thoracodorsal nerve
Long thoracic nerve

Lateral cutaneous nn. (T₄, T₅, post. branches)
Thoracoepigastric vein

Fig. 11: The Axilla: Superficial Vessels and Nerves (left)

OBSERVE: 1) that the boundaries of the axilla are, a) anteriorly, the pectoralis major muscle; b) posteriorly, the subscapularis, teres major and latissimus dorsi muscles; c) medially, the serratus anterior muscle covering the ribs, and; d) laterally, the bicipital groove of the humerus.

2) that the inferior portion of the serratus anterior muscle arises from the lower ribs as fleshy interdigitations with the external oblique muscle.

3) the serratus anterior is innervated by the long thoracic nerve (C 5, 6, 7) and the latissimus dorsi is innervated by the thoracodorsal nerve (C 5, 6, 7).

4) the axillary vein lies medial to the axillary artery and the cords of the brachial plexus.

5) the descending course of the thoracoepigastric vein and the lateral thoracic artery and vein.

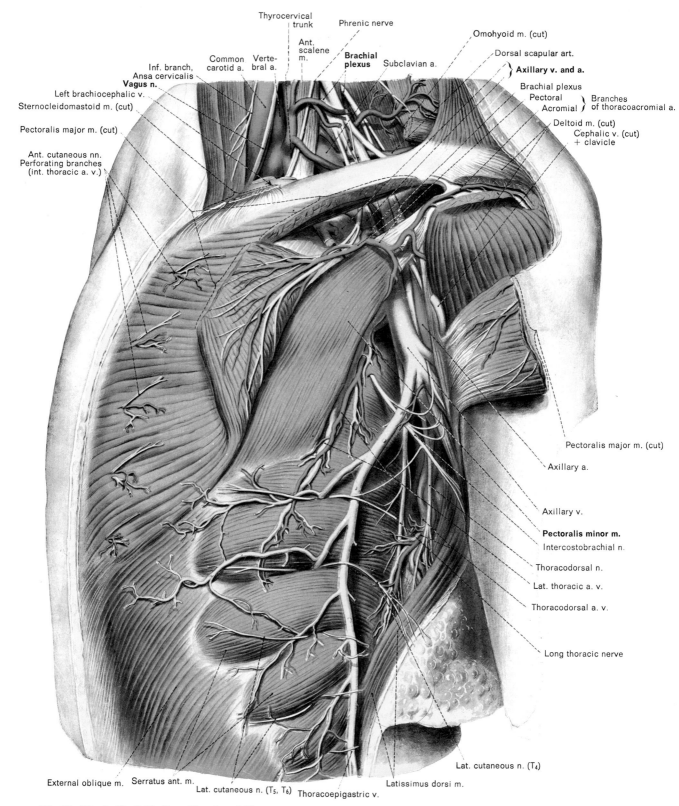

Fig. 12: The Axilla (left): Deep Vessels and Nerves

OBSERVE: 1) that the subclavian artery becomes the axillary artery as it passes beneath the clavicle;

2) that the pectoralis minor muscle is helpful in describing the underlying axillary artery in its course through the axilla, since the three parts of the axillary artery are medial, beneath and lateral to the pectoralis minor;

3) that the axillary vein courses medial to the axillary artery and it receives tributaries not only from the upper extremity but from the thorax as well;

4) that the axillary artery is surrounded by the three cords of the brachial plexus;

5) that the thoracoacromial artery divides into pectoral, acromial, deltoid and small clavicular branches (the latter are not shown in the figure);

6) that the intercostobrachial (T_2) nerve pierces the thoracic cage through the 2nd intercostal space in its course toward the axilla and arm.

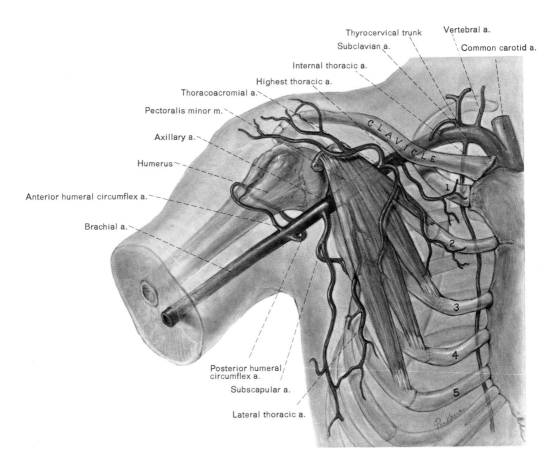

Fig. 13: The Branches of the Axillary Artery

NOTE: 1) as the subclavian artery passes beneath the clavicle, it becomes the axillary artery. The axillary artery becomes the brachial artery in the upper arm (at the level of the tendon of the teres major muscle). In the axilla the pectoralis minor muscle crosses anterior to the axillary artery, thereby, for description purposes, dividing the vessel into three parts.

2) from the 1st part of the axillary artery (medial to the pectoralis minor and lateral to the clavicle) branches one vessel, the supreme thoracic artery. From the 2nd part (beneath the muscle) branch two vessels, the thoracoacromial artery and the lateral thoracic. From the 3rd part of the axillary (lateral to the pectoralis minor muscle) are derived three branches, the subscapular artery and the anterior and posterior humeral circumflex arteries.

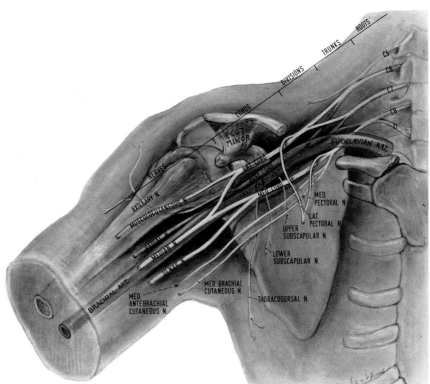

Fig. 14: The Brachial Plexus

Note: 1) five spinal roots form three trunks. Each trunk divides into anterior and posterior divisions. The three posterior divisions unite to form the posterior cord. The anterior divisions of the upper and middle trunks form the lateral cord while the anterior division of the lower trunk forms the medial cord.

2) the three cords of the brachial plexus lie posterior, lateral and medial to the axillary artery. Branches from the cords form the peripheral nerves of the pectoral girdle and the upper extremity.

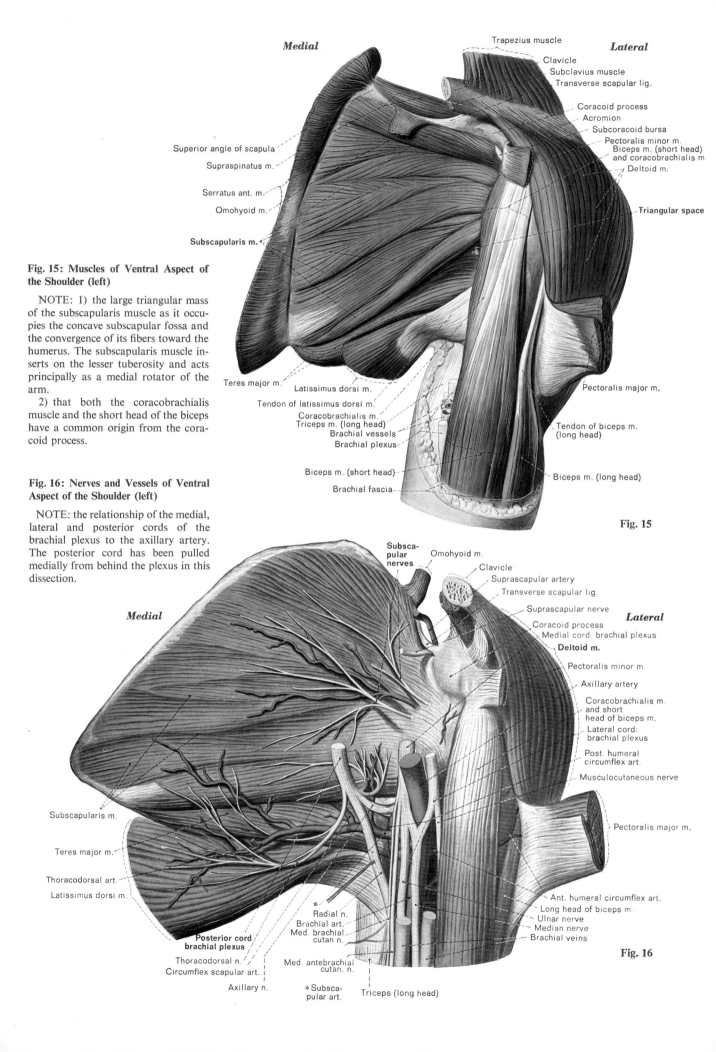

Medial   Trapezius muscle   **Lateral**

Clavicle
Subclavius muscle
Transverse scapular lig.

Coracoid process
Acromion
Subcoracoid bursa
Pectoralis minor m.
Biceps m. (short head)
and coracobrachialis m.
Deltoid m.

Superior angle of scapula

Supraspinatus m.

Serratus ant. m.

Omohyoid m.

Triangular space

Subscapularis m.

Fig. 15: Muscles of Ventral Aspect of the Shoulder (left)

NOTE: 1) the large triangular mass of the subscapularis muscle as it occupies the concave subscapular fossa and the convergence of its fibers toward the humerus. The subscapularis muscle inserts on the lesser tuberosity and acts principally as a medial rotator of the arm.

2) that both the coracobrachialis muscle and the short head of the biceps have a common origin from the coracoid process.

Teres major m.

Latissimus dorsi m.
Tendon of latissimus dorsi m.
Coracobrachialis m.
Triceps m. (long head)
Brachial vessels
Brachial plexus

Pectoralis major m.

Tendon of biceps m. (long head)

Biceps m. (short head)

Biceps m. (long head)

Brachial fascia

Fig. 15

Fig. 16: Nerves and Vessels of Ventral Aspect of the Shoulder (left)

NOTE: the relationship of the medial, lateral and posterior cords of the brachial plexus to the axillary artery. The posterior cord has been pulled medially from behind the plexus in this dissection.

Subscapular nerves

Omohyoid m.

Clavicle
Suprascapular artery
Transverse scapular lig.
Suprascapular nerve
Coracoid process
Medial cord: brachial plexus
Deltoid m.
Pectoralis minor m.
Axillary artery
Coracobrachialis m. and short head of biceps m.
Lateral cord: brachial plexus
Post. humeral circumflex art.
Musculocutaneous nerve

Medial   **Lateral**

Pectoralis major m.

Subscapularis m.

Teres major m.

Thoracodorsal art.
Latissimus dorsi m.

Ant. humeral circumflex art.
Long head of biceps m.
Ulnar nerve
Median nerve
Brachial veins

* Radial n.
Brachial art.
Med. brachial cutan. n.

Posterior cord brachial plexus

Thoracodorsal n.
Circumflex scapular art.

Med. antebrachial cutan. n.

Axillary n.

*Subscapular art.

Triceps (long head)

Fig. 16

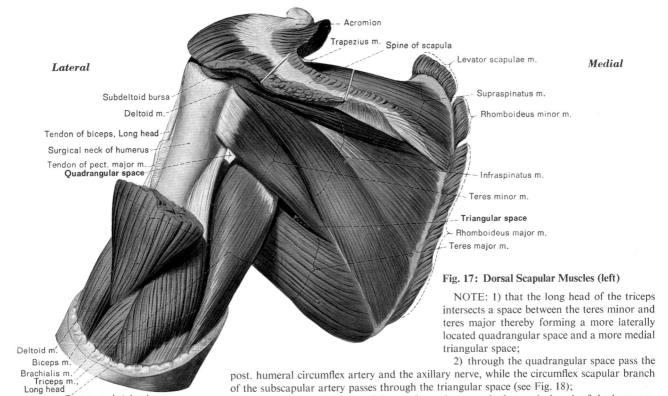

Fig. 17: **Dorsal Scapular Muscles (left)**

NOTE: 1) that the long head of the triceps intersects a space between the teres minor and teres major thereby forming a more laterally located quadrangular space and a more medial triangular space;

2) through the quadrangular space pass the post. humeral circumflex artery and the axillary nerve, while the circumflex scapular branch of the subscapular artery passes through the triangular space (see Fig. 18);

3) since the lateral border of the quadrangular space is the surgical neck of the humerus, the axillary nerve and post. humeral circumflex art. are in danger if the bone is fractured at this site.

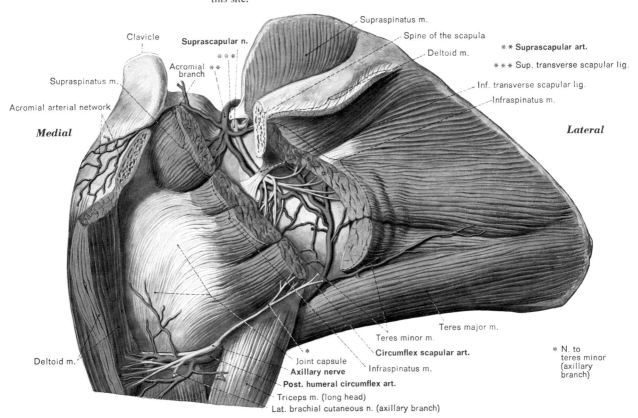

Fig. 18: **Nerves and Vessels of Dorsal Scapular Region (left)**

NOTE: 1) that the sup. transverse scapular lig. bridges across the scapular notch and the suprascapular nerve passes beneath the ligament while the suprascapular artery usually passes above it;

2) that the axillary nerve supplies four structures: the deltoid muscle, the teres minor muscle, the capsule of the shoulder joint and the skin over the shoulder joint;

3) that the axillary nerve and post. humeral circumflex artery achieve the dorsal aspect of the shoulder through the quadrangular space while the circumflex scapular artery reaches the infraspinatus fossa through the triangular space.

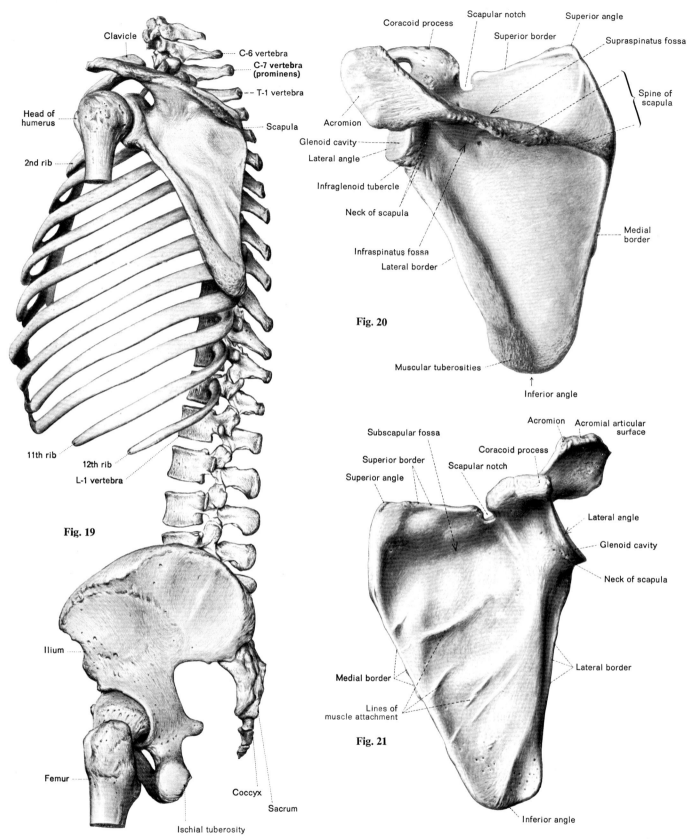

Fig. 19: Skeleton of Trunk with Scapula and Pelvis

Note that the flat triangular shaped scapula articulates with the head of the humerus and the clavicle and is also attached to the rib cage by muscles.

Fig. 20: The Left Scapula (Dorsal Surface)

Note that the socket for the head of the humerus is formed by the glenoid cavity and is further enlarged by the coracoid and acromial processes along with their related ligaments. The spine of the scapula separates the dorsal surface into supraspinatus and infraspinatus fossae.

Fig. 21: The Left Scapula (Ventral Surface)

Note that much of the ventral surface is a concave fossa within which lies the subscapularis muscle.

Fig. 22: Left Shoulder Joint and Acromioclavicular Joint (Anterior View)

NOTE: 1) that the clavicle is attached by ligaments to both the acromion (acromioclavicular lig) and the coracoid process (coracoclavicular lig.) of the scapula. The acromion and coracoid process are themselves connected by the coracoacromial ligament;

2) neither the acromion nor the clavicle articulates directly with the humerus, whereas the coracoid process and the glenoid labrum afford attachment of the scapula to the humerus;

3) the acromion, coracoid process and clavicle assist in the protection of the shoulder joint from above. Thus, the joint is weakest inferiorly and anteriorly, the directions in which most dislocations occur;

4) the glenohumeral ligaments are thickened bands which tend to strengthen somewhat the capsule of the joint anteriorly;

5) the position of the long tendon of the biceps traversing the articular cavity to its point of attachment on the supraglenoid tubercle.

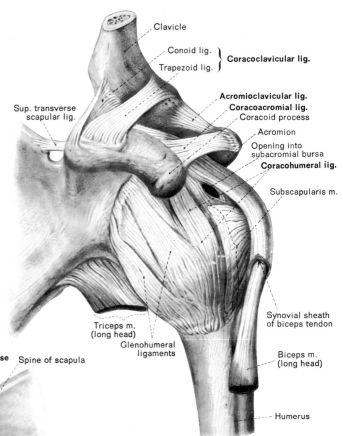

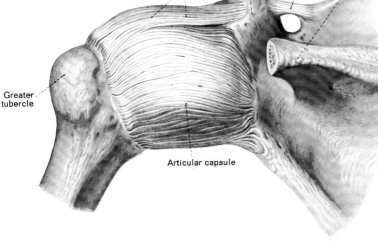

Fig. 23: Capsule of Left Shoulder Joint (Posterior View)

NOTE: 1) the articular capsule completely surrounds the joint, being attached beyond the glenoid cavity on the scapula above and to the anatomical neck of the humerus below;

2) the superior part of the capsule is further strengthened by the coracohumeral ligament.

Fig. 24: Left Shoulder Joint (Posterior View)

NOTE: 1) the shoulder joint is a freely moving ball and socket joint. The capsule of the joint is not drawn tightly between the humeral head and scapula but attached loosely over these bony structures;

2) the tendons of the supraspinatus, infraspinatus and teres minor blend superiorly and posteriorly with the capsule of the joint. These muscles along with the subscapularis anteriorly form a muscular encasement lending some support in the maintenance of the head of the humerus in its socket;

3) the close relationship of the long head of the triceps to the capsule of joint. When the arm is abducted the triceps is drawn even closer to the capsule to help prevent dislocation.

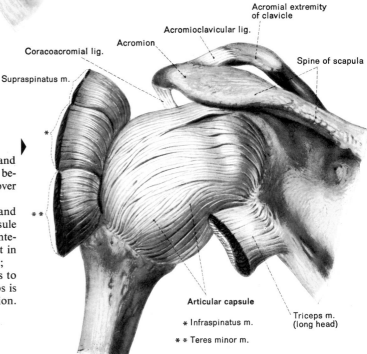

Fig. 25: The Left Glenoid Cavity and Scapuloclavicular Joint (Lateral View)

NOTE: 1) exposure of the glenoid cavity was achieved by removal of the articular capsule at the glenoid labrum;

2) the attachment of the tendon of the long head of the biceps muscle at the supraglenoid tubercle and that of the long head of the triceps at the infraglenoid tubercle have been left intact;

3) the shallowness of the glenoid cavity is slightly deepened (4 to 6 mm.) by the glenoid labrum;

4) the protection afforded to the shoulder joint superiorly by the acromion, coracoid process and clavicle and their ligamentous attachments and by the tendon of the long head of the biceps.

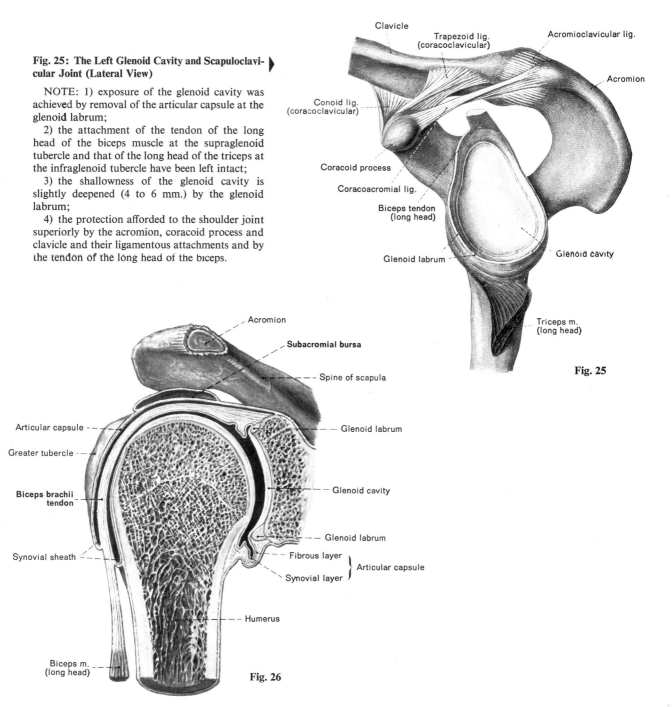

Fig. 25

Fig. 26

Fig. 26: Frontal Section through Right Shoulder Joint

NOTE: 1) that the tendon of the long head of the biceps arises from the supraglenoid tuberosity and is at once enclosed by a reflection of the synovial sheath. Thus, although the tendon passes through the joint, it is not contained within the synovial cavity of the joint;

2) the capsule of the joint is composed of a dense fibrous outer layer and a thin synovial inner layer. It is this thin inner layer which reflects itself around the biceps tendon in its course through the joint;

3) a bursa is a sac lined with a synovial-like membrane containing a small amount of fluid. Bursae are found at sites subjected to friction and normally do not communicate with the joint capsule. In the shoulder separate bursae are found between the capsule and the subscapularis, infraspinatus and deltoid tendons as well as other muscles, and between the capsule and the coracoid and acromial processes (subacromial bursa).

Superficial Veins and Cutaneous Nerves of Left Upper Limb (Anterior Surface)
Fig. 27: Arm

NOTE: 1) the basilic vein ascends on the medial (ulnar) aspect of the arm, pierces the deep fascia and at the lower border of the teres major joins the brachial vein to form the axillary vein. The cephalic vein ascends laterally in the arm in its course toward the axillary vein.

2) the principle sensory nerves of the anterior arm are the medial and lateral brachial cutaneous nerves and the intercostobrachial nerve.

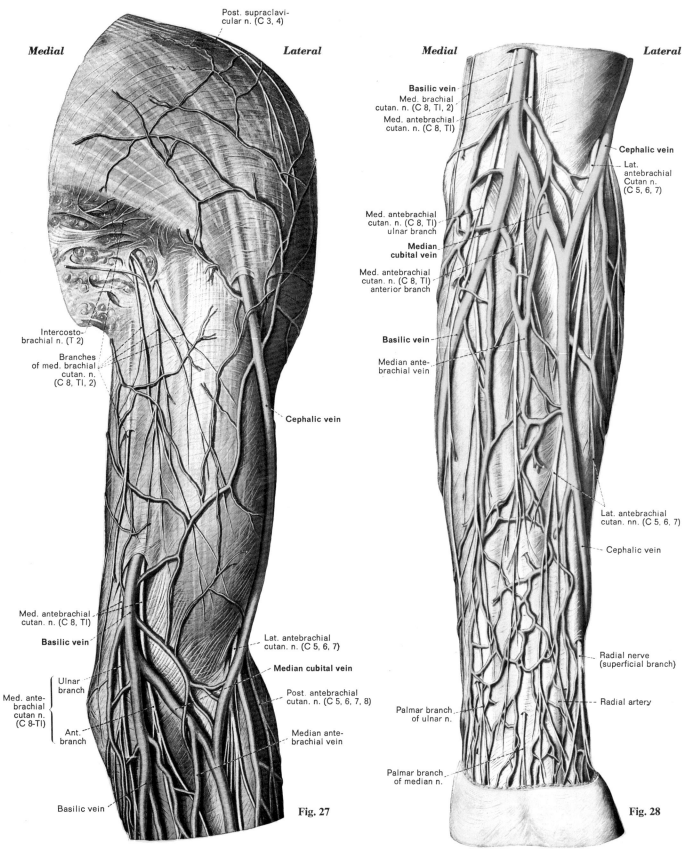

Superficial Veins and Cutaneous Nerves of Left Upper Limb (Anterior Surface)
Fig. 28: Forearm

NOTE: 1) the median cubital vein, interconnecting the cephalic and the basilic veins in the cubital fossa.

2) the main sensory nerves of the anterior forearm are the medial antebrachial cutaneous nerve (derived from the medial cord of the brachial plexus) and the lateral antebrachial cutaneous nerve which is the continuation of the musculocutaneous nerve.

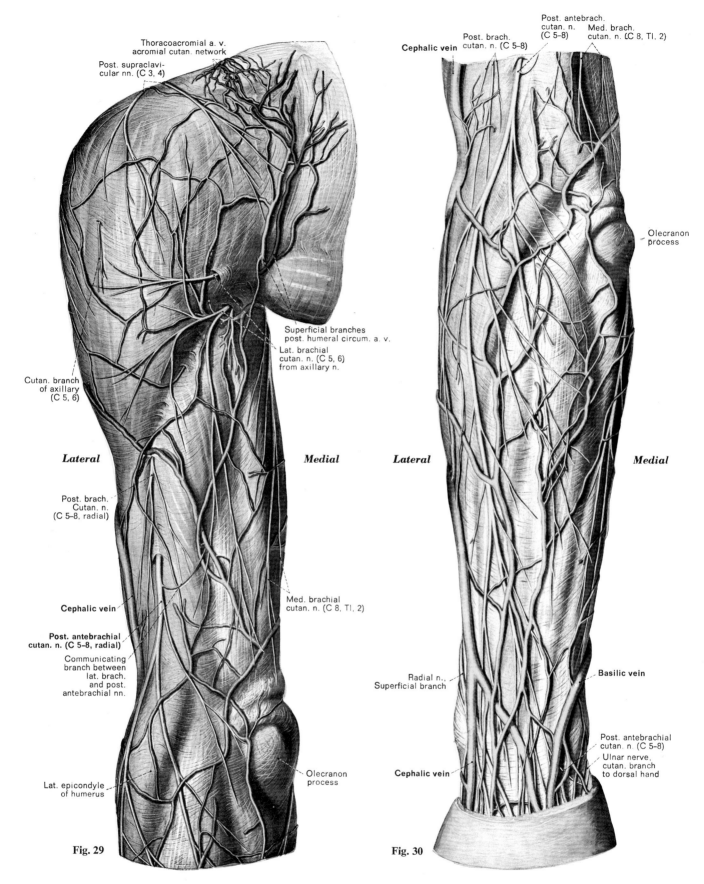

Superficial Veins and Cutaneous Nerves of Left Upper Limb (Posterior Surface)
Fig. 29: Arm

    NOTE: the posterior surface of the arm receives cutaneous innervation from branches of the radial (post. brachial cutan n)
and axillary (lat. brachial cutan. n) nerves, both of which are derived from the posterior cord of the brachial plexus.

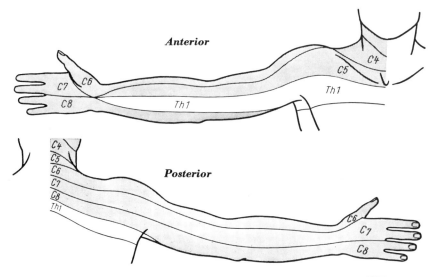

Anterior

Posterior

Fig. 31: Dermatomes of the Upper Limb

NOTE: the dermatomes of the upper limb are supplied by the 5th cervical to the 1st thoracic segments of the spinal cord. The boundary between the 5th cervical and the 1st thoracic dermatomes ventrally is called the ventral axial line of the upper limb. The 4th cervical dermatome lies in the neck. Commencing with the 5th cervical dermatome and proceeding radially around the upper limb the dermatomes can be followed sequentially to the 1st thoracic and thus, the ventral axial line.

The Left Humerus

NOTE: 1) the humerus consists of a body and two extremities. The head of the humerus is shaped as a hemisphere and articulates with the scapula at the glenoid cavity.

2) the anatomical neck is a constricted zone just distal to the head of the humerus, and the surgical neck, where fractures frequently occur, lies just below the two tubercles.

3) the greater and lesser tubercles are roughened prominences which allow the insertion of muscles: the supraspinatus, infraspinatus, and the teres minor on the greater tubercle and the subscapularis on the lesser.

4) within the tubercular sulcus passes the tendon of the long head of the biceps.

5) adjacent to the radial groove courses the radial nerve, which is therefore endangered by fractures of the humerus.

6) the distal extremity affords articulation with the radius and ulna.

◀ Superficial Veins and Cutaneous Nerves of Left Upper Limb (Posterior Surface)
Fig. 30: Forearm

NOTE: 1) branches of the radial n. (post. antebrach. cutan. and superficial radial) supply the principal cutaneous innervation to the posterior forearm.

2) the basilic (ulnar side) and cephalic (radial side) veins commence on the dorsum of the hand in their ascent up the forearm.

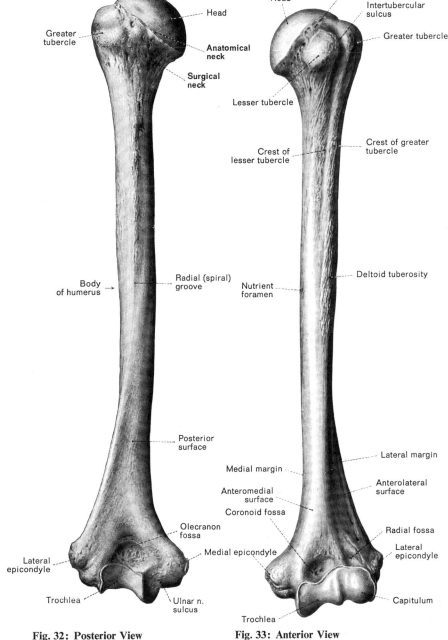

Fig. 32: Posterior View

Fig. 33: Anterior View

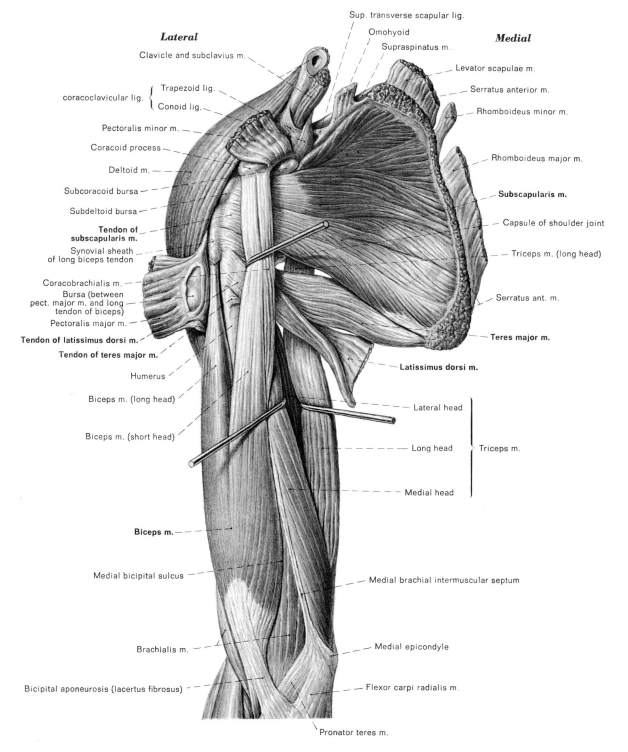

Lateral

Sup. transverse scapular lig.

Omohyoid

Suprapinatus m.

Medial

Clavicle and subclavius m.

coracoclavicular lig. { Trapezoid lig.
{ Conoid lig.

Pectoralis minor m.

Coracoid process

Deltoid m.

Subcoracoid bursa

Subdeltoid bursa

Tendon of subscapularis m.

Synovial sheath of long biceps tendon

Coracobrachialis m.

Bursa (between pect. major m. and long tendon of biceps)

Pectoralis major m.

Tendon of latissimus dorsi m.

Tendon of teres major m.

Humerus

Biceps m. (long head)

Biceps m. (short head)

Biceps m.

Medial bicipital sulcus

Brachialis m.

Bicipital aponeurosis (lacertus fibrosus)

Pronator teres m.

Levator scapulae m.

Serratus anterior m.

Rhomboideus minor m.

Rhomboideus major m.

Subscapularis m.

Capsule of shoulder joint

Triceps m. (long head)

Serratus ant. m.

Teres major m.

Latissimus dorsi m.

Lateral head

Long head } Triceps m.

Medial head

Medial brachial intermuscular septum

Medial epicondyle

Flexor carpi radialis m.

Fig. 34: Muscles of the Right Shoulder and Arm (Anterior View)

NOTE: 1) the insertion of the subscapularis muscle on the lesser tubercle of the humerus. Distal to this, from medial to lateral, insert the teres major, latissimus dorsi and pectoralis major muscles.

2) attaching to the coracoid process are the pectoralis minor m., coracobrachialis m. and the short head of the biceps m.

3) the insertion of the pectoralis major m. and the long tendon of the biceps muscle are frequently separated by a bursa.

4) in the arm the flexor compartment (biceps, coracobrachialis and brachialis) is separated from the extensor compartment (triceps) by an intermuscular septum of deep fascia.

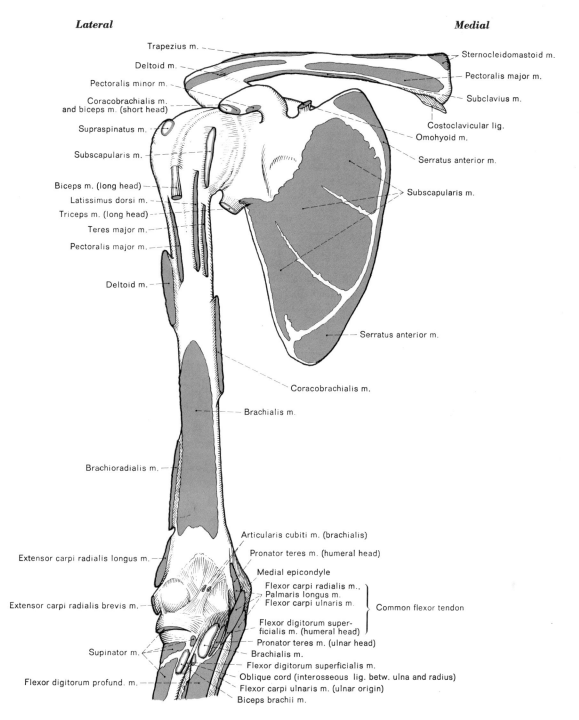

Lateral **Medial**

Trapezius m.

Deltoid m.

Pectoralis minor m.

Coracobrachialis m. and biceps m. (short head)

Supraspinatus m.

Subscapularis m.

Biceps m. (long head)

Latissimus dorsi m.

Triceps m. (long head)

Teres major m.

Pectoralis major m.

Deltoid m.

Brachioradialis m.

Extensor carpi radialis longus m.

Extensor carpi radialis brevis m.

Supinator m.

Flexor digitorum profund. m.

Sternocleidomastoid m.

Pectoralis major m.

Subclavius m.

Costoclavicular lig.

Omohyoid m.

Serratus anterior m.

Subscapularis m.

Serratus anterior m.

Coracobrachialis m.

Brachialis m.

Articularis cubiti m. (brachialis)

Pronator teres m. (humeral head)

Medial epicondyle

Flexor carpi radialis m.,
Palmaris longus m.
Flexor carpi ulnaris m.

Common flexor tendon

Flexor digitorum super- ficialis m. (humeral head)

Pronator teres m. (ulnar head)

Brachialis m.

Flexor digitorum superficialis m.

Oblique cord (interosseous lig. betw. ulna and radius)

Flexor carpi ulnaris m. (ulnar origin)

Biceps brachii m.

Fig. 35: Anterior View of Bones of the Upper Limb (Including Proximal End of Radius and Ulna) Showing Attachments of Muscles

NOTE: 1) the broad *origin* of the subscapularis in the subscapular fossa of the scapula and its *insertion* on the lesser tubercle of the humerus proximal to the insertions of the latissimus dorsi and teres major muscles. The subscapularis is an adductor and medial rotator of the arm.

2) the brachialis muscle *arises* from the distal three-fifths of the anterior surface of the humerus and *inserts* on the coronoid process of the ulna. This muscle is the strongest flexor of the forearm.

3) the short head of the biceps m. *arises* with the coracobrachialis m. from the coracoid process, while the long head *arises* from the supraglenoid tubercle of the scapula.

4) the coracobrachialis *inserts* onto the shaft of the humerus near its middle, while the biceps inserts onto the tuberosity of the radius and onto the deep fascia of the forearm by way of the bicipital aponeurosis.

5) the coracobrachialis flexes and adducts the arm at the shoulder joint, while the biceps flexes and supinates the forearm, with the long head assisting in flexion of the arm at the shoulder joint.

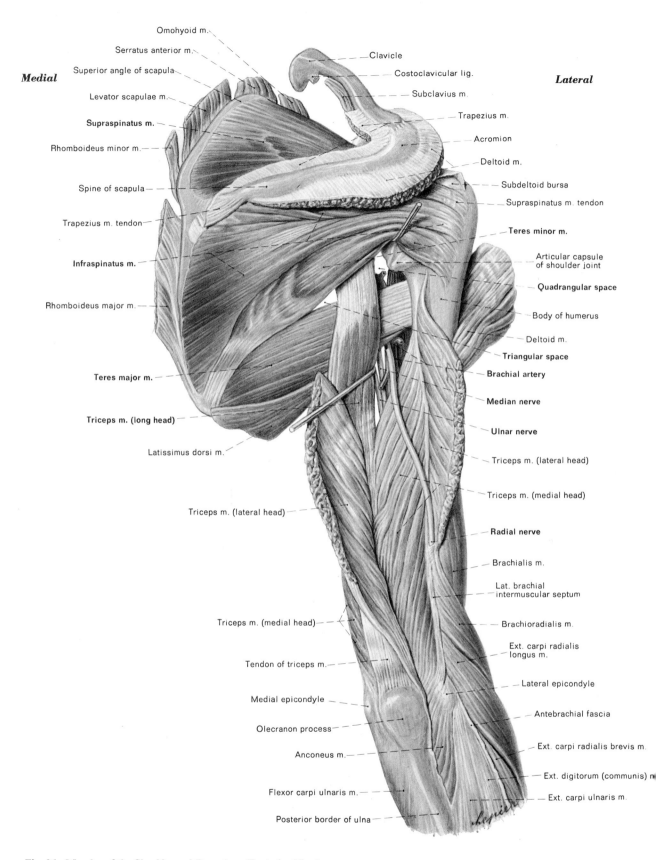

Omohyoid m.

Serratus anterior m.

Superior angle of scapula

Medial

Levator scapulae m.

Supraspinatus m.

Rhomboideus minor m.

Spine of scapula

Trapezius m. tendon

Infraspinatus m.

Rhomboideus major m.

Teres major m.

Triceps m. (long head)

Latissimus dorsi m.

Triceps m. (lateral head)

Triceps m. (medial head)

Tendon of triceps m.

Medial epicondyle

Olecranon process

Anconeus m.

Flexor carpi ulnaris m.

Posterior border of ulna

Clavicle

Costoclavicular lig.

Subclavius m.

Lateral

Trapezius m.

Acromion

Deltoid m.

Subdeltoid bursa

Supraspinatus m. tendon

Teres minor m.

Articular capsule of shoulder joint

Quadrangular space

Body of humerus

Deltoid m.

Triangular space

Brachial artery

Median nerve

Ulnar nerve

Triceps m. (lateral head)

Triceps m. (medial head)

Radial nerve

Brachialis m.

Lat. brachial intermuscular septum

Brachioradialis m.

Ext. carpi radialis longus m.

Lateral epicondyle

Antebrachial fascia

Ext. carpi radialis brevis m.

Ext. digitorum (communis) m.

Ext. carpi ulnaris m.

Fig. 36: Muscles of the Shoulder and Deep Arm (Posterior View)

NOTE: 1) that with the deltoid muscle and the lateral head of the triceps muscle severed, the course of the radial nerve in the upper arm is revealed.

2) the sequential insertions of the supraspinatus, infraspinatus and teres minor muscles on the greater tubercle of the humerus.

3) the boundaries of the quadrangular and triangular spaces.

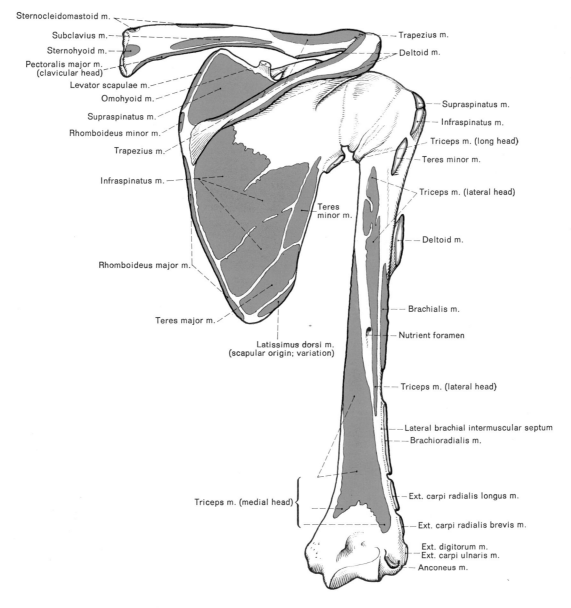

Fig. 37: Posterior View of the Clavicle, Scapula and Humerus Showing Muscle Attachments

NOTE: 1) that dorsally the vertebral border of the scapula is attached to the trunk by the levator scapulae and the rhomboideus major and minor muscles, whereas on the ventral scapular surface (see Fig. 35) the serratus anterior attaches along the vertebral border.

2) the supraspinatus muscle arising from the medial two-thirds of the supraspinatus fossa.

3) the origins of the teres major and teres minor muscles along the axillary border of the scapula and the broad origin of the infraspinatus muscle from the infraspinatus fossa.

4) that onto the spine of the scapula and extending to the lateral third of the clavicle are attached the trapezius and deltoid muscles.

5) most of the posterior surface of the humerus affords origin to the medial and lateral heads of the triceps muscle.

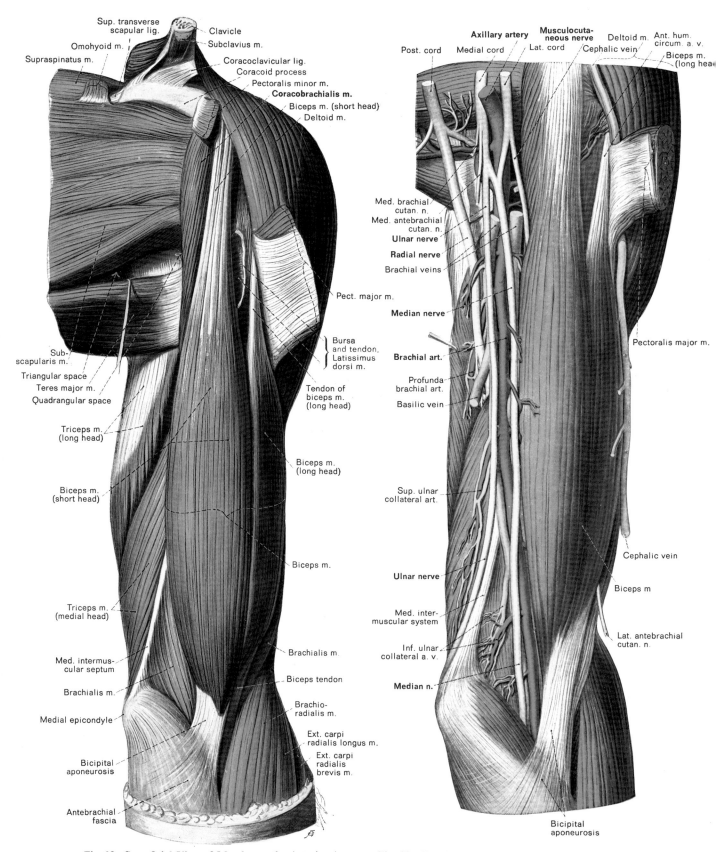

Fig. 38: Superficial View of Muscles on the Anterior Aspect of the Left Arm

NOTE: that the biceps muscle extends across both the shoulder and elbow joints, but that the coracobrachialis muscle extends only across the shoulder joint.

Fig. 39: Vessels and Nerves of the Anterior Arm (left)

NOTE: 1) the median nerve crosses the brachial artery anteriorly from lateral to medial just above the cubital fossa.

2) neither the ulnar nor median nerve gives off branches in the arm.

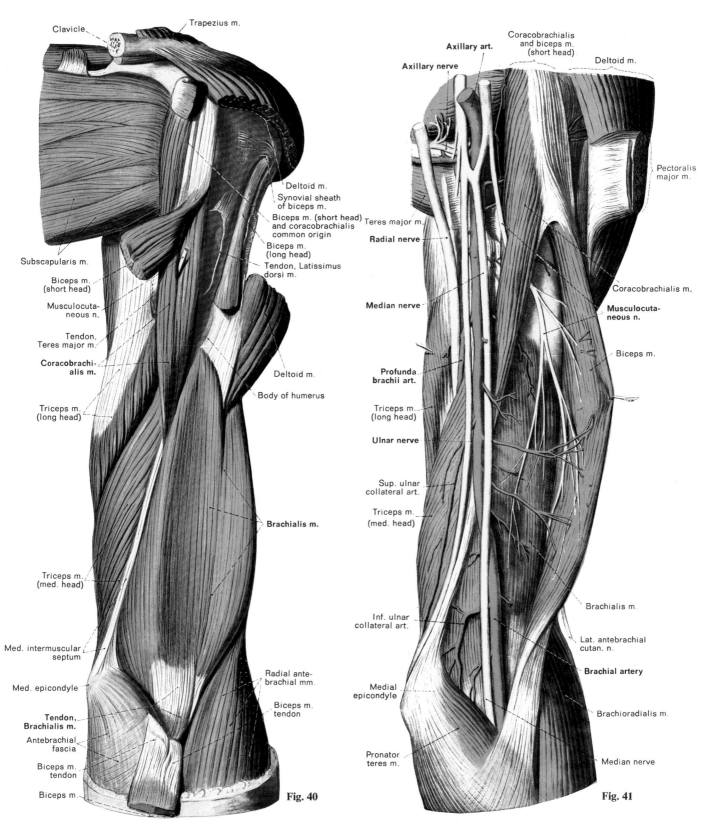

Clavicle

Trapezius m.

Deltoid m.

Synovial sheath
of biceps m.

Biceps m. (short head)
and coracobrachialis
common origin

Biceps m.
(long head)

Tendon, Latissimus
dorsi m.

Subscapularis m.

Biceps m.
(short head)

Musculocuta-
neous n.

Tendon,
Teres major m.

Coracobrachi-
alis m.

Deltoid m.

Body of humerus

Triceps m.
(long head)

Brachialis m.

Triceps m.
(med. head)

Med. intermuscular
septum

Med. epicondyle

Radial ante-
brachial mm.

Biceps m.
tendon

Tendon,
Brachialis m.

Antebrachial
fascia

Biceps m.
tendon

Biceps m.

Fig. 40

Axillary art.

Axillary nerve

Coracobrachialis
and biceps m.
(short head)

Deltoid m.

Pectoralis
major m.

Teres major m.

Radial nerve

Median nerve

Profunda
brachii art.

Triceps m.
(long head)

Ulnar nerve

Sup. ulnar
collateral art.

Triceps m.
(med. head)

Coracobrachialis m.

Musculocuta-
neous n.

Biceps m.

Brachialis m.

Lat. antebrachial
cutan. n.

Brachial artery

Brachioradialis m.

Inf. ulnar
collateral art.

Medial
epicondyle

Pronator
teres m.

Median nerve

Fig. 41

Fig. 40: Deep View of Muscles on the Anterior Aspect of the Left Arm

NOTE: In this dissection both the long head and short head of the biceps brachii muscle have been severed and reflected in order to reveal the underlying brachialis muscle. The coracobrachialis muscle has been left intact.

Fig. 41: The Nerves and Arteries of the Anterior Arm (left)

NOTE: 1) the short head of the biceps muscle has been pulled aside to reveal the musculocutaneous nerve which supplies the coracobrachialis, biceps and brachialis muscles. This nerve continues into the forearm as the lateral antebrachial cutaneous nerve.

2) the superficial course of the brachial artery in the arm. Its branches include the profunda brachii artery and the superior and inferior ulnar collateral arteries in addition to its muscular branches.

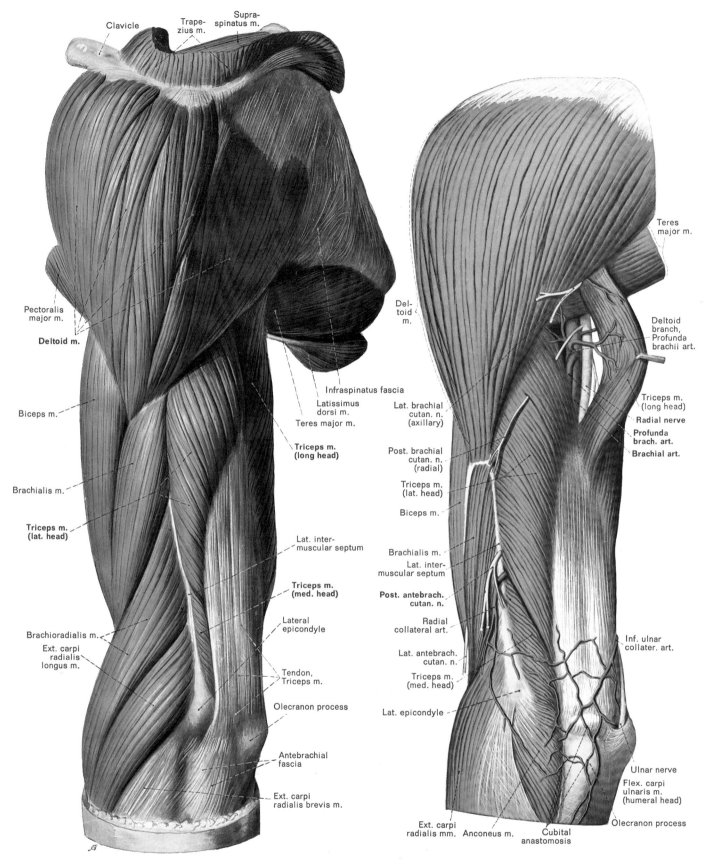

Fig. 42: The Muscles of the Arm (Lateral View)

NOTE: 1) the deltoid muscle acting as a whole abducts the arm. The clavicular portion flexes and medially rotates the arm, while the scapular portion extends and laterally rotates the arm.

2) the lateral intermuscular septum separates the anterior muscular compartment from the posterior muscular compartment.

Fig. 43: Nerves and Arteries of the Left Posterior Arm (Superficial Branches)

NOTE: 1) the origin of the profunda brachii artery from the brachial artery and its relationship to the radial nerve The long head of the triceps has been pulled medially.

2) the relationship of the ulnar nerve to the olecranon process and the vascular anastomosis around the elbow.

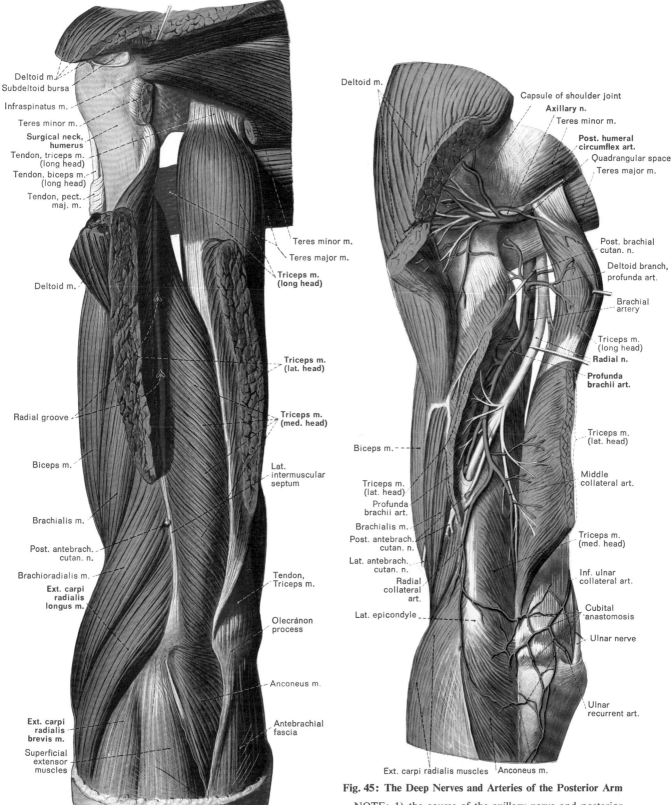

Fig. 44: Deep Muscles of the Arm and Shoulder (Postero-lateral View)

NOTE: in this dissection much of the deltoid and teres minor muscles was removed, and the lateral head of the triceps muscle was transected and reflected. Observe the radial groove between the medial and lateral heads of the triceps.

Fig. 45: The Deep Nerves and Arteries of the Posterior Arm

NOTE: 1) the course of the axillary nerve and posterior humeral circumflex artery through the quadrangular space to achieve the deltoid muscle and dorsal shoulder region.

2) the course of the radial nerve and profunda brachii artery along the musculospiral groove to the posterior brachial region. The groove lies along the body of the humerus between the origins of the lateral and medial heads of the triceps muscle.

3) the common insertion of the triceps muscle onto the olecranon process of the ulna.

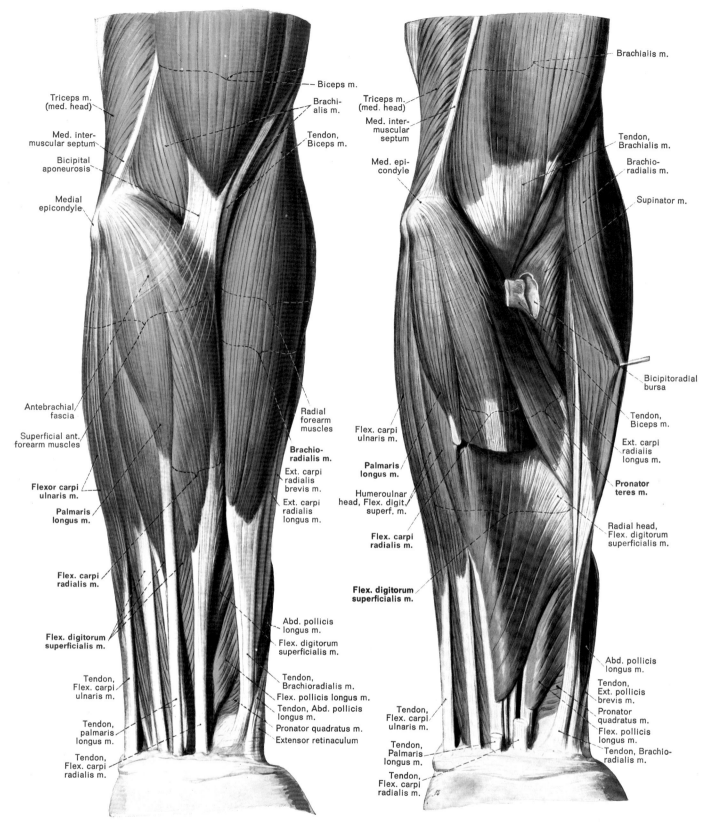

Fig. 46: The Left Anterior Forearm Muscles, Superficial Group

NOTE: 1) that the brachioradialis m. is studied with the posterior forearm muscles instead of the anterior muscles.

2) that the anterior forearm muscles arise from the medial epicondyle of the humerus and include the pronator teres (not labelled), flexor carpi radialis, palmaris longus and flexor carpi ulnaris. Beneath these is the flexor digitorum superficialis.

Fig. 47: The Flexor Digitorum Superficialis Muscle and Related Muscles (left)

NOTE: 1) the palmaris longus, flexor carpi radialis and tendon of the biceps have been cut to reveal the flexor digitorum superficialis and pronator teres.

2) the triangular cubital fossa is bounded medially by the superficial flexors and laterally by the extensors. Its floor is the brachialis m.

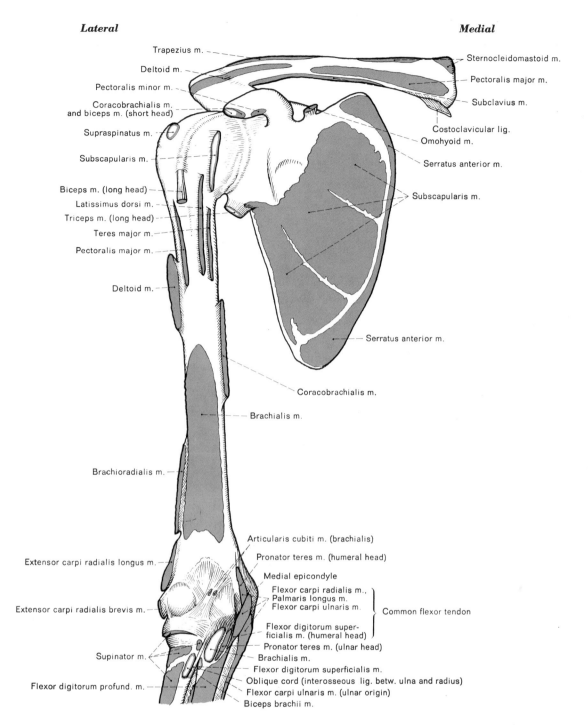

Lateral

Medial

Trapezius m.
Deltoid m.
Pectoralis minor m.
Coracobrachialis m. and biceps m. (short head)
Supraspinatus m.
Subscapularis m.
Biceps m. (long head)
Latissimus dorsi m.
Triceps m. (long head)
Teres major m.
Pectoralis major m.
Deltoid m.
Brachioradialis m.
Extensor carpi radialis longus m.
Extensor carpi radialis brevis m.
Supinator m.
Flexor digitorum profund. m.

Sternocleidomastoid m.
Pectoralis major m.
Subclavius m.
Costoclavicular lig.
Omohyoid m.
Serratus anterior m.
Subscapularis m.
Serratus anterior m.
Coracobrachialis m.
Brachialis m.

Articularis cubiti m. (brachialis)
Pronator teres m. (humeral head)
Medial epicondyle
Flexor carpi radialis m.,
Palmaris longus m.
Flexor carpi ulnaris m.
Flexor digitorum super-ficialis m. (humeral head)
Common flexor tendon
Pronator teres m. (ulnar head)
Brachialis m.
Flexor digitorum superficialis m.
Oblique cord (interosseous lig. betw. ulna and radius)
Flexor carpi ulnaris m. (ulnar origin)
Biceps brachii m.

Fig. 35: Anterior View of Bones of the Upper Limb (Including Proximal End of Radius and Ulna) Showing Attachments of Muscles

NOTE: 1) the broad *origin* of the subscapularis in the subscapular fossa of the scapula and its *insertion* on the lesser tubercle of the humerus proximal to the insertions of the latissimus dorsi and teres major muscles. The subscapularis is an adductor and medial rotator of the arm.

2) the brachialis muscle *arises* from the distal three-fifths of the anterior surface of the humerus and *inserts* on the coronoid process of the ulna. This muscle is the strongest flexor of the forearm.

3) the short head of the biceps m. *arises* with the coracobrachialis m. from the coracoid process, while the long head *arises* from the supraglenoid tubercle of the scapula.

4) the coracobrachialis *inserts* onto the shaft of the humerus near its middle, while the biceps inserts onto the tuberosity of the radius and onto the deep *fascia* of the forearm by way of the bicipital aponeurosis.

5) the coracobrachialis flexes and adducts the arm at the shoulder joint, while the biceps flexes and supinates the forearm, with the long head assisting in flexion of the arm at the shoulder joint.

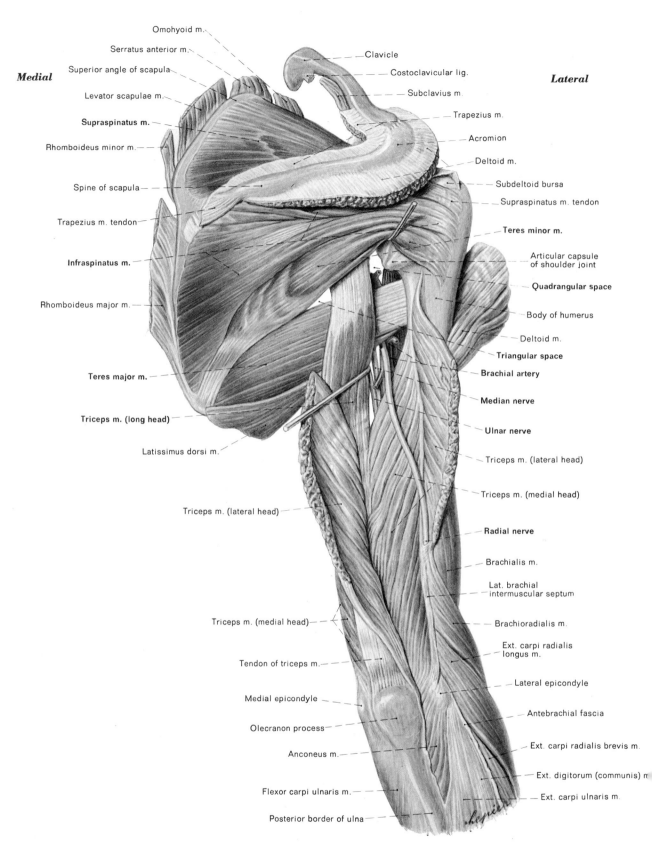

Medial   **Lateral**

Omohyoid m.

Serratus anterior m.

Superior angle of scapula

Levator scapulae m.

Supraspinatus m.

Rhomboideus minor m.

Spine of scapula

Trapezius m. tendon

Infraspinatus m.

Rhomboideus major m.

Teres major m.

Triceps m. (long head)

Latissimus dorsi m.

Triceps m. (lateral head)

Triceps m. (medial head)

Tendon of triceps m.

Medial epicondyle

Olecranon process

Anconeus m.

Flexor carpi ulnaris m.

Posterior border of ulna

Clavicle

Costoclavicular lig.

Subclavius m.

Trapezius m.

Acromion

Deltoid m.

Subdeltoid bursa

Supraspinatus m. tendon

Teres minor m.

Articular capsule of shoulder joint

Quadrangular space

Body of humerus

Deltoid m.

Triangular space

Brachial artery

Median nerve

Ulnar nerve

Triceps m. (lateral head)

Triceps m. (medial head)

Radial nerve

Brachialis m.

Lat. brachial intermuscular septum

Brachioradialis m.

Ext. carpi radialis longus m.

Lateral epicondyle

Antebrachial fascia

Ext. carpi radialis brevis m.

Ext. digitorum (communis) m

Ext. carpi ulnaris m.

Fig. 36: Muscles of the Shoulder and Deep Arm (Posterior View)

NOTE: 1) that with the deltoid muscle and the lateral head of the triceps muscle severed, the course of the radial nerve in the upper arm is revealed.

2) the sequential insertions of the supraspinatus, infraspinatus and teres minor muscles on the greater tubercle of the humerus.

3) the boundaries of the quadrangular and triangular spaces.

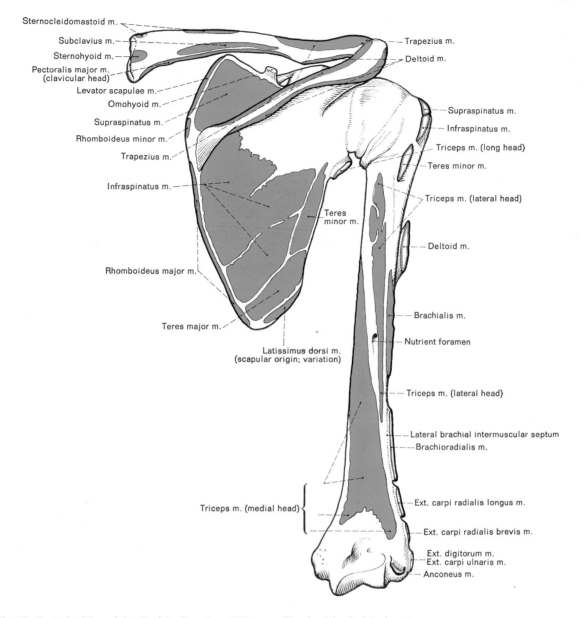

Sternocleidomastoid m.
Subclavius m.
Sternohyoid m.
Pectoralis major m. (clavicular head)
Levator scapulae m.
Omohyoid m.
Supraspinatus m.
Rhomboideus minor m.
Trapezius m.
Infraspinatus m.
Rhomboideus major m.
Teres major m.
Latissimus dorsi m. (scapular origin; variation)
Triceps m. (medial head)
Teres minor m.

Trapezius m.
Deltoid m.
Supraspinatus m.
Infraspinatus m.
Triceps m. (long head)
Teres minor m.
Triceps m. (lateral head)
Deltoid m.
Brachialis m.
Nutrient foramen
Triceps m. (lateral head)
Lateral brachial intermuscular septum
Brachioradialis m.
Ext. carpi radialis longus m.
Ext. carpi radialis brevis m.
Ext. digitorum m.
Ext. carpi ulnaris m.
Anconeus m.

Fig. 37: Posterior View of the Clavicle, Scapula and Humerus Showing Muscle Attachments

NOTE: 1) that dorsally the vertebral border of the scapula is attached to the trunk by the levator scapulae and the rhomboideus major and minor muscles, whereas on the ventral scapular surface (see Fig. 35) the serratus anterior attaches along the vertebral border.

2) the supraspinatus muscle arising from the medial two-thirds of the supraspinatus fossa.

3) the origins of the teres major and teres minor muscles along the axillary border of the scapula and the broad origin of the infraspinatus muscle from the infraspinatus fossa.

4) that onto the spine of the scapula and extending to the lateral third of the clavicle are attached the trapezius and deltoid muscles.

5) most of the posterior surface of the humerus affords origin to the medial and lateral heads of the triceps muscle.

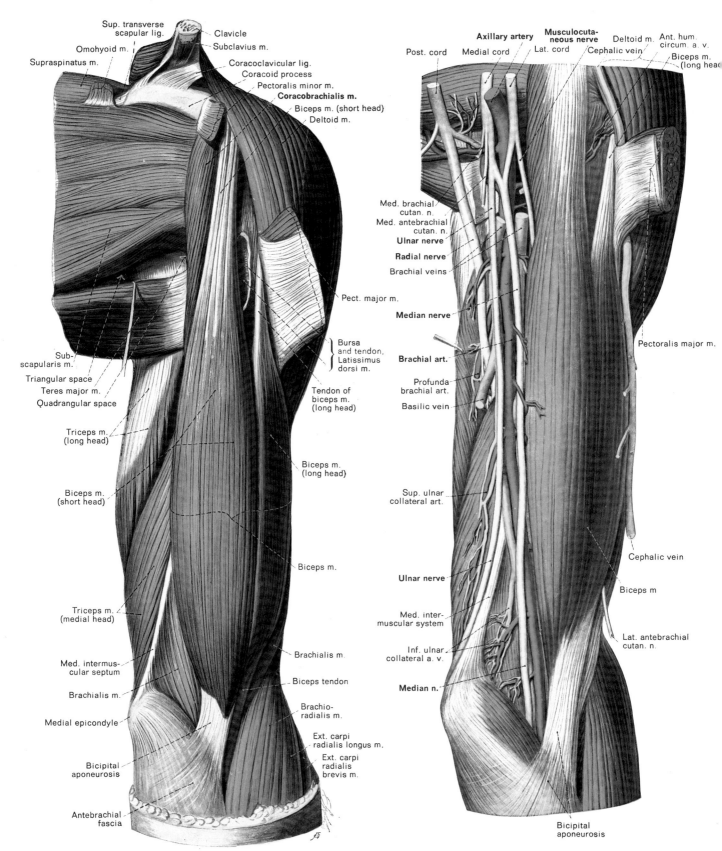

Fig. 38: Superficial View of Muscles on the Anterior Aspect of the Left Arm

NOTE: that the biceps muscle extends across both the shoulder and elbow joints, but that the coracobrachialis muscle extends only across the shoulder joint.

Fig. 39: Vessels and Nerves of the Anterior Arm (left)

NOTE: 1) the median nerve crosses the brachial artery anteriorly from lateral to medial just above the cubital fossa.

2) neither the ulnar nor median nerve gives off branches in the arm.

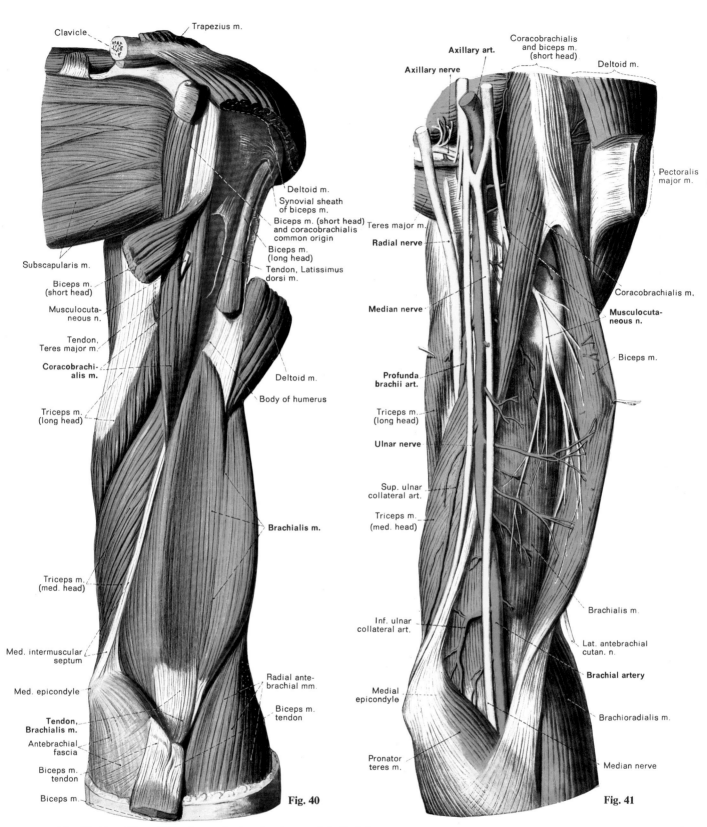

Fig. 40: Deep View of Muscles on the Anterior Aspect of the Left Arm

NOTE: In this dissection both the long head and short head of the biceps brachii muscle have been severed and reflected in order to reveal the underlying brachialis muscle. The coracobrachialis muscle has been left intact.

Fig. 41: The Nerves and Arteries of the Anterior Arm (left)

NOTE: 1) the short head of the biceps muscle has been pulled aside to reveal the musculocutaneous nerve which supplies the coracobrachialis, biceps and brachialis muscles. This nerve continues into the forearm as the lateral antebrachial cutaneous nerve.

2) the superficial course of the brachial artery in the arm. Its branches include the profunda brachii artery and the superior and inferior ulnar collateral arteries in addition to its muscular branches.

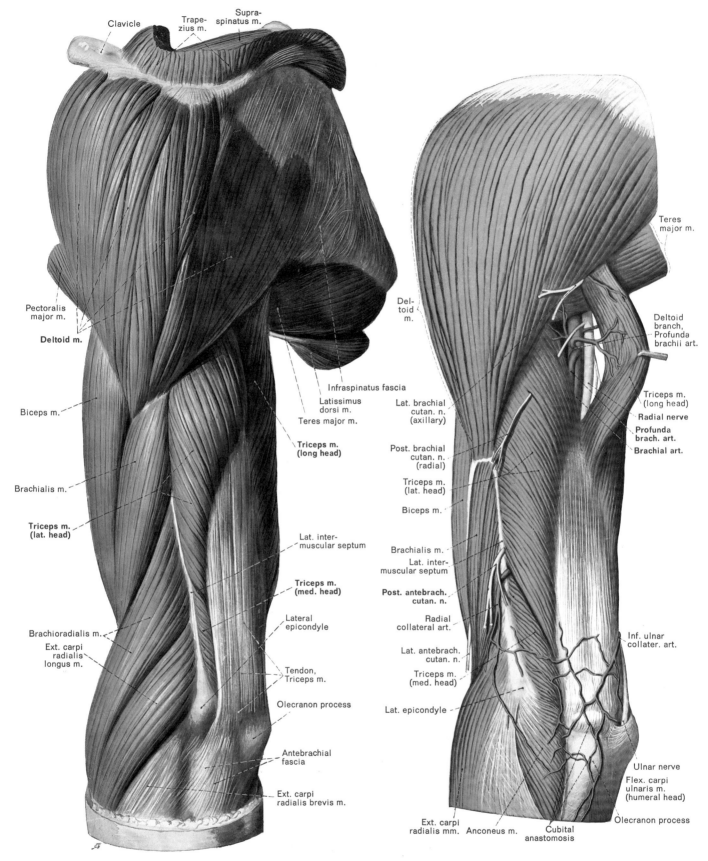

Fig. 42: The Muscles of the Arm (Lateral View)

NOTE: 1) the deltoid muscle acting as a whole abducts the arm. The clavicular portion flexes and medially rotates the arm, while the scapular portion extends and laterally rotates the arm.

2) the lateral intermuscular septum separates the anterior muscular compartment from the posterior muscular compartment.

Fig. 43: Nerves and Arteries of the Left Posterior Arm (Superficial Branches)

NOTE: 1) the origin of the profunda brachii artery from the brachial artery and its relationship to the radial nerve The long head of the triceps has been pulled medially.

2) the relationship of the ulnar nerve to the olecranon process and the vascular anastomosis around the elbow.

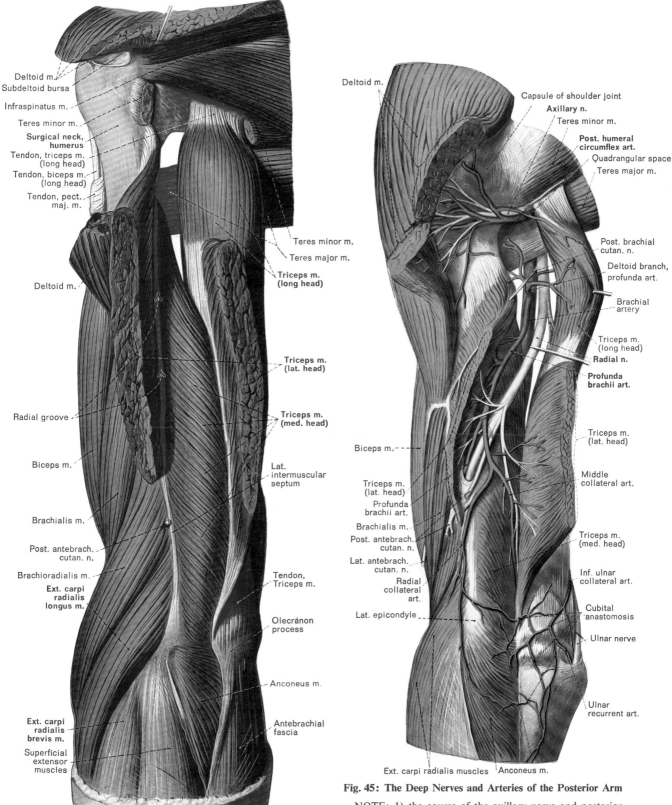

Fig. 44: Deep Muscles of the Arm and Shoulder (Postero-lateral View)

NOTE: in this dissection much of the deltoid and teres minor muscles was removed, and the lateral head of the triceps muscle was transected and reflected. Observe the radial groove between the medial and lateral heads of the triceps.

Fig. 45: The Deep Nerves and Arteries of the Posterior Arm

NOTE: 1) the course of the axillary nerve and posterior humeral circumflex artery through the quadrangular space to achieve the deltoid muscle and dorsal shoulder region.

2) the course of the radial nerve and profunda brachii artery along the musculospiral groove to the posterior brachial region. The groove lies along the body of the humerus between the origins of the lateral and medial heads of the triceps muscle.

3) the common insertion of the triceps muscle onto the olecranon process of the ulna.

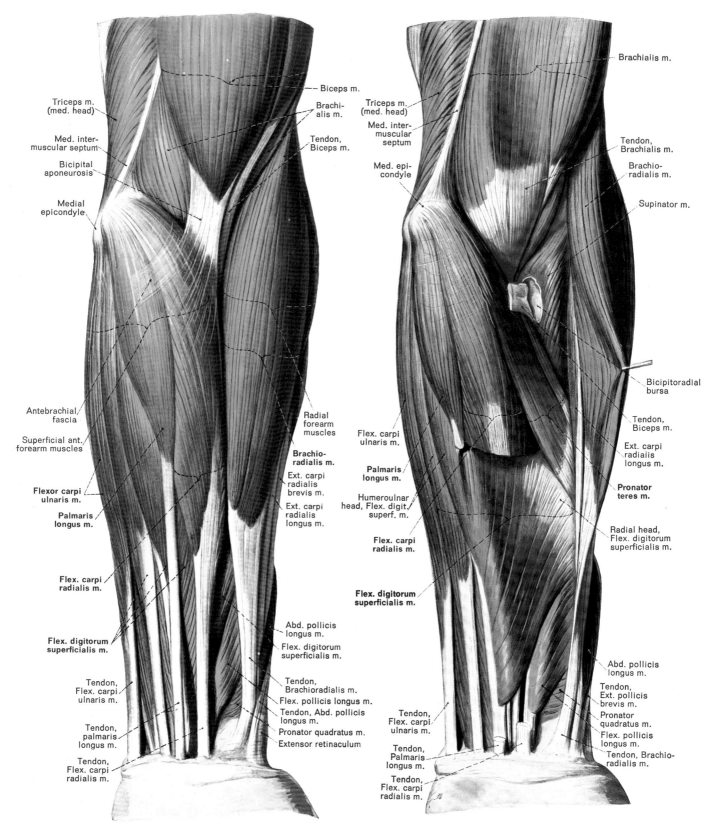

Fig. 46: The Left Anterior Forearm Muscles, Superficial Group

NOTE: 1) that the brachioradialis m. is studied with the posterior forearm muscles instead of the anterior muscles.

2) that the anterior forearm muscles arise from the medial epicondyle of the humerus and include the pronator teres (not labelled), flexor carpi radialis, palmaris longus and flexor carpi ulnaris. Beneath these is the flexor digitorum superficialis.

Fig. 47: The Flexor Digitorum Superficialis Muscle and Related Muscles (left)

NOTE: 1) the palmaris longus, flexor carpi radialis and tendon of the biceps have been cut to reveal the flexor digitorum superficialis and pronator teres.

2) the triangular cubital fossa is bounded medially by the superficial flexors and laterally by the extensors. Its floor is the brachialis m.

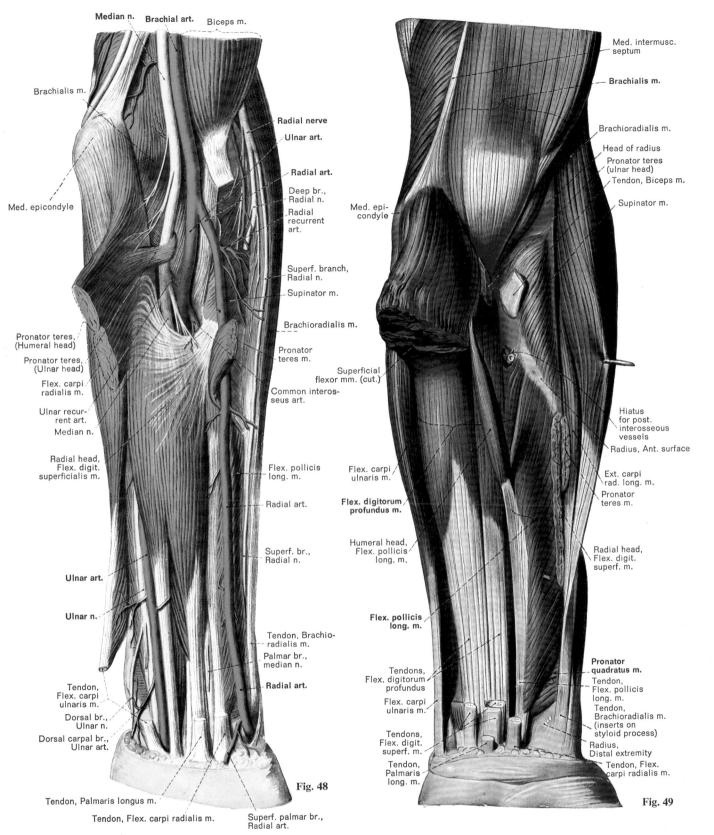

Fig. 48: Median n.   Brachial art.   Biceps m.   Brachialis m.   Med. epicondyle   Radial nerve   Ulnar art.   Radial art.   Deep br., Radial n.   Radial recurrent art.   Superf. branch, Radial n.   Supinator m.   Brachioradialis m.   Pronator teres m.   Common interosseus art.   Flex. pollicis long. m.   Radial art.   Superf. br., Radial n.   Tendon, Brachioradialis m.   Palmar br., median n.   Radial art.   Superf. palmar br., Radial art.   Tendon, Flex. carpi radialis m.   Tendon, Palmaris longus m.   Dorsal carpal br., Ulnar art.   Dorsal br., Ulnar n.   Tendon, Flex. carpi ulnaris m.   Ulnar n.   Ulnar art.   Radial head, Flex. digit. superficialis m.   Median n.   Ulnar recurrent art.   Flex. carpi radialis m.   Pronator teres, (Ulnar head)   Pronator teres, (Humeral head)   Med. epicondyle   Brachialis m.

Fig. 48: Nerves and Arteries, Anterior Aspect of Left Forearm

NOTE: 1) the pronator teres and flexor carpi radialis muscles are reflected just below the cubital fossa to reveal the origins of the ulnar and radial arteries.

2) at the wrist, the flexor carpi ulnaris muscle is severed to expose the ulnar nerve and artery.

Fig. 49: The Left Anterior Forearm Muscles, Deep Group

NOTE: 1) the superficial anterior forearm muscles have been removed to reveal the three muscles of the deep group. These include the flexor digitorum profundus, the flexor pollicis longus and the pronator quadratus.

2) the pronator quadratus is a small quadrangular muscle situated at the distal end of the forearm beneath the tendons of the flexor digitorum profundus and flexor pollicis longus. It is only partially shown in this dissection and can better be seen in Fig. 79.

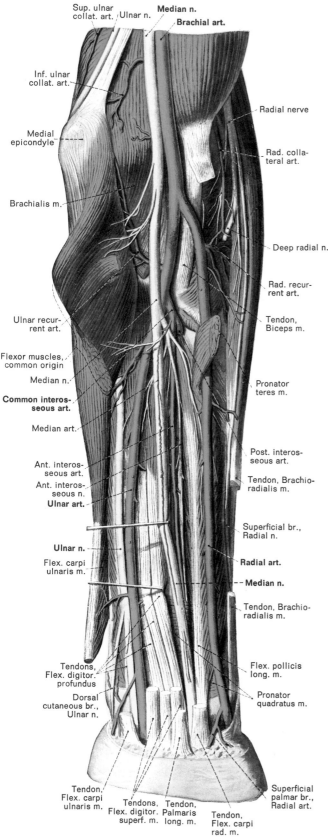

Fig. 50: Nerves and Arteries of Left Anterior Forearm (Deep Dissection)

Note the division of the brachial artery into the radial and ulnar. The common interosseous artery branches from the ulnar artery and divides immediately into anterior and posterior interosseous arteries. Observe the courses of the median and ulnar nerves.

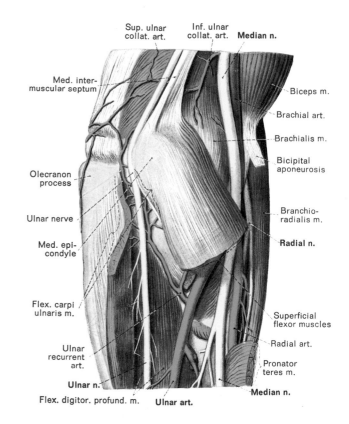

Fig. 51: Nerves and Arteries at the Elbow (Medial View)

NOTE: the ulnar nerve enters the forearm directly behind the medial epicondyle.

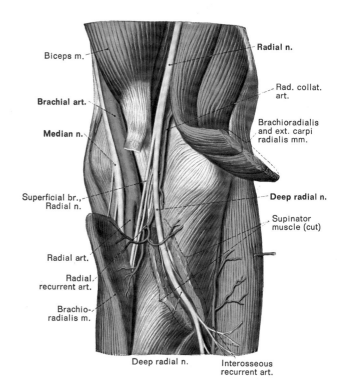

Fig. 52: Nerves and Arteries at the Elbow (Lateral View)

NOTE: the deep radial nerve passes into the forearm in front of the lateral part of the elbow joint. It then courses dorsally through the supinator muscle to supply the posterior forearm muscles.

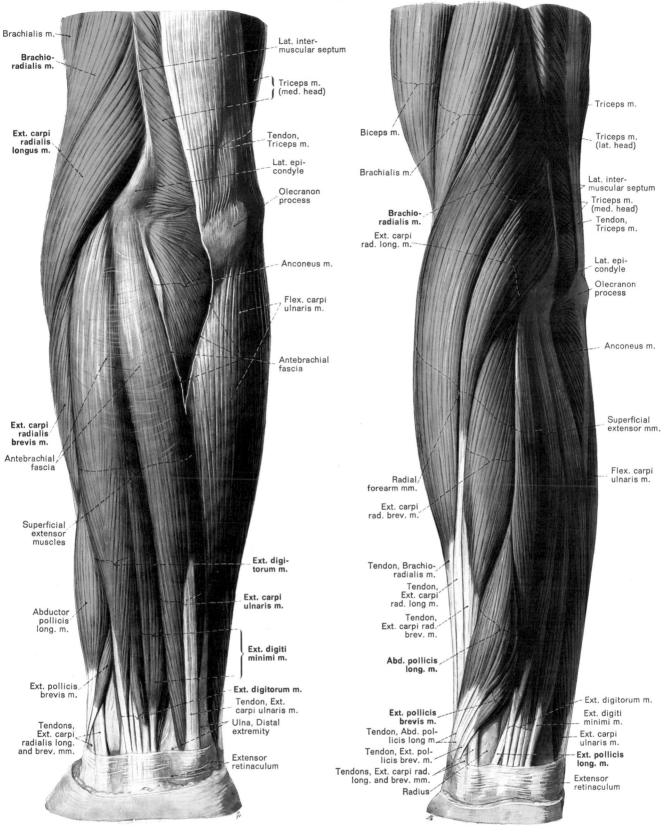

Fig. 53: Posterior Muscles of the Left Forearm, Superficial Group

Note that most of the superficial extensor muscles arise from the lateral epicondyle of the humerus. These are the extensor carpi radialis brevis, the extensor digitorum, the extensor digiti minimi and the extensor carpi ulnaris. The brachioradialis and extensor carpi radialis longus arise from the supracondylar ridge.

Fig. 54: Posterior Muscles (Superficial) of the Left Forearm, Lateral View

NOTE: 1) the superficial location of the brachioradialis muscle.

2) three muscles of the thumb: extensor pollicis longus, extensor pollicis brevis and abductor pollicis longus.

3) the closely investing extensor retinaculum under which the extensor tendons pass into the dorsum of the hand.

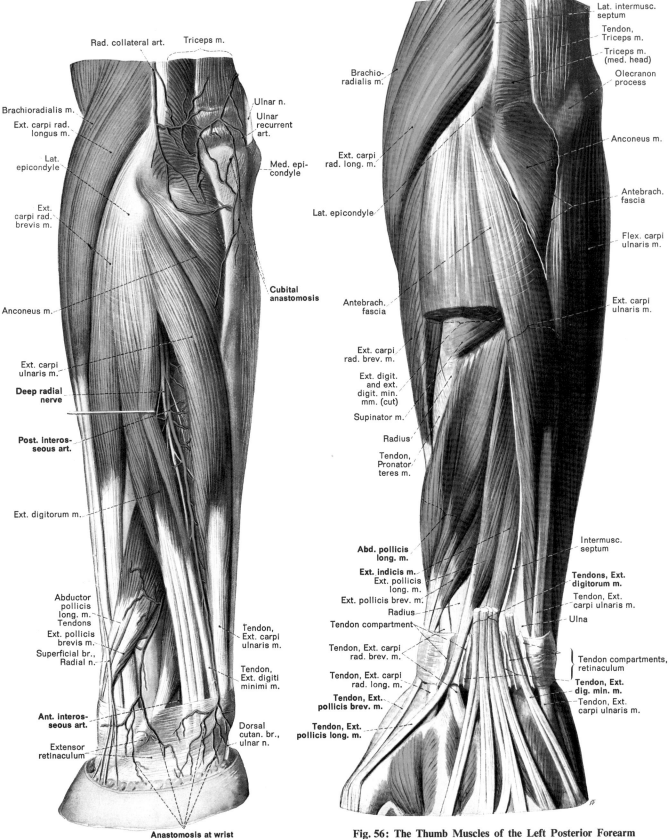

Fig. 55: Nerves and Arteries of the Left Posterior Forearm

NOTE: 1) the extensor digiti minimi and extensor digitorum have been separated from the extensor carpi ulnaris to expose the deep radial nerve and posterior interosseous artery coursing inferiorly in the posterior forearm.

2) the anastomoses at the elbow and wrist.

Fig. 56: The Thumb Muscles of the Left Posterior Forearm

NOTE: 1) that the three thumb muscles (abductor pollicis longus and extensors pollicis brevis and longus) are exposed when the extensor digitorum and extensor digiti minimi muscles are partially removed. Observe also the extensor indicis muscle inserting onto the index finger.

2) the tendon compartments formed by the extensor retinaculum at the wrist.

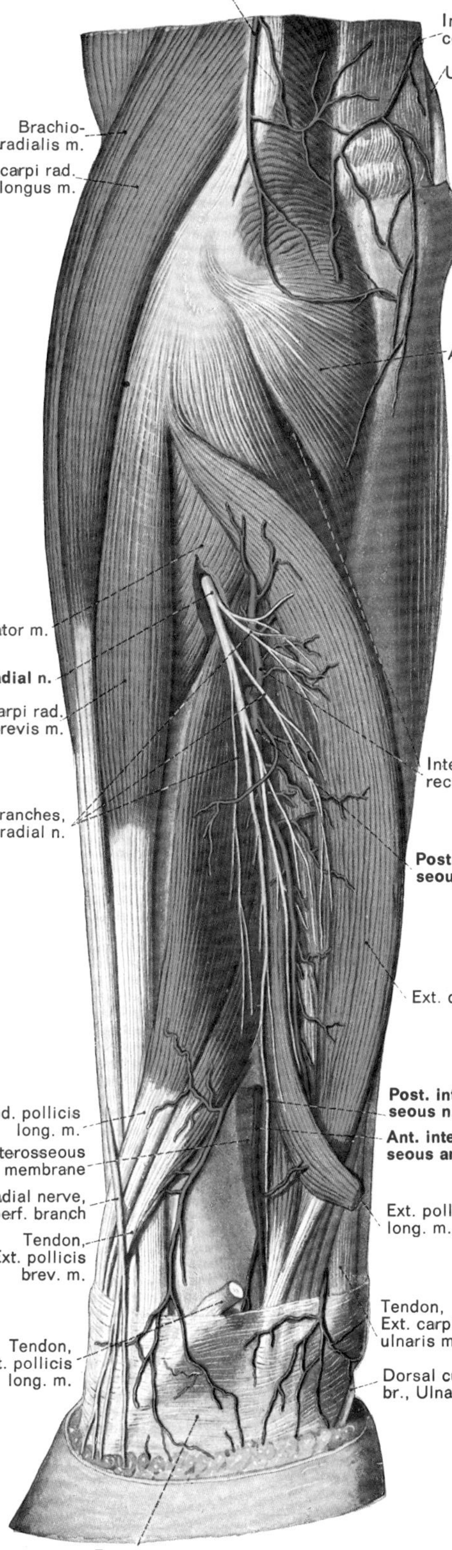

Fig. 57: Nerves and Arteries of the Left Posterior Forearm (Deep Dissection)

NOTE: 1) the extensor digitorum muscle is separated from the extensor carpi radialis brevis and pulled medially to reveal the posterior interosseous artery and deep radial nerve.

2) the emergence of the deep radial nerve to the posterior forearm through the supinator muscle.

3) the posterior interosseous nerve is a continuation inferiorly of the deep radial nerve and may be seen coursing deep to the extensor pollicis longus muscle. This muscle has been cut at the wrist in this dissection.

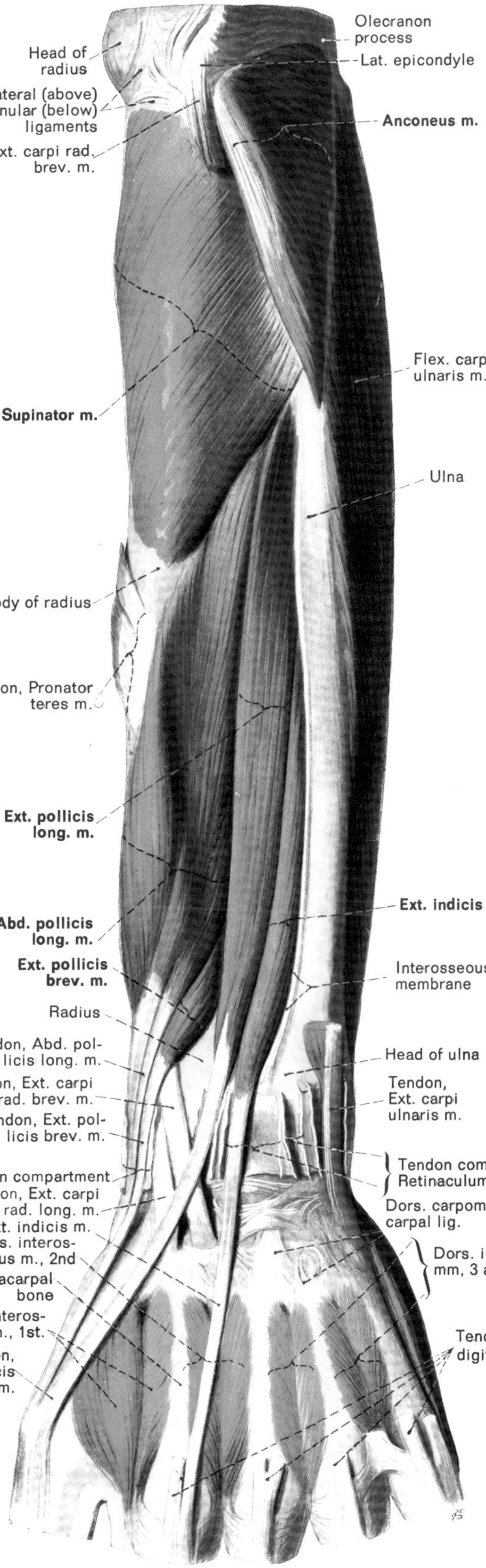

Fig. 58: The Left Posterior Forearm Muscles, Deep Group

NOTE: 1) all of the superficial posterior forearm muscles have been removed except the anconeus. The five deep muscles are the supinator, abductor pollicis longus, extensors pollicis brevis and longus and extensor indicis.

2) the supinator is a broad muscle, arising from the lateral epicondyle of the humerus and from the ridge of the ulna. It courses obliquely to insert around the upper third of the radius.

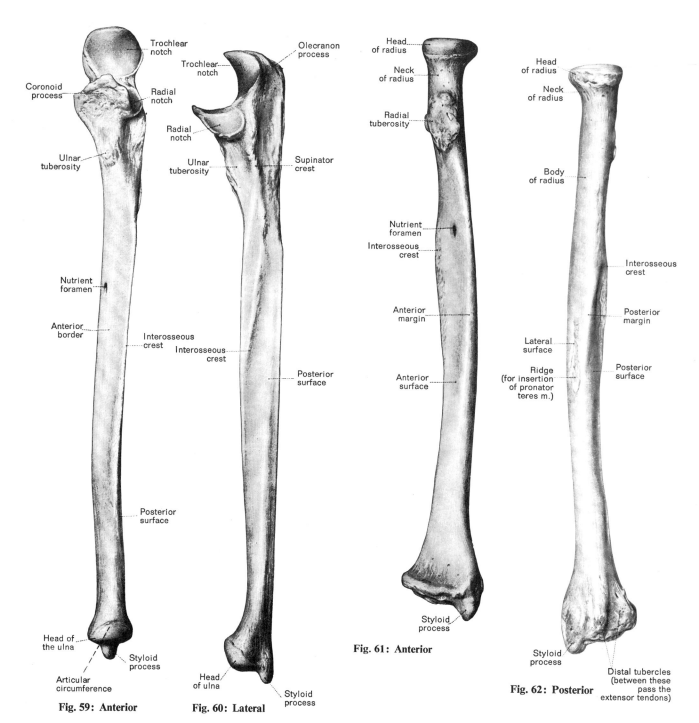

Fig. 59: Anterior **Fig. 60: Lateral**

Fig. 61: Anterior

Fig. 62: Posterior

The Left Ulna

NOTE: 1) the ulna is the medial bone of the forearm. It presents a superior extremity, a body or shaft and an inferior extremity.

2) the superior extremity is marked by two processes, the olecranon and coronoid processes and two concave cavities, the radial notch for articulation with the radius, and the trochlear notch which serves for articulation with the trochlea of the humerus. The brachialis muscle inserts on the tuberosity of the ulna.

3) the tapering body of the ulna affords attachment of the interosseous membrane. The distal extremity is marked by the ulnar head laterally, and the styloid process postero-medially. The head of the ulna is attached to an articular disc which, in turn, articulates with the triquetral bone. Onto the styloid process of the ulna is attached the ulnar collateral ligament of the wrist joint.

The Left Radius

NOTE: 1) the radius is situated lateral to the ulna in the forearm. It has a body and two extremities. The proximal extremity articulates with both the humerus and ulna. The larger distal extremity articulates inferiorly with the carpal bones (scaphoid, lunate and triquetrum) and medially with the ulna.

2) the proximal extremity is marked by a cylindrical head which articulates with both the capitulum of the humerus and the radial notch of the ulna. Just beneath the neck on the anteromedial aspect is found the radial tuberosity on which is inserted the biceps tendon.

3) the interosseous membrane is attached along the interosseous crest of the shaft.

4) the styloid process distally gives attachment to the brachioradialis muscle and the radial collateral ligament of the radiocarpal joint.

Fig. 63: The Left Elbow Joint, Anterior View

NOTE: 1) the elbow joint is a hinge (ginglymus) joint in which the trochlear notch of the ulna receives the trochlea of the humerus, and the shallow fovea on the head of radius articulates with the capitulum of the humerus.

2) the entire joint is encased by an articular capsule which tends to be loose to allow flexion and extension of the forearm. The capsule is thickened medially by the ulnar collateral ligament and laterally by the radial collateral ligament.

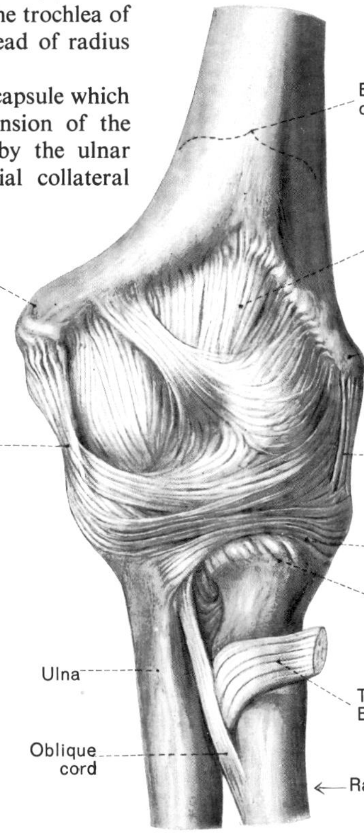

Fig. 63

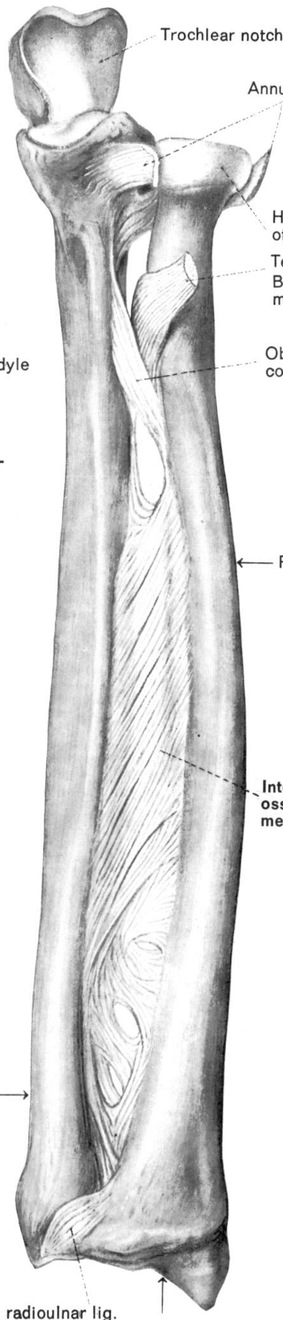

Fig. 65

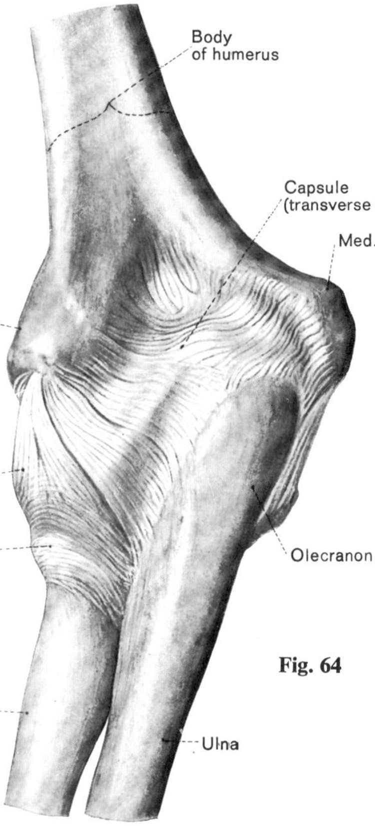

Fig. 64

Fig. 64: The Left Elbow Joint, Posterolateral View

NOTE: 1) the fan-shaped form of the radial collateral ligament. It attaches superiorly to the lateral epicondyle and blends inferiorly with the capsule of the joint.

2) the superior portion of the radial annular ligament also blends with the articular capsule.

3) the transverse fibers of the articular capsule forming a band between the medial and lateral epicondyles and bridging the olecranon fossa.

Fig. 65: Radioulnar Joints, Anterior View (left)

NOTE: 1) articulations between the radius and ulna occur proximally, along the shafts of the two bones and distally.

2) the proximal joint is a pivot (trochoid) type joint and consists of the head of the radius which rotates within the radial notch of the ulna. This joint is protected by the lower part of the capsule of the elbow joint and by an underlying annular ligament attached at both ends to the ulna and forming a circular band around the head of the radius.

3) the broad, fibrous interosseous membrane extends obliquely between the bones while distally the head of the ulna articulates with the ulnar notch of the radius.

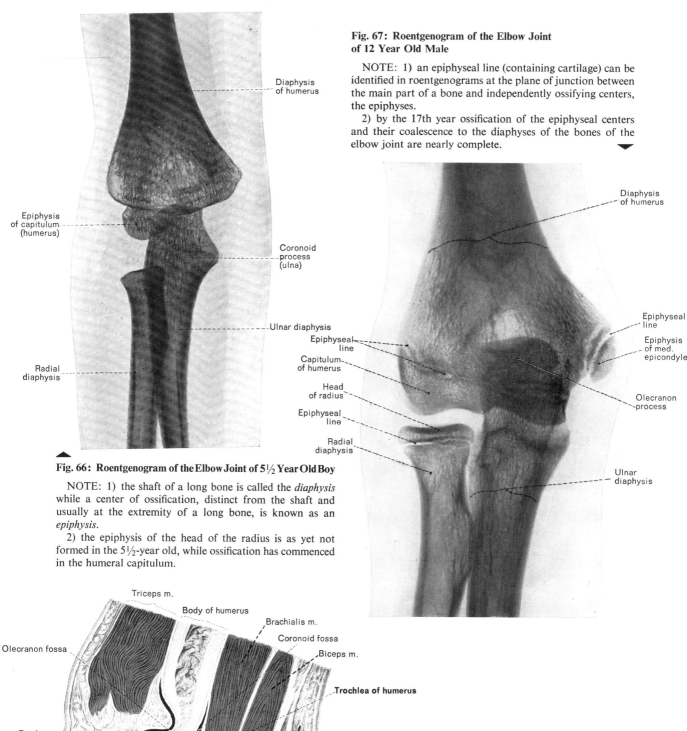

Fig. 67: Roentgenogram of the Elbow Joint of 12 Year Old Male

NOTE: 1) an epiphyseal line (containing cartilage) can be identified in roentgenograms at the plane of junction between the main part of a bone and independently ossifying centers, the epiphyses.

2) by the 17th year ossification of the epiphyseal centers and their coalescence to the diaphyses of the bones of the elbow joint are nearly complete. ▼

Diaphysis of humerus

Epiphysis of capitulum (humerus)

Coronoid process (ulna)

Ulnar diaphysis

Radial diaphysis

Diaphysis of humerus

Epiphyseal line

Epiphyseal line

Epiphysis of med. epicondyle

Capitulum of humerus

Head of radius

Olecranon process

Epiphyseal line

Radial diaphysis

Ulnar diaphysis

Fig. 66: Roentgenogram of the Elbow Joint of 5½ Year Old Boy

NOTE: 1) the shaft of a long bone is called the *diaphysis* while a center of ossification, distinct from the shaft and usually at the extremity of a long bone, is known as an *epiphysis*.

2) the epiphysis of the head of the radius is as yet not formed in the 5½-year old, while ossification has commenced in the humeral capitulum.

Triceps m.

Body of humerus

Brachialis m.

Coronoid fossa

Biceps m.

Olecranon fossa

Trochlea of humerus

Median cubital vein

Tendon, Triceps m.

Olecranon bursa

Joint cavity

Brachial artery

Ulna

Fig. 68: Sagittal Section of the Left Elbow Joint

NOTE: 1) the trochlea of the humerus articulates with the trochlear notch of the ulna to form a ginglymus or hinge joint. The adaptation of these two articular surfaces is such that only flexion and extension can take place and not lateral displacement.

2) the posterior aspect of the olecranon process is separated from the skin by a subcutaneous bursa.

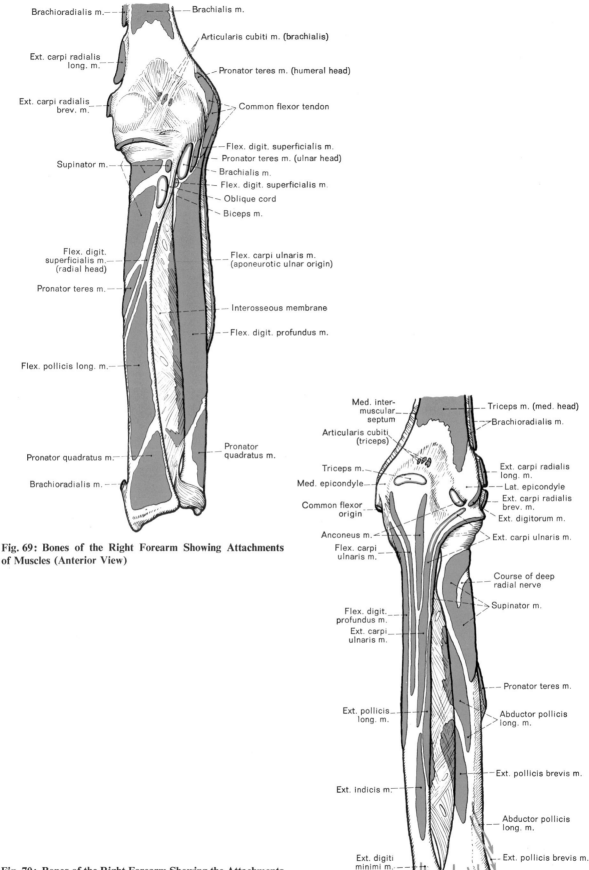

Brachioradialis m.

Brachialis m.

Articularis cubiti m. (brachialis)

Ext. carpi radialis long. m.

Pronator teres m. (humeral head)

Ext. carpi radialis brev. m.

Common flexor tendon

Flex. digit. superficialis m.

Pronator teres m. (ulnar head)

Supinator m.

Brachialis m.

Flex. digit. superficialis m.

Oblique cord

Biceps m.

Flex. digit. superficialis m. (radial head)

Flex. carpi ulnaris m. (aponeurotic ulnar origin)

Pronator teres m.

Interosseous membrane

Flex. digit. profundus m.

Flex. pollicis long. m.

Pronator quadratus m.

Pronator quadratus m.

Brachioradialis m.

Fig. 69: Bones of the Right Forearm Showing Attachments of Muscles (Anterior View)

Med. intermuscular septum

Triceps m. (med. head)

Brachioradialis m.

Articularis cubiti (triceps)

Ext. carpi radialis long. m.

Triceps m.

Lat. epicondyle

Med. epicondyle

Ext. carpi radialis brev. m.

Common flexor origin

Ext. digitorum m.

Anconeus m.

Ext. carpi ulnaris m.

Flex. carpi ulnaris m.

Course of deep radial nerve

Supinator m.

Flex. digit. profundus m.

Ext. carpi ulnaris m.

Pronator teres m.

Abductor pollicis long. m.

Ext. pollicis long. m.

Ext. pollicis brevis m.

Ext. indicis m.

Abductor pollicis long. m.

Ext. pollicis brevis m.

Ext. digiti minimi m.

Ext. pollicis long. m.

Ext. digitorum m.

Ext. carpi radialis long. m.

Ext. carpi ulnaris m.

Ext. carpi radialis brevis m.

Fig. 70: Bones of the Right Forearm Showing the Attachments of Muscles (Posterior View)

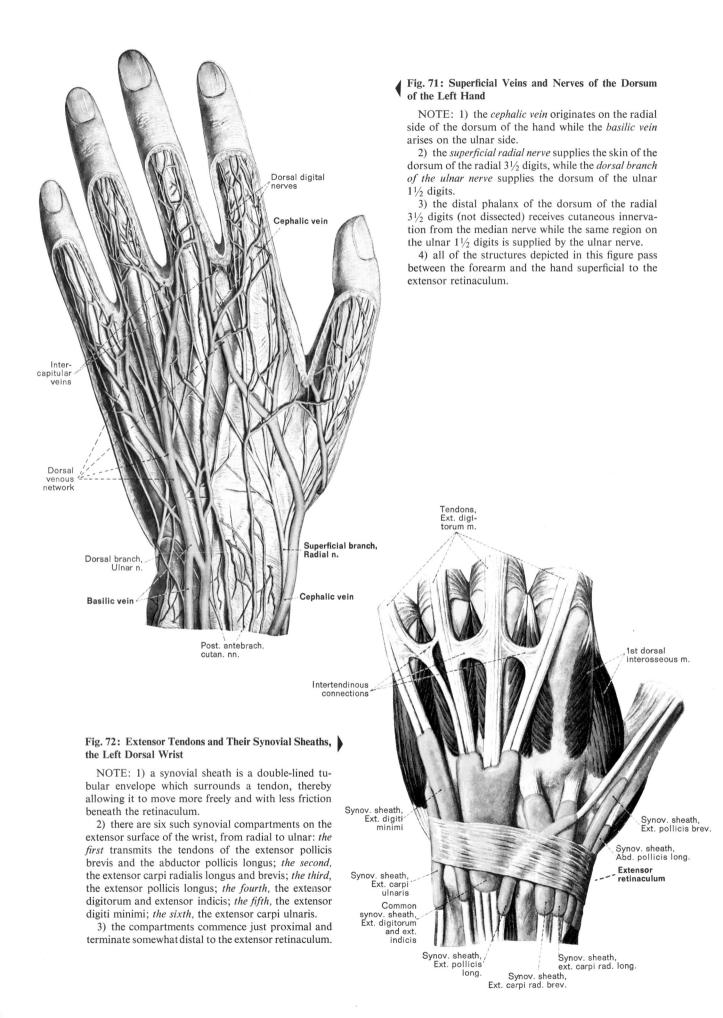

Fig. 71: Superficial Veins and Nerves of the Dorsum of the Left Hand

NOTE: 1) the *cephalic vein* originates on the radial side of the dorsum of the hand while the *basilic vein* arises on the ulnar side.

2) the *superficial radial nerve* supplies the skin of the dorsum of the radial 3½ digits, while the *dorsal branch of the ulnar nerve* supplies the dorsum of the ulnar 1½ digits.

3) the distal phalanx of the dorsum of the radial 3½ digits (not dissected) receives cutaneous innervation from the median nerve while the same region on the ulnar 1½ digits is supplied by the ulnar nerve.

4) all of the structures depicted in this figure pass between the forearm and the hand superficial to the extensor retinaculum.

Dorsal digital nerves

Cephalic vein

Inter-capitular veins

Dorsal venous network

Dorsal branch, Ulnar n.

Basilic vein

Superficial branch, Radial n.

Cephalic vein

Post. antebrach. cutan. nn.

Tendons, Ext. digitorum m.

1st dorsal interosseous m.

Intertendinous connections

Fig. 72: Extensor Tendons and Their Synovial Sheaths, the Left Dorsal Wrist

NOTE: 1) a synovial sheath is a double-lined tubular envelope which surrounds a tendon, thereby allowing it to move more freely and with less friction beneath the retinaculum.

2) there are six such synovial compartments on the extensor surface of the wrist, from radial to ulnar: *the first* transmits the tendons of the extensor pollicis brevis and the abductor pollicis longus; *the second,* the extensor carpi radialis longus and brevis; *the third,* the extensor pollicis longus; *the fourth,* the extensor digitorum and extensor indicis; *the fifth,* the extensor digiti minimi; *the sixth,* the extensor carpi ulnaris.

3) the compartments commence just proximal and terminate somewhat distal to the extensor retinaculum.

Synov. sheath, Ext. digiti minimi

Synov. sheath, Ext. pollicis brev.

Synov. sheath, Abd. pollicis long.

Extensor retinaculum

Synov. sheath, Ext. carpi ulnaris

Synov. sheath, Ext. digitorum and ext. indicis

Synov. sheath, Ext. pollicis long.

Synov. sheath, ext. carpi rad. long.

Synov. sheath, Ext. carpi rad. brev.

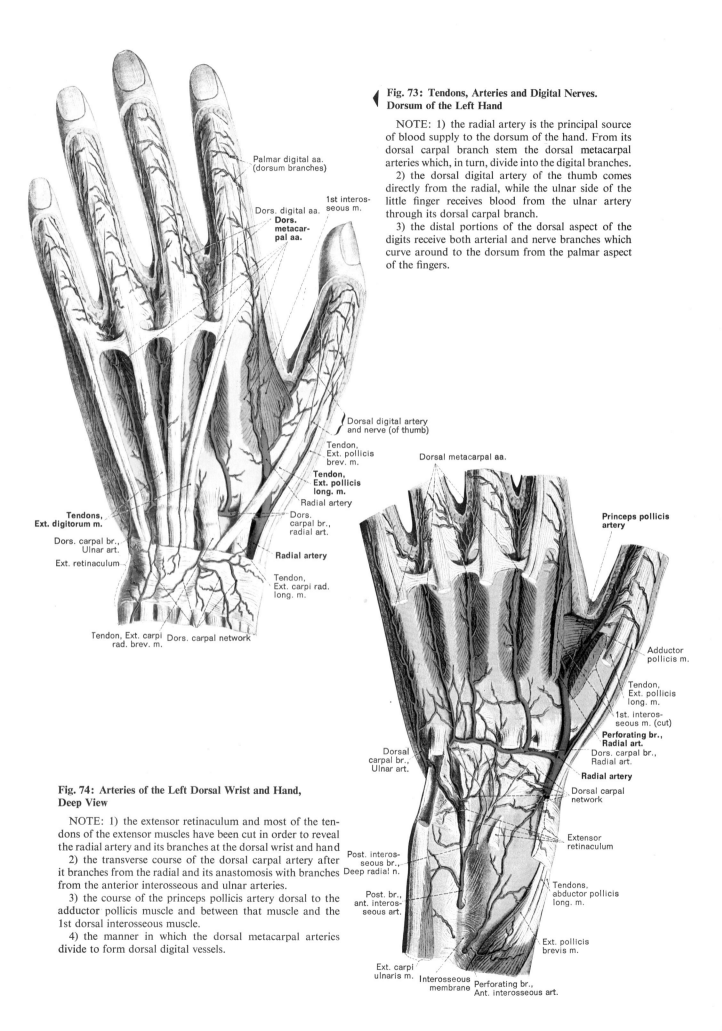

Palmar digital aa.
(dorsum branches)

1st interos-
seous m.

Dors. digital aa.
**Dors.
metacar-
pal aa.**

Dorsal digital artery
and nerve (of thumb)

Tendon,
Ext. pollicis
brev. m.

**Tendon,
Ext. pollicis
long. m.**

Radial artery

Dors.
carpal br.,
radial art.

Radial artery

**Tendons,
Ext. digitorum m.**

Dors. carpal br.,
Ulnar art.

Ext. retinaculum

Tendon,
Ext. carpi rad.
long. m.

Tendon, Ext. carpi
rad. brev. m.

Dors. carpal network

Fig. 73: Tendons, Arteries and Digital Nerves. Dorsum of the Left Hand

NOTE: 1) the radial artery is the principal source of blood supply to the dorsum of the hand. From its dorsal carpal branch stem the dorsal metacarpal arteries which, in turn, divide into the digital branches.

2) the dorsal digital artery of the thumb comes directly from the radial, while the ulnar side of the little finger receives blood from the ulnar artery through its dorsal carpal branch.

3) the distal portions of the dorsal aspect of the digits receive both arterial and nerve branches which curve around to the dorsum from the palmar aspect of the fingers.

Dorsal metacarpal aa.

**Princeps pollicis
artery**

Adductor
pollicis m.

Tendon,
Ext. pollicis
long. m.

1st. interos-
seous m. (cut)

**Perforating br.,
Radial art.**

Dors. carpal br.,
Radial art.

Radial artery

Dorsal carpal
network

Extensor
retinaculum

Tendons,
abductor pollicis
long. m.

Ext. pollicis
brevis m.

Dorsal
carpal br.,
Ulnar art.

Post. interos-
seous br.,
Deep radial n.

Post. br.,
ant. interos-
seous art.

Ext. carpi
ulnaris m.

Interosseous
membrane

Perforating br.,
Ant. interosseous art.

Fig. 74: Arteries of the Left Dorsal Wrist and Hand, Deep View

NOTE: 1) the extensor retinaculum and most of the tendons of the extensor muscles have been cut in order to reveal the radial artery and its branches at the dorsal wrist and hand

2) the transverse course of the dorsal carpal artery after it branches from the radial and its anastomosis with branches from the anterior interosseous and ulnar arteries.

3) the course of the princeps pollicis artery dorsal to the adductor pollicis muscle and between that muscle and the 1st dorsal interosseous muscle.

4) the manner in which the dorsal metacarpal arteries divide to form dorsal digital vessels.

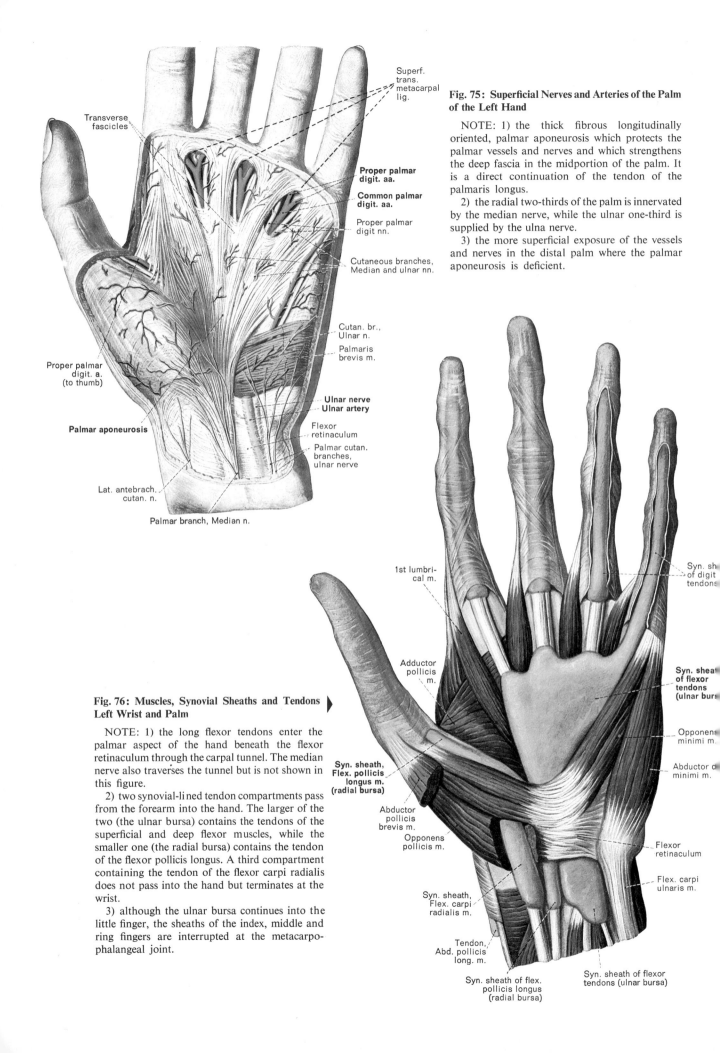

Transverse fascicles

Superf. trans. metacarpal lig.

Proper palmar digit. aa.

Common palmar digit. aa.

Proper palmar digit nn.

Cutaneous branches, Median and ulnar nn.

Cutan. br., Ulnar n.

Palmaris brevis m.

Ulnar nerve
Ulnar artery

Flexor retinaculum

Palmar cutan. branches, ulnar nerve

Proper palmar digit. a. (to thumb)

Palmar aponeurosis

Lat. antebrach. cutan. n.

Palmar branch, Median n.

Fig. 75: Superficial Nerves and Arteries of the Palm of the Left Hand

NOTE: 1) the thick fibrous longitudinally oriented, palmar aponeurosis which protects the palmar vessels and nerves and which strengthens the deep fascia in the midportion of the palm. It is a direct continuation of the tendon of the palmaris longus.

2) the radial two-thirds of the palm is innervated by the median nerve, while the ulnar one-third is supplied by the ulna nerve.

3) the more superficial exposure of the vessels and nerves in the distal palm where the palmar aponeurosis is deficient.

1st lumbrical m.

Adductor pollicis m.

Syn. sheath, Flex. pollicis longus m. (radial bursa)

Abductor pollicis brevis m.

Opponens pollicis m.

Syn. sheath, Flex. carpi radialis m.

Tendon, Abd. pollicis long. m.

Syn. sheath of flex. pollicis longus (radial bursa)

Syn. sh of digit tendons

Syn. sheath of flexor tendons (ulnar bursa)

Opponens minimi m.

Abductor d minimi m.

Flexor retinaculum

Flex. carpi ulnaris m.

Syn. sheath of flexor tendons (ulnar bursa)

Fig. 76: Muscles, Synovial Sheaths and Tendons Left Wrist and Palm

NOTE: 1) the long flexor tendons enter the palmar aspect of the hand beneath the flexor retinaculum through the carpal tunnel. The median nerve also traverses the tunnel but is not shown in this figure.

2) two synovial-lined tendon compartments pass from the forearm into the hand. The larger of the two (the ulnar bursa) contains the tendons of the superficial and deep flexor muscles, while the smaller one (the radial bursa) contains the tendon of the flexor pollicis longus. A third compartment containing the tendon of the flexor carpi radialis does not pass into the hand but terminates at the wrist.

3) although the ulnar bursa continues into the little finger, the sheaths of the index, middle and ring fingers are interrupted at the metacarpophalangeal joint.

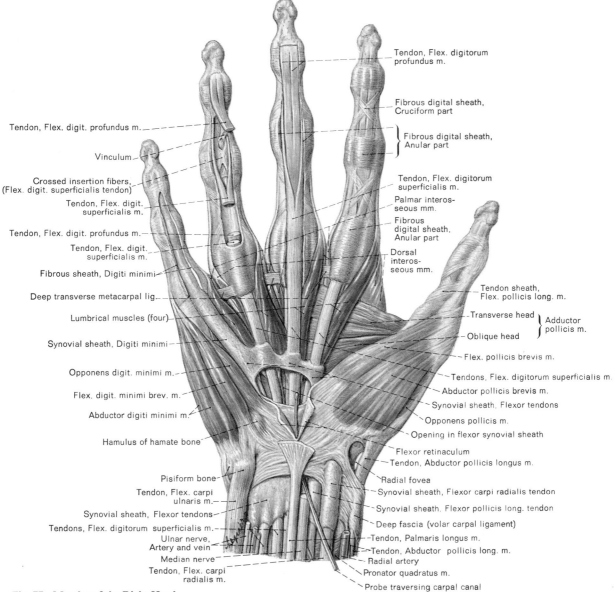

Tendon, Flex. digitorum profundus m.

Fibrous digital sheath, Cruciform part

Fibrous digital sheath, Anular part

Tendon, Flex. digit. profundus m.

Vinculum

Crossed insertion fibers, (Flex. digit. superficialis tendon)

Tendon, Flex. digit. superficialis m.

Tendon, Flex. digit. profundus m.

Tendon, Flex. digit. superficialis m.

Fibrous sheath, Digiti minimi

Deep transverse metacarpal lig.

Lumbrical muscles (four)

Synovial sheath, Digiti minimi

Opponens digit. minimi m.

Flex. digit. minimi brev. m.

Abductor digiti minimi m.

Hamulus of hamate bone

Pisiform bone

Tendon, Flex. carpi ulnaris m.

Synovial sheath, Flexor tendons

Tendons, Flex. digitorum superficialis m.

Ulnar nerve, Artery and vein

Median nerve

Tendon, Flex. carpi radialis m.

Tendon, Flex. digitorum superficialis m.

Palmar interosseous mm.

Fibrous digital sheath, Anular part

Dorsal interosseous mm.

Tendon sheath, Flex. pollicis long. m.

Transverse head } Adductor
Oblique head   } pollicis m.

Flex. pollicis brevis m.

Tendons, Flex. digitorum superficialis m.

Abductor pollicis brevis m.

Synovial sheath, Flexor tendons

Opponens pollicis m.

Opening in flexor synovial sheath

Flexor retinaculum

Tendon, Abductor pollicis longus m.

Radial fovea

Synovial sheath, Flexor carpi radialis tendon

Synovial sheath, Flexor pollicis long. tendon

Deep fascia (volar carpal ligament)

Tendon, Palmaris longus m.

Tendon, Abductor pollicis long. m.

Radial artery

Pronator quadratus m.

Probe traversing carpal canal

Fig. 77: Muscles of the Right Hand

NOTE: 1) how the flexor digit. profundus achieves its insertion on the distal phalanx. The tendon of the flexor digit. superficialis divides into two slips, allowing the corresponding deep flexor tendon to pass.

2) that along the fingers, the tendons are encased in a synovial sheath and then they are bound by both crossed and transverse (cruciate and annular) fibrous sheaths.

3) the muscles of the thenar eminence: abductor pollicis brevis, flexor pollicis brevis and the underlying opponens pollicis muscle.

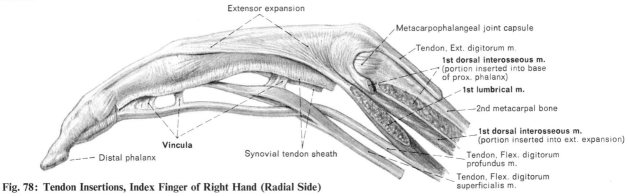

Extensor expansion

Metacarpophalangeal joint capsule

Tendon, Ext. digitorum m.

1st dorsal interosseous m. (portion inserted into base of prox. phalanx)

1st lumbrical m.

2nd metacarpal bone

1st dorsal interosseous m. (portion inserted into ext. expansion)

Tendon, Flex. digitorum profundus m.

Tendon, Flex. digitorum superficialis m.

Vincula

Distal phalanx

Synovial tendon sheath

Fig. 78: Tendon Insertions, Index Finger of Right Hand (Radial Side)

NOTE: 1) the flexor digit. superficialis inserts on the middle phalanx while the flexor digit. profundus inserts on the distal phalanx.

2) the dorsal interosseous and lumbrical muscles join the diverging extensor fibers in the formation of the extensor expansion on the dorsum of the finger.

3) the vincula are remnants of mesotendons and attach both superficial and deep flexor tendons to the digital sheath.

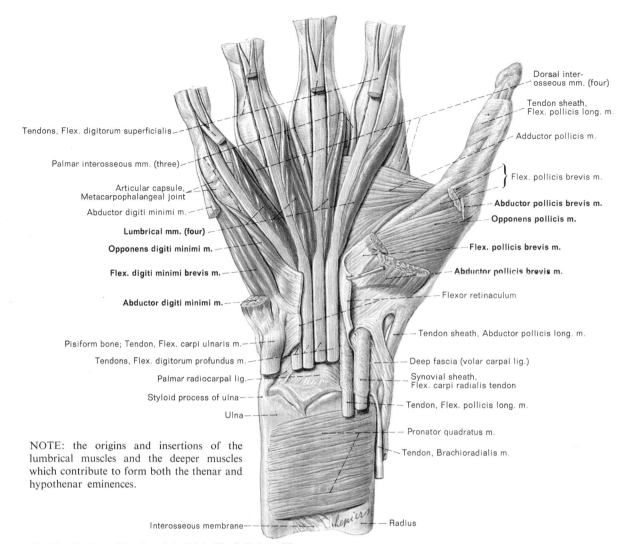

Dorsal inter-osseous mm. (four)

Tendon sheath, Flex. pollicis long. m.

Adductor pollicis m.

} Flex. pollicis brevis m.

Abductor pollicis brevis m.

Opponens pollicis m.

Flex. pollicis brevis m.

Abductor pollicis brevis m.

Flexor retinaculum

Tendon sheath, Abductor pollicis long. m.

Deep fascia (volar carpal lig.)

Synovial sheath, Flex. carpi radialis tendon

Tendon, Flex. pollicis long. m.

Pronator quadratus m.

Tendon, Brachioradialis m.

Tendons, Flex. digitorum superficialis

Palmar interosseous mm. (three)

Articular capsule, Metacarpophalangeal joint

Abductor digiti minimi m.

Lumbrical mm. (four)

Opponens digiti minimi m.

Flex. digiti minimi brevis m.

Abductor digiti minimi m.

Pisiform bone; Tendon, Flex. carpi ulnaris m.

Tendons, Flex. digitorum profundus m.

Palmar radiocarpal lig.

Styloid process of ulna

Ulna

NOTE: the origins and insertions of the lumbrical muscles and the deeper muscles which contribute to form both the thenar and hypothenar eminences.

Interosseous membrane

Radius

Fig. 79: The Deep Muscles of the Right Hand, Palmar View

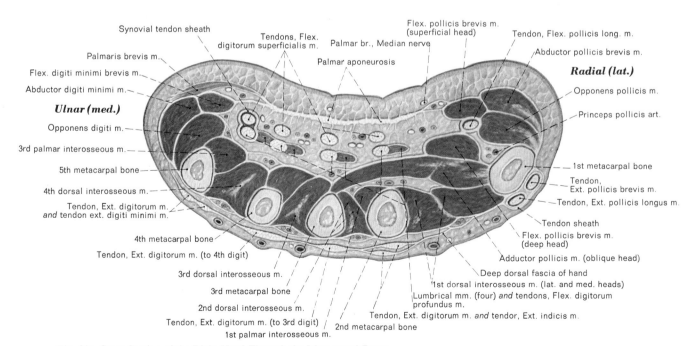

Synovial tendon sheath

Tendons, Flex. digitorum superficialis m.

Palmar br., Median nerve

Flex. pollicis brevis m. (superficial head)

Tendon, Flex. pollicis long. m.

Abductor pollicis brevis m.

Palmaris brevis m.

Flex. digiti minimi brevis m.

Abductor digiti minimi m.

Palmar aponeurosis

Radial (lat.)

Opponens pollicis m.

Ulnar (med.)

Princeps pollicis art.

Opponens digiti m.

3rd palmar interosseous m.

5th metacarpal bone

1st metacarpal bone

4th dorsal interosseous m.

Tendon, Ext. pollicis brevis m.

Tendon, Ext. pollicis longus m.

Tendon, Ext. digitorum m. *and* tendon ext. digiti minimi m.

Tendon sheath

Flex. pollicis brevis m. (deep head)

4th metacarpal bone

Adductor pollicis m. (oblique head)

Tendon, Ext. digitorum m. (to 4th digit)

Deep dorsal fascia of hand

3rd dorsal interosseous m.

1st dorsal interosseous m. (lat. and med. heads)

3rd metacarpal bone

Lumbrical mm. (four) *and* tendons, Flex. digitorum profundus m.

2nd dorsal interosseous m.

Tendon, Ext. digitorum m. (to 3rd digit)

Tendon, Ext. digitorum m. *and* tendor, Ext. indicis m.

2nd metacarpal bone

1st palmar interosseous m.

Fig. 80: Cross Section of the Right Hand Through the Metacarpal Bones

IDENTIFY a) the four dorsal interossei which act as abductors of the fingers and which fill the intervals between the metacarpal bones, b) the three palmar interossei which act as adductors of the fingers, c) the thenar and hypothenar muscles and d) the tendons and lumbrical muscles in the palmar compartment.

Fig. 81: Nerves and Arteries of the Left Palm, Superficial Palmar Arch

NOTE: 1) the median nerve enters the palm beneath the flexor retinaculum and supplies the muscles of the thenar eminence: abductor pollicis brevis, opponens pollicis and flexor pollicis brevis (superficial head). Additionally, it supplies the two most lateral lumbrical muscles and the palmar surface of the lateral three and one-half fingers.

2) the superficial location of the small but important "recurrent" branch of the median nerve which supplies several of the thenar muscles. Its location, just below the deep fascia on the thenar eminence, makes it vulnerable to injury.

3) the ulnar nerve enters the palm superficial to the flexor retinaculum, supplies the medial one and one-half fingers and all the remaining musculature of the hand: three hypothenar muscles, seven interosseous muscles, two medial lumbrical muscles, the adductor pollicis and the flexor pollicis brevis (deep head).

4) the superficial palmar arch is derived principally from the ulnar artery. It crosses the palm to the radial side superficial to the nerves and tendons and is joined by a palmar branch of the radial artery. Three or four common palmar digital arteries arise from the arch, proceed distally and divide into proper palmar digital arteries which course along the fingers with corresponding digital nerves.

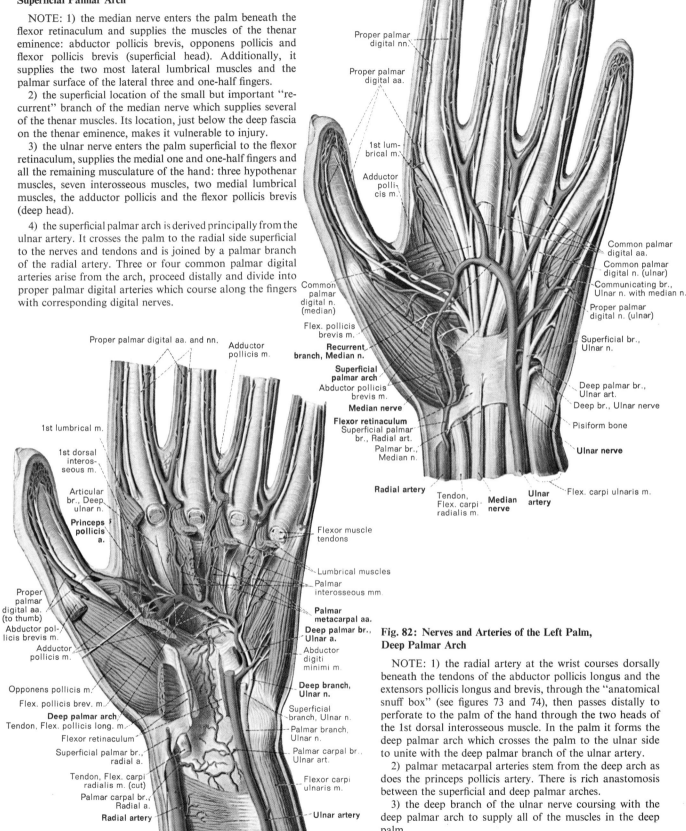

Fig. 82: Nerves and Arteries of the Left Palm, Deep Palmar Arch

NOTE: 1) the radial artery at the wrist courses dorsally beneath the tendons of the abductor pollicis longus and the extensors pollicis longus and brevis, through the "anatomical snuff box" (see figures 73 and 74), then passes distally to perforate to the palm of the hand through the two heads of the 1st dorsal interosseous muscle. In the palm it forms the deep palmar arch which crosses the palm to the ulnar side to unite with the deep palmar branch of the ulnar artery.

2) palmar metacarpal arteries stem from the deep arch as does the princeps pollicis artery. There is rich anastomosis between the superficial and deep palmar arches.

3) the deep branch of the ulnar nerve coursing with the deep palmar arch to supply all of the muscles in the deep palm.

4) the palmar carpal anastomosis between the ulnar and radial arteries.

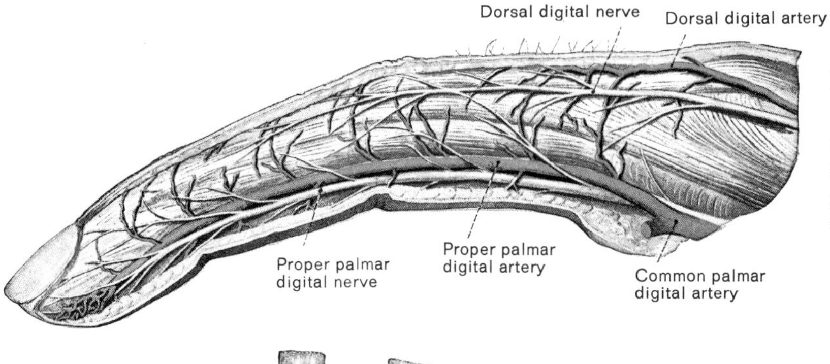

Fig. 83: Nerves and Arteries of the Index Finger

NOTE: the dorsal digital nerve and artery extend only two-thirds the length of the finger. The palmar digital nerve and artery supply not only the entire palmar surface but also the distal one-third of the dorsal surface.

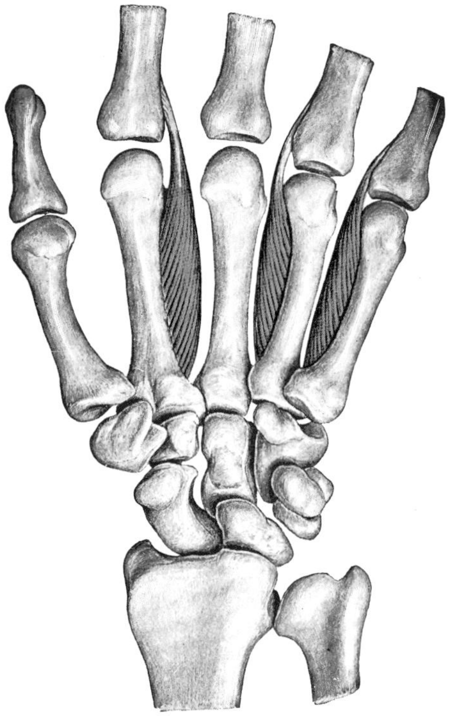

Fig. 84: The Three Palmar Interosseus Muscles (left, Palmar View)

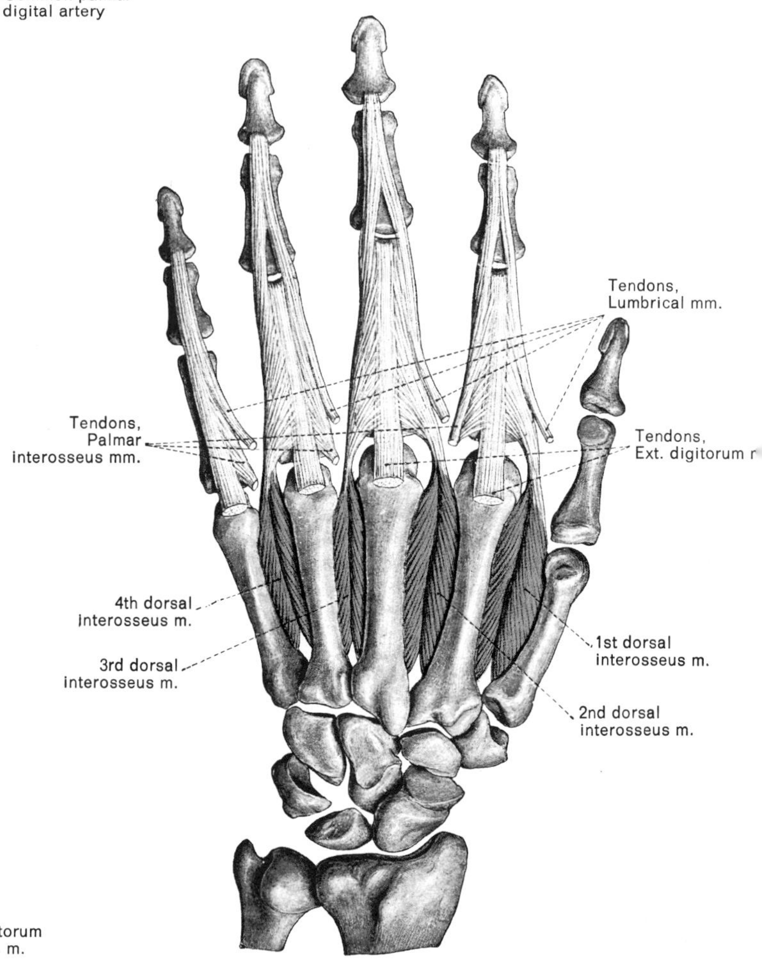

Fig. 85: The Four Dorsal Interosseus Muscles (left, Dorsal View)

NOTE: whereas the three palmar interosseus muscles (figure 84) are adductors of the fingers, the four dorsal interosseus muscles are abductors. All of the interossei flex the metacarpophalangeal joint and extend the interphalangeal joints, and they are all supplied by the ulnar nerve.

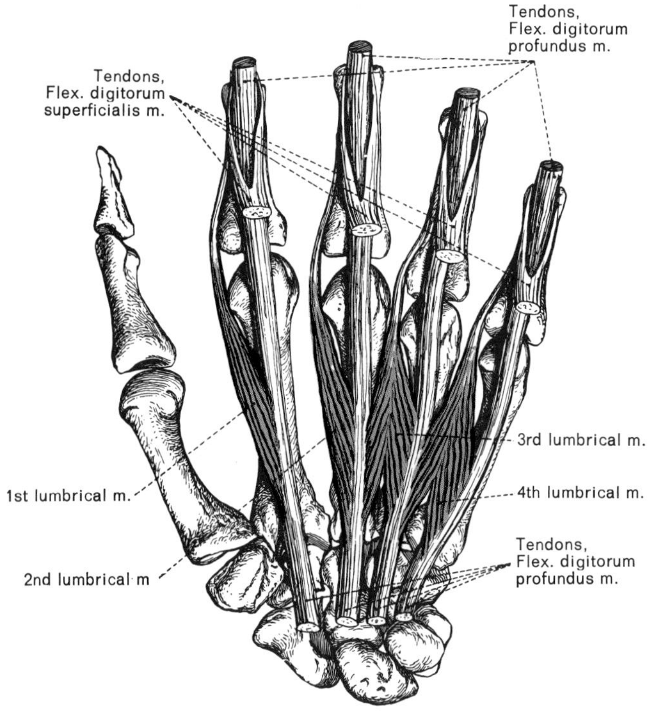

Fig. 86: The Four Lumbrical Muscles (left, Palmar View)

NOTE: The four lumbrical muscles arise from the tendons of the flexor digitorum profundus at the level of the metacarpal bones and course distally to insert on the extensor expansions beyond the metacarpophalangeal joint. They flex the metacarpophalangeal joint and extend the distal phalanges.

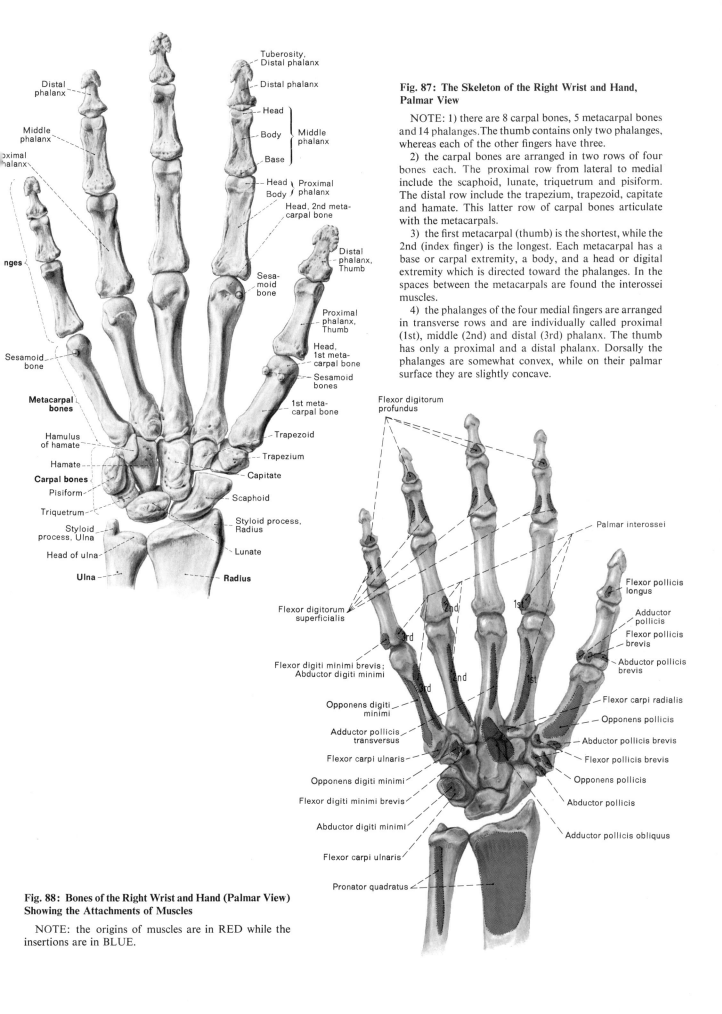

Tuberosity, Distal phalanx

Distal phalanx

Distal phalanx

Head
Body } Middle phalanx
Base

Middle phalanx

Head } Proximal phalanx
Body

Head, 2nd metacarpal bone

Proximal phalanx

Distal phalanx, Thumb

Sesamoid bone

Proximal phalanx, Thumb

Head, 1st metacarpal bone

Sesamoid bones

1st metacarpal bone

Trapezoid

Trapezium

Capitate

Scaphoid

Styloid process, Radius

Lunate

Radius

Distal phalanx

Middle phalanx

Proximal phalanx

nges

Sesamoid bone

Metacarpal bones

Hamulus of hamate

Hamate

Carpal bones

Pisiform

Triquetrum

Styloid process, Ulna

Head of ulna

Ulna

Fig. 87: The Skeleton of the Right Wrist and Hand, Palmar View

NOTE: 1) there are 8 carpal bones, 5 metacarpal bones and 14 phalanges. The thumb contains only two phalanges, whereas each of the other fingers have three.

2) the carpal bones are arranged in two rows of four bones each. The proximal row from lateral to medial include the scaphoid, lunate, triquetrum and pisiform. The distal row include the trapezium, trapezoid, capitate and hamate. This latter row of carpal bones articulate with the metacarpals.

3) the first metacarpal (thumb) is the shortest, while the 2nd (index finger) is the longest. Each metacarpal has a base or carpal extremity, a body, and a head or digital extremity which is directed toward the phalanges. In the spaces between the metacarpals are found the interossei muscles.

4) the phalanges of the four medial fingers are arranged in transverse rows and are individually called proximal (1st), middle (2nd) and distal (3rd) phalanx. The thumb has only a proximal and a distal phalanx. Dorsally the phalanges are somewhat convex, while on their palmar surface they are slightly concave.

Flexor digitorum profundus

Palmar interossei

Flexor pollicis longus

Adductor pollicis

Flexor pollicis brevis

Abductor pollicis brevis

Flexor digitorum superficialis

Flexor digiti minimi brevis; Abductor digiti minimi

Opponens digiti minimi

Adductor pollicis transversus

Flexor carpi ulnaris

Opponens digiti minimi

Flexor digiti minimi brevis

Abductor digiti minimi

Flexor carpi ulnaris

Pronator quadratus

Flexor carpi radialis

Opponens pollicis

Abductor pollicis brevis

Flexor pollicis brevis

Opponens pollicis

Abductor pollicis

Adductor pollicis obliquus

Fig. 88: Bones of the Right Wrist and Hand (Palmar View) Showing the Attachments of Muscles

NOTE: the origins of muscles are in RED while the insertions are in BLUE.

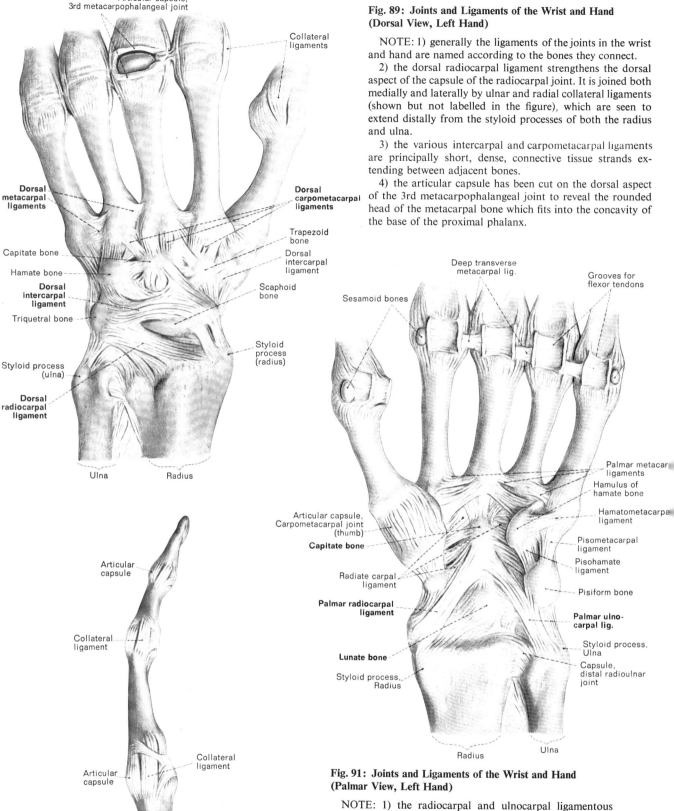

Fig. 89: Joints and Ligaments of the Wrist and Hand (Dorsal View, Left Hand)

NOTE: 1) generally the ligaments of the joints in the wrist and hand are named according to the bones they connect.

2) the dorsal radiocarpal ligament strengthens the dorsal aspect of the capsule of the radiocarpal joint. It is joined both medially and laterally by ulnar and radial collateral ligaments (shown but not labelled in the figure), which are seen to extend distally from the styloid processes of both the radius and ulna.

3) the various intercarpal and carpometacarpal ligaments are principally short, dense, connective tissue strands extending between adjacent bones.

4) the articular capsule has been cut on the dorsal aspect of the 3rd metacarpophalangeal joint to reveal the rounded head of the metacarpal bone which fits into the concavity of the base of the proximal phalanx.

Fig. 90: Joints and Ligaments of the Middle Finger

NOTE: the articular capsules of the metacarpophalangeal and interphalangeal joints are strengthened by longitudinally oriented collateral ligaments.

Fig. 91: Joints and Ligaments of the Wrist and Hand (Palmar View, Left Hand)

NOTE: 1) the radiocarpal and ulnocarpal ligamentous bands strengthening the palmar aspect of the radiocarpal joint.

2) identify several strong ligaments in the palmar hand including the pisohamate, pisometacarpal and the radiate ligament surrounding the capitate bone.

3) the bases of the metacarpal bones are joined by the palmar metacarpal ligaments, while the more distal heads of these bones are interconnected by the deep transverse metacarpal ligament.

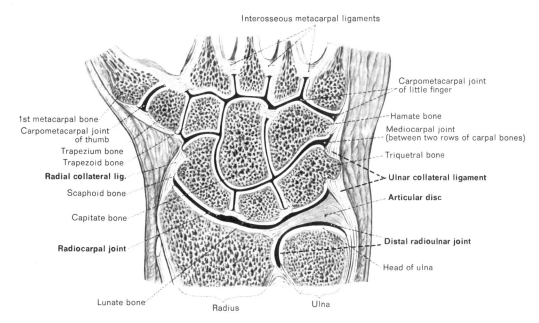

Interosseous metacarpal ligaments

Carpometacarpal joint of little finger

1st metacarpal bone

Carpometacarpal joint of thumb

Trapezium bone

Trapezoid bone

Radial collateral lig.

Scaphoid bone

Capitate bone

Radiocarpal joint

Lunate bone

Radius

Ulna

Hamate bone

Mediocarpal joint (between two rows of carpal bones)

Triquetral bone

Ulnar collateral ligament

Articular disc

Distal radioulnar joint

Head of ulna

Fig. 92: Coronal (Frontal) Section Through the Left Wrist Joints

NOTE: 1) the articular disc situated at the distal end of the ulna. Thus, the radiocarpal joint consists of the radius and articular disc proximally and the scaphoid, lunate and triquetrum distally.

2) the ulnar and radial collateral ligaments which provide the wrist joints with strong longitudinally oriented fibrous bands both laterally and medially.

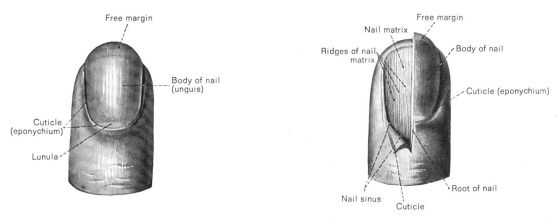

Free margin

Body of nail (unguis)

Cuticle (eponychium)

Lunula

Fig. 93: Finger Nail, Normal Position (Dorsal View)

Free margin

Nail matrix

Ridges of nail matrix

Body of nail

Cuticle (eponychium)

Nail sinus

Cuticle

Root of nail

Fig. 94: Left Half of Finger Nail Bed Exposed

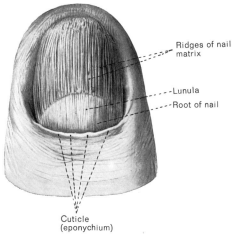

Ridges of nail matrix

Lunula

Root of nail

Cuticle (eponychium)

Fig. 95: Nail Bed of Thumb after Removal of Nail

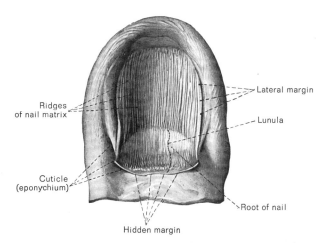

Ridges of nail matrix

Lateral margin

Lunula

Cuticle (eponychium)

Root of nail

Hidden margin

Fig. 96: Nail Bed of Thumb and Reflection of Cuticle

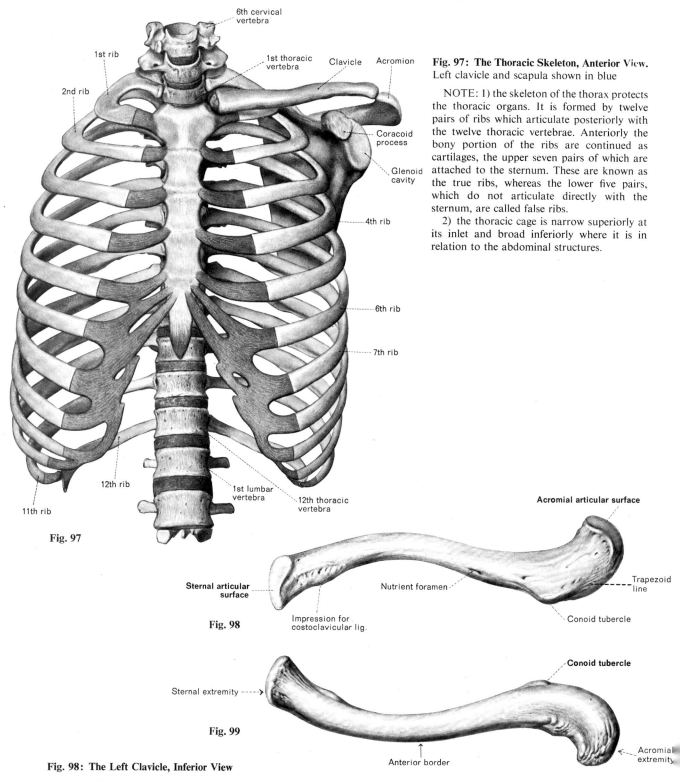

6th cervical vertebra

1st rib

2nd rib

1st thoracic vertebra

Clavicle

Acromion

Coracoid process

Glenoid cavity

4th rib

6th rib

7th rib

12th rib

1st lumbar vertebra

12th thoracic vertebra

11th rib

Fig. 97

Fig. 97: The Thoracic Skeleton, Anterior View. Left clavicle and scapula shown in blue

NOTE: 1) the skeleton of the thorax protects the thoracic organs. It is formed by twelve pairs of ribs which articulate posteriorly with the twelve thoracic vertebrae. Anteriorly the bony portion of the ribs are continued as cartilages, the upper seven pairs of which are attached to the sternum. These are known as the true ribs, whereas the lower five pairs, which do not articulate directly with the sternum, are called false ribs.

2) the thoracic cage is narrow superiorly at its inlet and broad inferiorly where it is in relation to the abdominal structures.

Acromial articular surface

Sternal articular surface

Nutrient foramen

Trapezoid line

Conoid tubercle

Fig. 98

Impression for costoclavicular lig.

Conoid tubercle

Sternal extremity

Fig. 99

Anterior border

Acromial extremity

Fig. 98: The Left Clavicle, Inferior View

NOTE: 1) the clavicle is a double-curved bone which articulates medially with the sternum just above the first rib and laterally with the acromion of the scapula.

2) the inferior surface has roughened areas for the attachment of costoclavicular ligament medially and the conoid and trapezoid fascicles of the coracoclavicular ligament laterally. The subclavius muscle attaches along the middle third of the inferior surface.

Fig. 99: The Left Clavicle, Superior View

NOTE: 1) the superior surface of the clavicle affords attachment of the pectoralis major and sternocleidomastoid muscles medially and the deltoid and trapezius muscles laterally.

2) the claviculoacromial articulation associates the clavicle with all the movements of the scapula, while the sternal articulation of the clavicle is a more secure and less movable joint.

Fig. 100: The Sternum, Anterior View

NOTE: 1) the sternum consists of three parts: the manubrium, the body and the xiphoid process and forms the middle portion of the anterior wall of the thorax.

2) the manubrium articulates with the body of the sternum at somewhat of an angle called the sternal angle. The xiphoid process is thin and usually cartilaginous.

Fig. 101: The Sternum, Lateral View

NOTE: 1) the clavicle and the 1st rib articulate with the manubrium. The 2nd rib articulates at the sternal angle where the sternal manubrium and body join. The 3rd to the 6th ribs articulate with the body of the sternum, while the 7th joins the sternum inferiorly at the junction of the xiphoid process.

2) A line projected posteriorly through the sternal angle would meet the vertebral column at the 4th thoracic vertebral level, while the xiphisternal junction lies at vertebral level T-9.

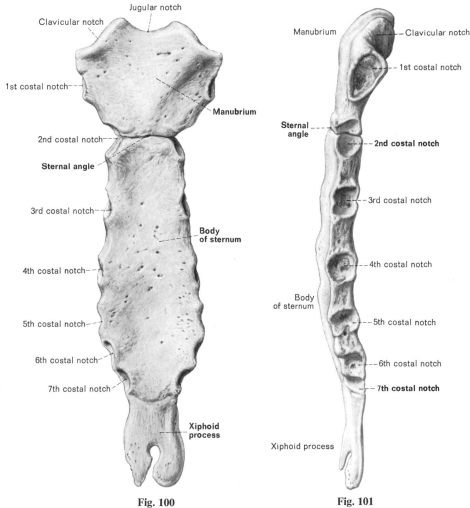

Fig. 100

Fig. 101

Fig. 102: The Sternoclavicular and the First Two Sternocostal Joints

NOTE: 1) the sternoclavicular joint is formed by the junction of the clavicle with a) the upper lateral aspect of the manubrium and b) the cartilage of the first rib. A flat articular disc is interposed between the clavicle and the sternum. An articular capsule and fibrous ligamentous bands protect the joint.

2) the cartilages of the 2nd through the 7th ribs articulate with the sternum by means of movable diarthrodial joints, whereas the cartilage of the 1st rib is directly joined to the sternum and, without a joint cavity, to form an immovable articulation (synarthrosis).

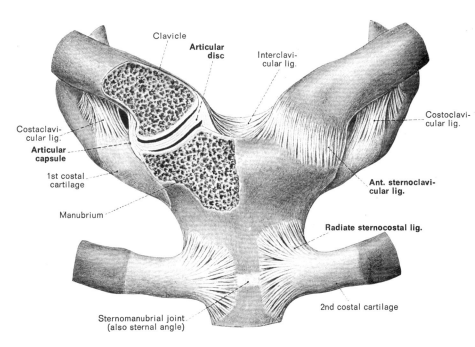

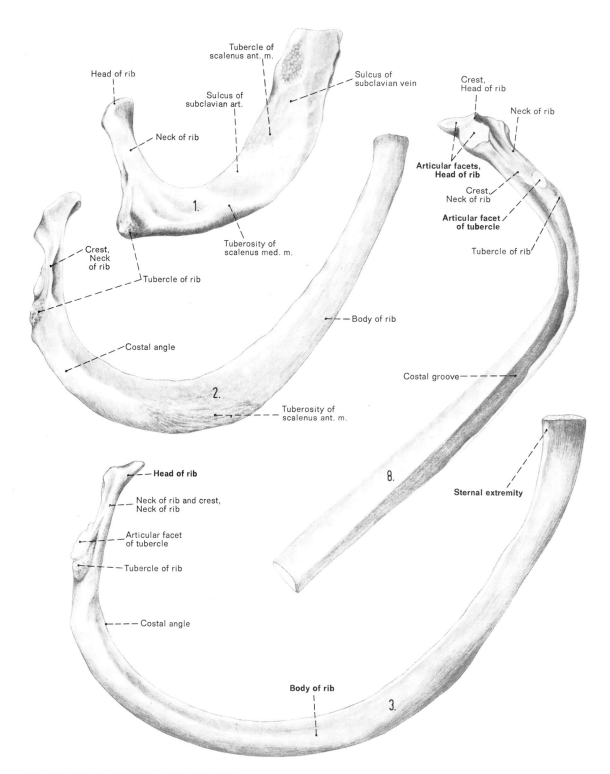

Fig. 103: The 1st, 2nd, 3rd and 8th Right Ribs

NOTE: 1) the superior surfaces of the first, second and third ribs are illustrated in this figure, while the inferior surface of the eighth rib is shown.

2) each rib has a vertebral extremity directed posteriorly and a sternal extremity directed anteriorly. The body of the rib is the shaft which stretches between these two extremities.

3) the vertebral extremity is marked by a head, a neck and a tubercle. The head contains two facets for articulation with the bodies of the thoracic vertebrae, while the tubercle consists of a non-articular roughened elevation and an articular facet for connection with the transverse process of the thoracic vertebrae.

4) the 1st, 2nd, 10th, 11th and 12th ribs present somewhat different structural characteristics from the 3rd through the 9th ribs. The 1st rib is the most curved of all the ribs and has only a single articular facet on the head of the rib. The 10th, 11th and 12th ribs also have only a single facet on the rib head. The 2nd rib is shaped similar to the 1st rib but is longer.

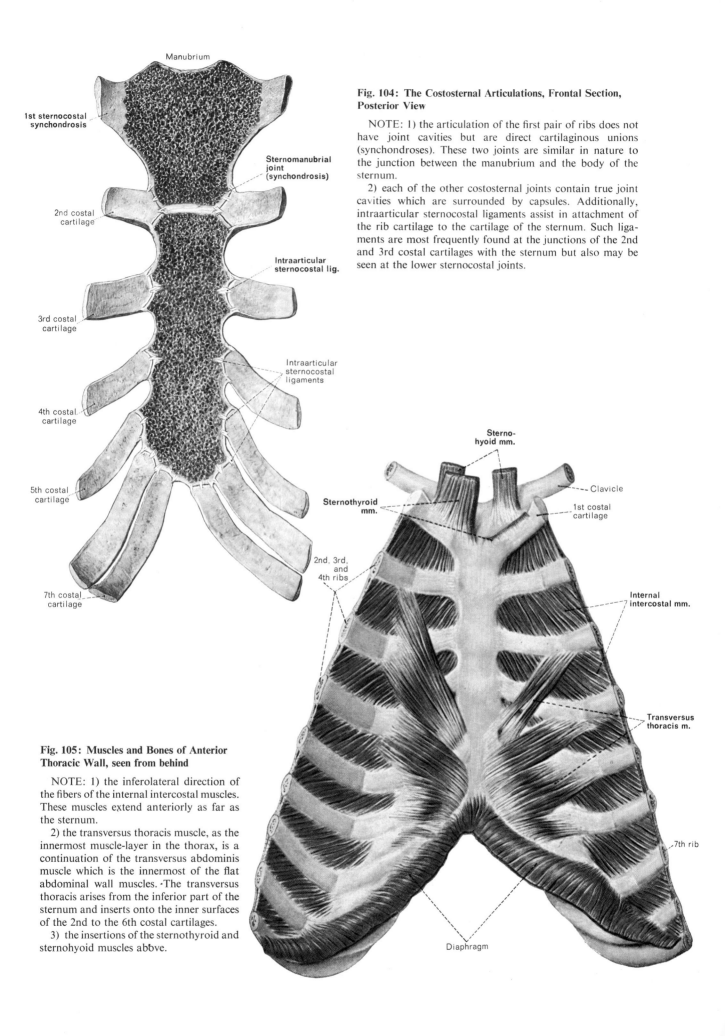

Manubrium

1st sternocostal synchondrosis

Sternomanubrial joint (synchondrosis)

2nd costal cartilage

Intraarticular sternocostal lig.

3rd costal cartilage

Intraarticular sternocostal ligaments

4th costal cartilage

5th costal cartilage

7th costal cartilage

Fig. 104: The Costosternal Articulations, Frontal Section, Posterior View

NOTE: 1) the articulation of the first pair of ribs does not have joint cavities but are direct cartilaginous unions (synchondroses). These two joints are similar in nature to the junction between the manubrium and the body of the sternum.

2) each of the other costosternal joints contain true joint cavities which are surrounded by capsules. Additionally, intraarticular sternocostal ligaments assist in attachment of the rib cartilage to the cartilage of the sternum. Such ligaments are most frequently found at the junctions of the 2nd and 3rd costal cartilages with the sternum but also may be seen at the lower sternocostal joints.

Sterno-hyoid mm.

Clavicle

Sternothyroid mm.

1st costal cartilage

2nd, 3rd, and 4th ribs

Internal intercostal mm.

Transversus thoracis m.

7th rib

Diaphragm

Fig. 105: Muscles and Bones of Anterior Thoracic Wall, seen from behind

NOTE: 1) the inferolateral direction of the fibers of the internal intercostal muscles. These muscles extend anteriorly as far as the sternum.

2) the transversus thoracis muscle, as the innermost muscle-layer in the thorax, is a continuation of the transversus abdominis muscle which is the innermost of the flat abdominal wall muscles. The transversus thoracis arises from the inferior part of the sternum and inserts onto the inner surfaces of the 2nd to the 6th costal cartilages.

3) the insertions of the sternothyroid and sternohyoid muscles above.

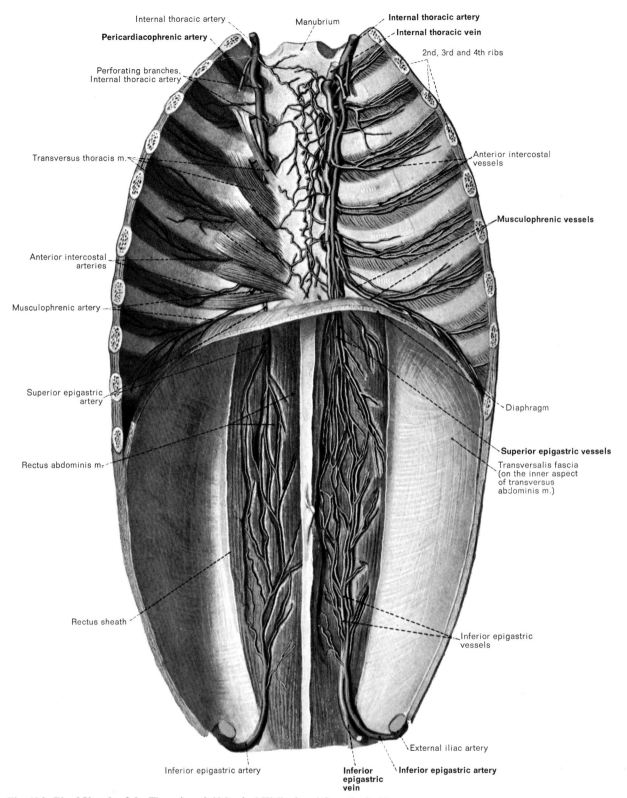

Internal thoracic artery

Pericardiacophrenic artery

Perforating branches,
Internal thoracic artery

Manubrium

Internal thoracic artery

Internal thoracic vein

2nd, 3rd and 4th ribs

Transversus thoracis m.

Anterior intercostal
arteries

Musculophrenic artery

Superior epigastric
artery

Rectus abdominis m.

Rectus sheath

Anterior intercostal
vessels

Musculophrenic vessels

Diaphragm

Superior epigastric vessels

Transversalis fascia
(on the inner aspect
of transversus
abdominis m.)

Inferior epigastric
vessels

External iliac artery

Inferior epigastric artery

**Inferior
epigastric
vein**

Inferior epigastric artery

Fig. 106: Blood Vessels of the Thoracic and Abdominal Wall, viewed from the inside

NOTE: 1) the principal vessels dissected have been the internal thoracic and inferior epigastric arteries and veins and their terminal branches.

2) the internal thoracic artery branches from the subclavian artery and descends behind the costal cartilages on the inner aspect of the anterior thoracic wall parallel to the lateral margin of the sternum. In its course the internal thoracic artery gives rise to the pericardiacophrenic artery, small anterior mediastinal vessels to the thymus and bronchial structures, perforating branches to the chest wall, anterior intercostal branches which anastomose with the intercostal arteries, and finally it terminates as the musculophrenic and superior epigastric arteries.

3) the superior epigastric artery anastomoses with the inferior epigastric artery, which is a branch of the external iliac artery and which ascends in the abdominal wall from below. The anastomosis occurs in the substance of the rectus abdominis muscle.

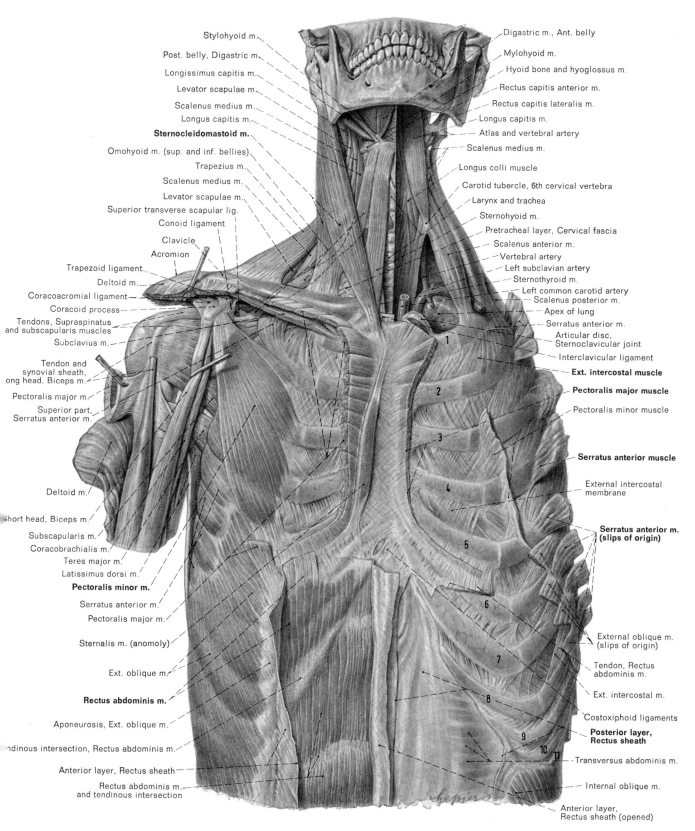

Fig. 107: Anterior Cervical, Thoracic and Abdominal Musculature

NOTE: 1) on the right side the muscles of the shoulder and upper arm are demonstrated following the removal of the pectoralis major muscle. The anterior layer of the rectus sheath has been opened.

2) on the left side the upper limb has been removed, as have all of the more superficial trunk and cervical musculature, revealing the thoracic cage and the deeper soft tissues.

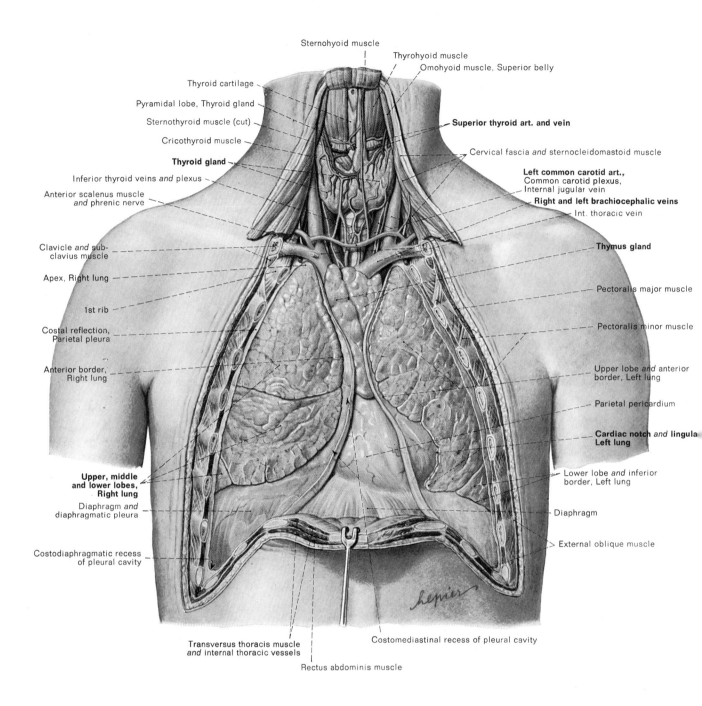

Sternohyoid muscle

Thyrohyoid muscle

Omohyoid muscle, Superior belly

Thyroid cartilage

Pyramidal lobe, Thyroid gland

Sternothyroid muscle (cut)

Cricothyroid muscle

Superior thyroid art. and vein

Thyroid gland

Cervical fascia *and* sternocleidomastoid muscle

Inferior thyroid veins *and* plexus

Left common carotid art.,
Common carotid plexus,
Internal jugular vein

Anterior scalenus muscle
and phrenic nerve

Right and left brachiocephalic veins

Int. thoracic vein

Clavicle *and* sub-
clavius muscle

Thymus gland

Apex, Right lung

Pectoralis major muscle

1st rib

Pectoralis minor muscle

Costal reflection,
Parietal pleura

Anterior border,
Right lung

Upper lobe *and* anterior
border, Left lung

Parietal pericardium

**Cardiac notch *and* lingula
Left lung**

**Upper, middle
and lower lobes,
Right lung**

Lower lobe *and* inferior
border, Left lung

Diaphragm *and*
diaphragmatic pleura

Diaphragm

External oblique muscle

Costodiaphragmatic recess
of pleural cavity

Transversus thoracis muscle
and internal thoracic vessels

Costomediastinal recess of pleural cavity

Rectus abdominis muscle

Fig. 108: The Thoracic Viscera and the Root of the Neck, Anterior Exposure

NOTE: 1) the anterior thoracic wall has been removed along with the medial portion of both clavicles to reveal the normal position of the heart, lungs, thymus and thyroid gland. The great vessels at the superior aperture to the thorax are also exposed.

2) the parietal pleura, likewise, has been removed arteriorly. The thymus is situated between the two lungs superiorly, whereas inferiorly is found the bare area of the heart. With the heart's apex directed more toward the left, a deficiency can be observed along the border of the left lung. This is called the cardiac notch.

3) the basal surface of both lungs and the inferior aspect of the heart rest on the diaphragm. Superiorly, the apex of each lung extends slightly above the level of the first rib.

4) at the root of the neck, the common carotid artery and internal jugular vein lie lateral and somewhat posterior to the thyroid gland.

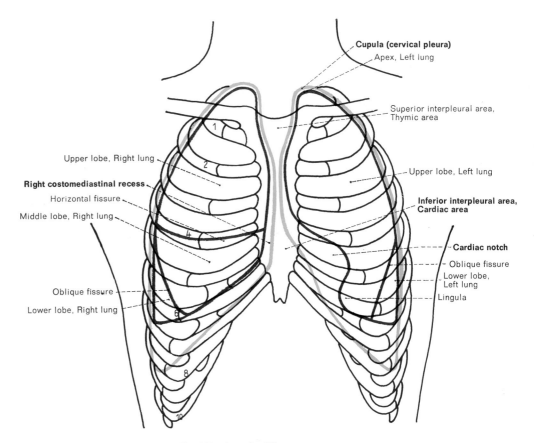

Fig. 109: Anterior View

Cupula (cervical pleura)
Apex, Left lung

Superior interpleural area, Thymic area

Upper lobe, Right lung

Right costomediastinal recess

Horizontal fissure

Middle lobe, Right lung

Upper lobe, Left lung

Inferior interpleural area, Cardiac area

Cardiac notch

Oblique fissure

Lower lobe, Left lung

Lingula

Oblique fissure

Lower lobe, Right lung

Pleural Reflections (blue) and Lungs (red) Projected onto Thoracic Wall

NOTE: 1) each lung is invested by two layers of pleural membranes which are continuous with each other at the hilum of the lung, thereby forming an invaginated sac. The parietal layer of pleura (represented in blue) is the outermost of the two layers and lines the inner surface of the thoracic wall and the superior surface of the diaphragm. The visceral, innermost layer of pleura closely invests and adheres to the surfaces of the lungs (represented in red).

2) the potential space between the two pleural layers is called the pleural cavity and contains only a small amount of serous fluid in the healthy individual but may contain considerable fluid and blood in pathological conditions.

3) although the parietal pleura is a continuous sheet for each lung, portions of it are described in relation to their adjacent surfaces. Thus, lining the inner surface of the ribs is the costal pleura, while the diaphragmatic and mediastinal pleurae are applied onto the surfaces of the diaphragm and mediastinal structures. Superiorly, the apex of each lung extends above the clavicle into the root of the neck. This is covered by the cupula, or cervical pleura.

4) because of the curvature of the diaphragm, a narrow recess is formed around its periphery into which the surface of the lung (visceral pleura) does not extend. This potential space, lying between reflections of the costal and diaphragmatic pleurae, is called the costodiaphragmatic recess and is of clinical importance since it may be punctured and drained without damage to lung tissue.

5) similarly, the costomediastinal recess is another pleural space which is situated anterior to the heart and which is formed at that site by the reflections of the costal and mediastinal pleurae.

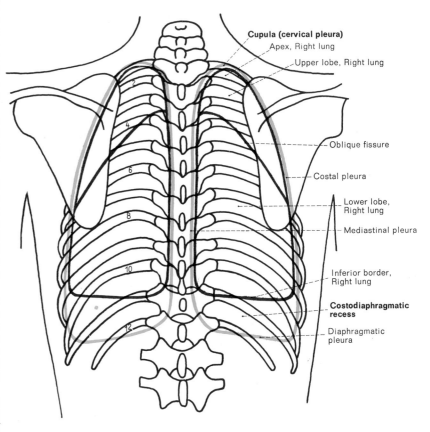

Cupula (cervical pleura)
Apex, Right lung

Upper lobe, Right lung

Oblique fissure

Costal pleura

Lower lobe, Right lung

Mediastinal pleura

Inferior border, Right lung

Costodiaphragmatic recess

Diaphragmatic pleura

Fig. 110: Posterior View

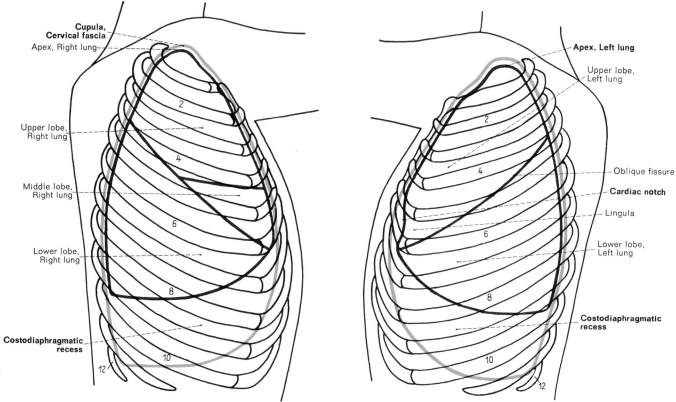

Fig. 111: Right Lateral View   **Fig. 112: Left Lateral View**
Pleural Reflections (blue) and Lungs (red) Projected onto Thoracic Wall

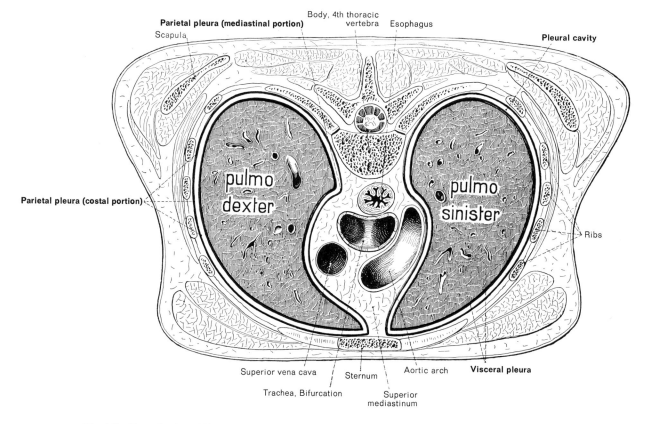

Fig. 113: Cross Section of Thorax at the Level of the Tracheal Bifurcation and the 4th Thoracic Vertebra (Pleura is shown in red)

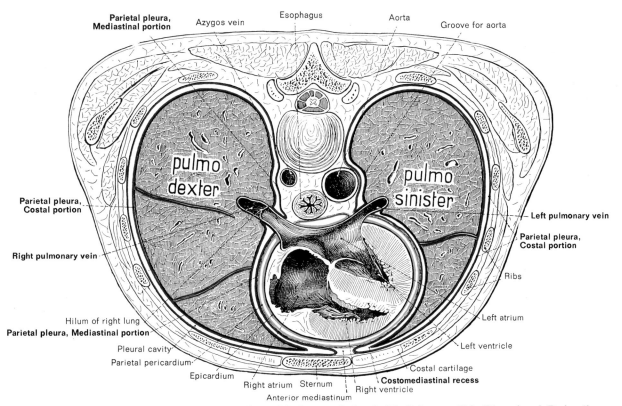

Fig. 114: Cross Section of Thorax Through the Hilum of the Lung at the Level of the Pulmonary Vein (Pleura in red, Pericardium in blue)

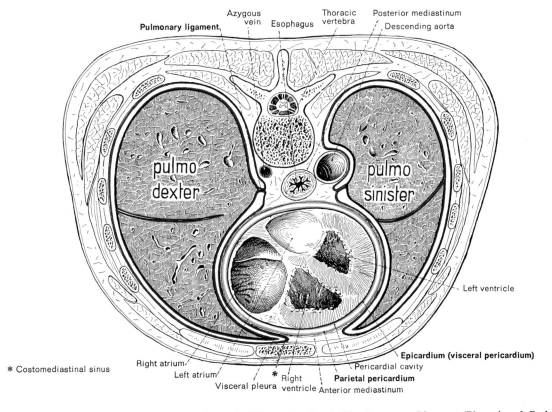

Fig. 115: Cross Section of the Thorax Inferior to the Hilum at the Level of the Pulmonary Ligament (Pleura in red, Pericardium in blue)

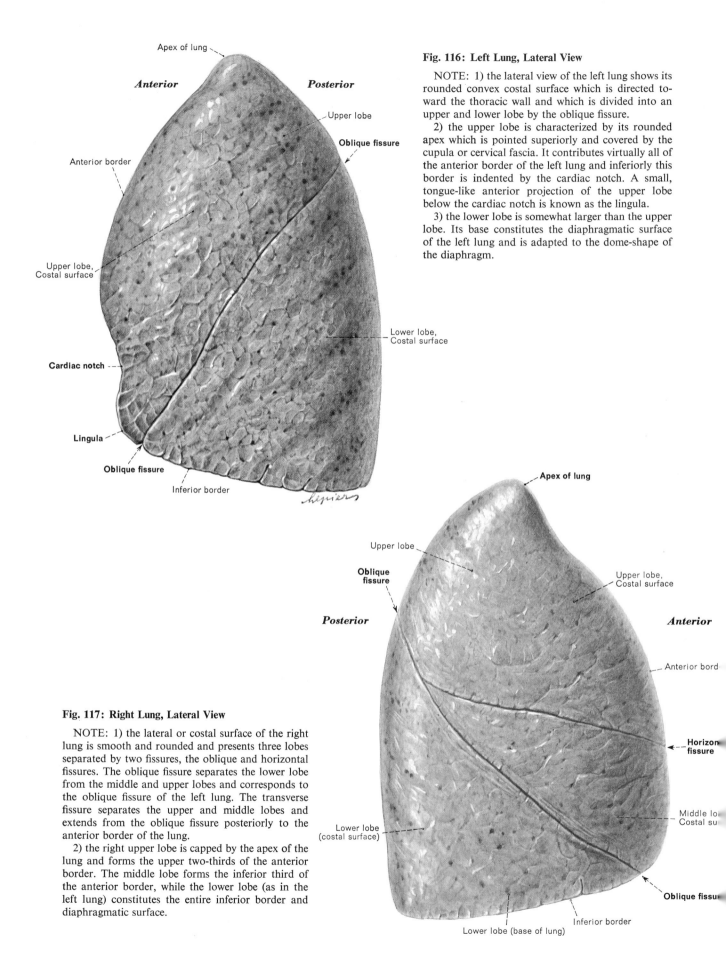

Apex of lung

Anterior

Posterior

Upper lobe

Oblique fissure

Anterior border

Upper lobe,
Costal surface

Cardiac notch

Lingula

Oblique fissure

Inferior border

Lower lobe,
Costal surface

Fig. 116: Left Lung, Lateral View

NOTE: 1) the lateral view of the left lung shows its rounded convex costal surface which is directed toward the thoracic wall and which is divided into an upper and lower lobe by the oblique fissure.

2) the upper lobe is characterized by its rounded apex which is pointed superiorly and covered by the cupula or cervical fascia. It contributes virtually all of the anterior border of the left lung and inferiorly this border is indented by the cardiac notch. A small, tongue-like anterior projection of the upper lobe below the cardiac notch is known as the lingula.

3) the lower lobe is somewhat larger than the upper lobe. Its base constitutes the diaphragmatic surface of the left lung and is adapted to the dome-shape of the diaphragm.

Apex of lung

Upper lobe

Upper lobe,
Costal surface

Oblique
fissure

Posterior

Anterior

Anterior bord

Horizon
fissure

Middle lo
Costal su

Lower lobe
(costal surface)

Oblique fissu

Inferior border

Lower lobe (base of lung)

Fig. 117: Right Lung, Lateral View

NOTE: 1) the lateral or costal surface of the right lung is smooth and rounded and presents three lobes separated by two fissures, the oblique and horizontal fissures. The oblique fissure separates the lower lobe from the middle and upper lobes and corresponds to the oblique fissure of the left lung. The transverse fissure separates the upper and middle lobes and extends from the oblique fissure posteriorly to the anterior border of the lung.

2) the right upper lobe is capped by the apex of the lung and forms the upper two-thirds of the anterior border. The middle lobe forms the inferior third of the anterior border, while the lower lobe (as in the left lung) constitutes the entire inferior border and diaphragmatic surface.

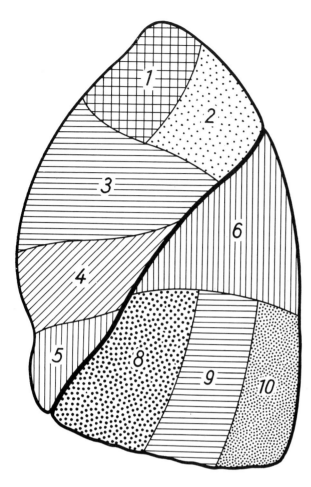

Fig. 118: Left Lung, Bronchopulmonary Segments – Lateral View

NOTE: 1) bronchopulmonary segments are anatomical subdivisions of the lung, each of which is supplied by its own segmental tertiary bronchus and artery, and drained by intersegmental veins.

2) the trachea divides into two primary bronchi, each of which supplies an entire lung. Each primary bronchus divides into secondary or lobar bronchi. There are two lobar bronchi on the left and three on the right, each supplying a single lobe. The secondary bronchi divide into the segmental or tertiary bronchi, which are distributed to the bronchopulmonary segments. Usual descriptions of the bronchopulmonary segments enumerate 8 to 10 segments in the left lung.

3) the bronchopulmonary segments of the left lung are numbered and named as follows:

Upper lobe

1	Apical	Frequently considered
2	Posterior	as a single broncho-
		pulmonary segment
3	Anterior	
4	Superior	Lingular
5	Inferior	

Lower lobe

6	Superior	(Cannot be seen
7	Medial basal	from lateral view)
8	Anterior basal	Usually considered
9	Lateral basal	as a single
10	Posterior basal	bronchopulmonary segment

4) in the left lower lobe the medial basal bronchus arises separate from the anterior basal in only about 13% of humans studied. Thus, in most instances the medial basal and anterior basal segments combine as an anteromedial basal segment.

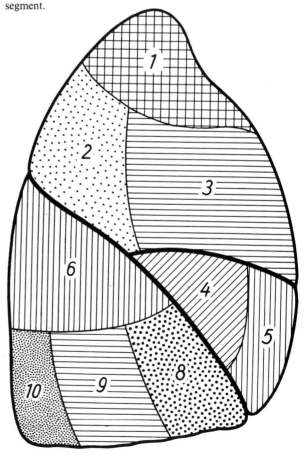

Fig. 119: Right Lung, Bronchopulmonary Segments, Lateral View

NOTE: 1) the concept of subdividing the lungs into functional bronchopulmonary segments allows the surgeon to determine whether segments of lung might be resected in operations in preference to entire lobes.

2) although minor variations exist in the division of the bronchial tree, a significant consistency has become recognized in the bronchopulmonary segmentation. The nomenclature utilized here was offered by Jackson and Huber in 1943 (Dis. of Chest **9**: 319–326) and has now become generally accepted because it is the simplest and most straightforward of the many suggested.

3) the bronchopulmonary segments of the right lung are numbered and named as follows:

Upper lobe	Middle lobe
1 Apical	4 Lateral
2 Posterior	5 Medial
3 Anterior	

Lower lobe

6 Superior
7 Medial basal (cannot be seen from lateral view)
8 Anterior basal
9 Lateral basal
10 Posterior basal

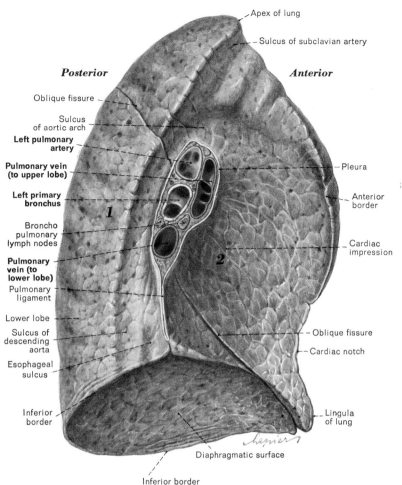

Apex of lung

Sulcus of subclavian artery

Posterior   *Anterior*

Oblique fissure

Sulcus of aortic arch

Left pulmonary artery

Pulmonary vein (to upper lobe)

Left primary bronchus

Broncho pulmonary lymph nodes

Pulmonary vein (to lower lobe)

Pulmonary ligament

Lower lobe

Sulcus of descending aorta

Esophageal sulcus

Inferior border

1

2

Pleura

Anterior border

Cardiac impression

Oblique fissure

Cardiac notch

Lingula of lung

Diaphragmatic surface

Inferior border

Fig. 120: Left Lung, Mediastinal and Diaphragmatic surfaces

NOTE: 1) the pulmonary arteries are shown in blue since their blood contains less oxygen than that in the pulmonary veins which are shown in red.

2) the concave diaphragmatic surface of the left lung is shaped to cover most of the convex dome of the diaphragm which is completely covered by diaphragmatic pleura. However, the lung does not completely fill the peripheral rim of the diaphragm, thereby forming the costodiaphragmatic recess.

3) the mediastinal (or medial) surface of the left lung is also concave and presents the contours of the adjacent organs in the mediastinum. The large anterior concavity is the cardiac impression. Also found are grooves for the aortic arch and the descending aorta as well as the subclavian artery superiorly and the esophagus inferiorly.

4) the structures which form the root of the left lung at the hilum include the left pulmonary artery, found most superior and below which is found the left bronchus. The left pulmonary veins lie anterior and inferior to the artery and bronchus. The oblique fissure extends across the mediastinal surface from the costal surface to the diaphragm, completely dividing the lung into its two lobes.

Fig. 121: Right Lung, Mediastinal and Diaphragmatic Surfaces

NOTE: 1) the diaphragmatic surface of the right lung, similar to that on the left, is shaped to the contour of the diaphragm, while the mediastinal surface superiorly shows grooves for the superior vena cava and subclavian artery. Just above the hilum of the right lung is the arched sulcus for the azygos vein, and this is continued inferiorly behind the root of the lung. The cardiac impression on the right lung is somewhat more shallow than on the left.

2) since the right bronchus frequently branches before the right pulmonary artery it is not unusual for the most superior structure at the root of the right lung to be the bronchus to the upper lobe (eparterial bronchus). The pulmonary artery lies anterior to the bronchus, while the pulmonary veins are located anterior and inferior to these structures.

3) the hilum of the lung is ensheathed by parietal pleura, the layers of which come into contact inferiorly to form the pulmonary ligament. It extends from the inferior border of the hilum to a point just above the diaphragm.

4) the numbers 1 and 2 on this figure refer to the costal and diaphragmatic portions of the medial surface of the lung.

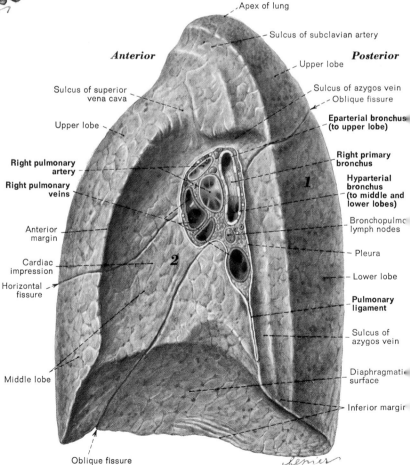

Apex of lung

Sulcus of subclavian artery

Anterior   *Posterior*

Upper lobe

Sulcus of azygos vein

Oblique fissure

Eparterial bronchus (to upper lobe)

Sulcus of superior vena cava

Upper lobe

Right primary bronchus

Hyparterial bronchus (to middle and lower lobes)

Right pulmonary artery

Right pulmonary veins

Bronchopulmo[nary] lymph nodes

Pleura

Lower lobe

Anterior margin

Cardiac impression

Pulmonary ligament

Horizontal fissure

Sulcus of azygos vein

1

2

Diaphragmati[c] surface

Inferior margi[n]

Middle lobe

Oblique fissure

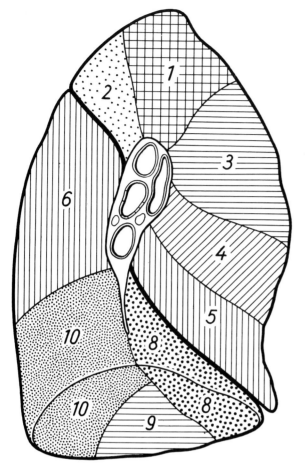

Fig. 122: Left Lung, Bronchopulmonary Segments, Medial View

NOTE: the bronchopulmonary segments of the left lung have been identified as follows:

Upper lobe

1	Apical	⎫ Frequently
2	Posterior	⎬ considered as one segment
3	Anterior	
4	Superior	⎫ Lingular
5	Inferior	⎭

Lower lobe

6 Superior
7 Medial basal *
8 Anterior basal *
9 Lateral basal
10 Posterior basal

* the medial basal and anterior basal segments were at one time frequently considered as a single bronchopulmonary segment. Today, however, they have been recognized as separate segments in a majority of left lungs. Therefore, on this figure that portion of segment 8 just inferior to the oblique fissure should be marked 7 and identified as medial basal.

Fig. 123: Right Lung, Bronchopulmonary Segments, Medial View

NOTE: the bronchopulmonary segments of the right lung have been identified as follows:

Upper lobe
1 Apical
2 Posterior
3 Anterior

Middle lobe
4 Lateral (not seen from this view)
5 Medial

Lower lobe
6 Superior
7 Medial basal
8 Anterior basal
9 Lateral basal
10 Posterior basal

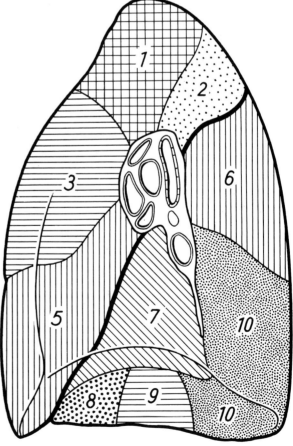

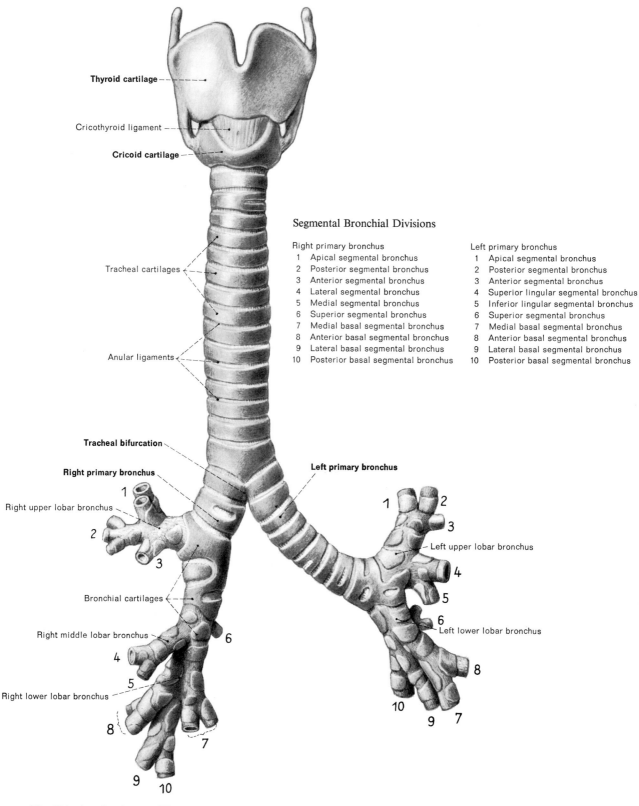

Segmental Bronchial Divisions

Right primary bronchus
1 Apical segmental bronchus
2 Posterior segmental bronchus
3 Anterior segmental bronchus
4 Lateral segmental bronchus
5 Medial segmental bronchus
6 Superior segmental bronchus
7 Medial basal segmental bronchus
8 Anterior basal segmental bronchus
9 Lateral basal segmental bronchus
10 Posterior basal segmental bronchus

Left primary bronchus
1 Apical segmental bronchus
2 Posterior segmental bronchus
3 Anterior segmental bronchus
4 Superior lingular segmental bronchus
5 Inferior lingular segmental bronchus
6 Superior segmental bronchus
7 Medial basal segmental bronchus
8 Anterior basal segmental bronchus
9 Lateral basal segmental bronchus
10 Posterior basal segmental bronchus

Thyroid cartilage

Cricothyroid ligament

Cricoid cartilage

Tracheal cartilages

Anular ligaments

Tracheal bifurcation

Right primary bronchus

Right upper lobar bronchus

Bronchial cartilages

Right middle lobar bronchus

Right lower lobar bronchus

Left primary bronchus

Left upper lobar bronchus

Left lower lobar bronchus

Fig. 124: Anterior Aspect of Larynx, Trachea, and Bronchi

NOTE: 1) the trachea bifurcates into two principal (primary) bronchi. These then divide into lobar (secondary) bronchi which in turn give rise to segmental (tertiary) bronchi.

2) the larynx is located in the anterior aspect of the neck, and its thyroid and cricoid cartilages can be felt through the skin.

3) the thyroid cartilage, projected posteriorly, lies at the level of the 4th and 5th cervical vertebrae, while the cricoid cartilage is at the 6th cervical level. The trachea commences at the lower end of the cricoid and extends slightly more than four inches before bifurcating into the two primary bronchi at the level of T-4. Two inches of trachea lie above the suprasternal notch in the neck, while about two inches of trachea are intrathoracic above its bifurcation.

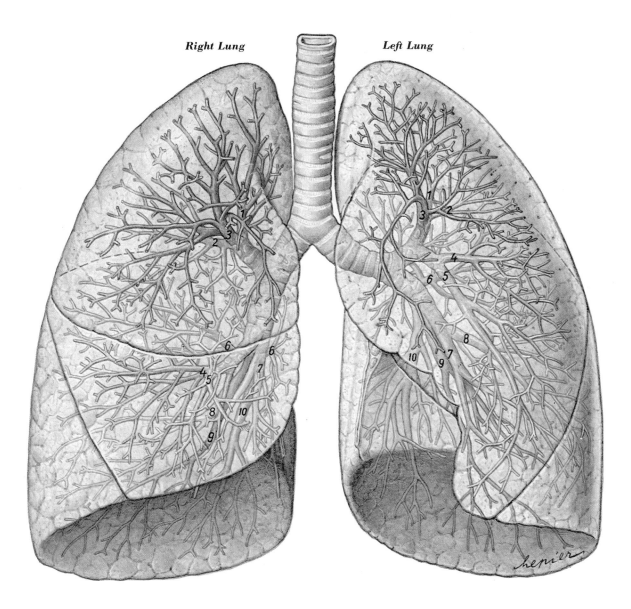

Right Lung   **Left Lung**

Fig. 125: Diagram of the Bronchial Tree and its Lobar and Bronchopulmonary Divisions, Anterior View

NOTE: 1) as the trachea divides, the left primary bronchus diverges at a more abrupt angle than the right primary bronchus to reach their respective lungs. Thus the left bronchus is directed more transversely and the right bronchus more inferiorly

2) on the right side the upper lobar bronchus branches from the primary bronchus almost immediately, even above the pulmonary artery (eparterial), while the bronchus directed toward the middle and lower lobes branches below the position of the main stem of the pulmonary artery (hyparterial).

3) on the left side the initial lobar bronchus, branching from the primary bronchus, is directed upward and lateralward to the upper lobe segments and its lingular segments. The remaining lobar bronchus is directed inferiorly and soon divides into the segmental bronchi of the lower lobe.

4) the segmental bronchi numbered above are as follows:

Right lung:

1	Apical	6	Superior
2	Posterior	7	Medial basal
3	Anterior	8	Anterior basal
4	Lateral	9	Lateral basal
5	Medial	10	Posterior basal

Left lung:

1	Apical	6	Superior
2	Posterior	7	Medial basal
3	Anterior	8	Anterior basal
4	Superior lingular	9	Lateral basal
5	Inferior lingular	10	Posterior basal

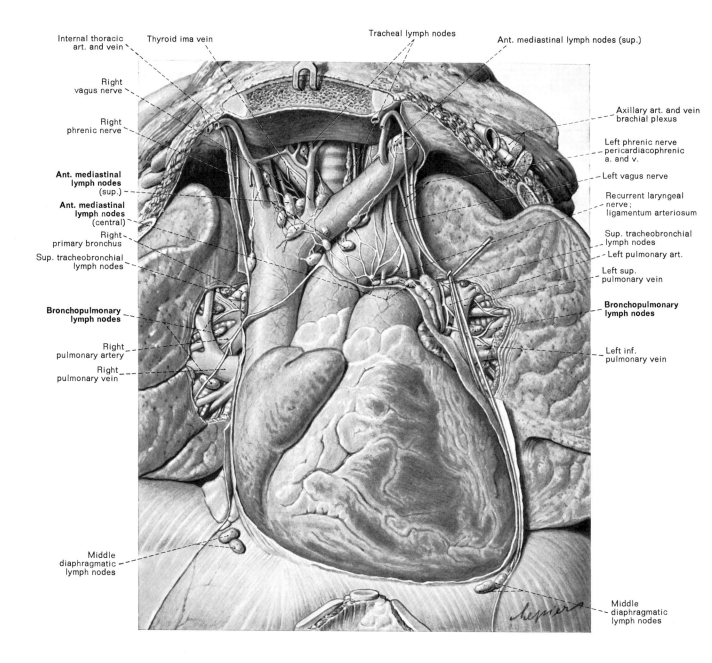

Internal thoracic art. and vein

Thyroid ima vein

Tracheal lymph nodes

Ant. mediastinal lymph nodes (sup.)

Right vagus nerve

Right phrenic nerve

Axillary art. and vein brachial plexus

Left phrenic nerve pericardiacophrenic a. and v.

Ant. mediastinal lymph nodes (sup.)

Left vagus nerve

Ant. mediastinal lymph nodes (central)

Recurrent laryngeal nerve; ligamentum arteriosum

Right primary bronchus

Sup. tracheobronchial lymph nodes

Sup. tracheobronchial lymph nodes

Left pulmonary art.

Left sup. pulmonary vein

Bronchopulmonary lymph nodes

Bronchopulmonary lymph nodes

Right pulmonary artery

Right pulmonary vein

Left inf. pulmonary vein

Middle diaphragmatic lymph nodes

Middle diaphragmatic lymph nodes

Fig. 126: Lymphatics of the Thorax, Anterior Aspect

NOTE: 1) in this dissection the anterior thoracic wall was removed along with the ventral portion of the pericardium. Further, the anterior borders of the lungs have been pulled laterally to reveal the lymphatic channels at the roots of the lungs. The thymus has also been removed and the manubrium reflected superiorly to expose the organs at the thoracic inlet and their associated lymphatics.

2) the lymph nodes in the anterior aspect of the thoracic cavity might be divided into those associated with the thoracic cage (parietal) and those associated with the organs (visceral). Probably all of the nodes indicated in this figure are visceral nodes.

3) situated ventrally are the *anterior mediastinal nodes* which include a superior group lying ventral to the brachiocephalic veins along their course in the superior mediastinum and at their junction to form the superior vena cava. A more centrally located group lies ventral to the arch of the aorta. Inferiorly, anterior diaphragmatic nodes are sometimes also classified as part of the anterior mediastinal nodes.

4) large numbers of lymph nodes are associated with the trachea, the bronchi and the other structures at the root of the lung. These nodes have been aptly named tracheal, tracheobronchial, bronchopulmonary and pulmonary.

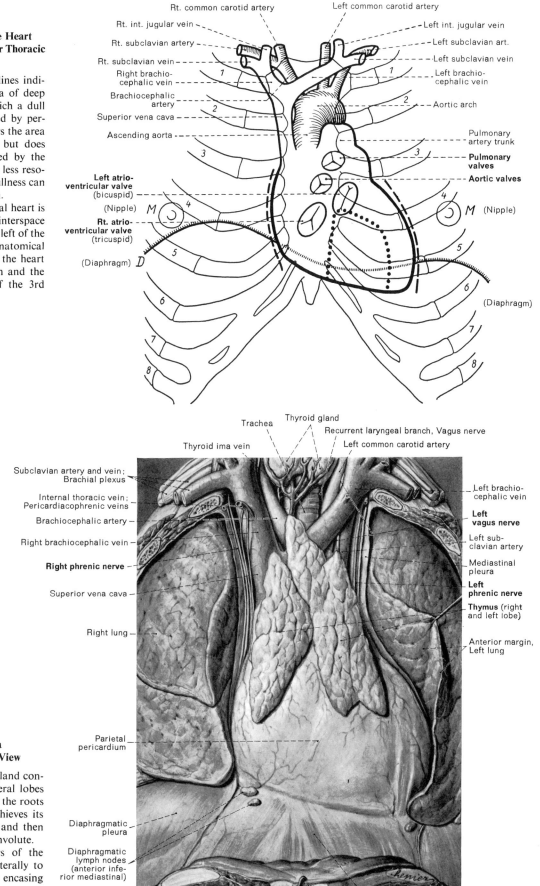

Fig. 127: Projection of the Heart and its Valves onto Anterior Thoracic Wall

NOTE: 1) the broken lines indicate the limits of the area of deep cardiac dullness from which a dull resonance can be obtained by percussion. Lung tissue covers the area of deep cardiac dullness but does not cover the area limited by the dotted lines from which a less resonant superficial cardiac dullness can be obtained by percussion.

2) the apex of the normal heart is usually found in the 5th interspace about 9 centimeters to the left of the midline. Observe the anatomical positions of the valves of the heart in relation to the sternum and the left sternocostal joints of the 3rd and 4th ribs.

Rt. common carotid artery
Left common carotid artery
Rt. int. jugular vein
Left int. jugular vein
Rt. subclavian artery
Left subclavian art.
Rt. subclavian vein
Left subclavian vein
Right brachio-cephalic vein
Left brachio-cephalic vein
Brachiocephalic artery
Aortic arch
Superior vena cava
Ascending aorta
Pulmonary artery trunk
Pulmonary valves
Aortic valves
Left atrio-ventricular valve (bicuspid)
(Nipple) M
M (Nipple)
Rt. atrio-ventricular valve (tricuspid)
(Diaphragm) D
(Diaphragm)

Fig. 128: Thoracic Viscera of a Young Boy, Anterior View

NOTE: 1) the thymus gland consists of two lobulated lateral lobes and is situated anterior to the roots of the great vessels. It achieves its largest weight at puberty and then commences gradually to involute.

2) the anterior borders of the lungs have been pulled laterally to reveal the pericardial sac encasing the heart.

Trachea
Thyroid gland
Thyroid ima vein
Recurrent laryngeal branch, Vagus nerve
Left common carotid artery
Subclavian artery and vein; Brachial plexus
Left brachio-cephalic vein
Internal thoracic vein; Pericardiacophrenic veins
Left vagus nerve
Brachiocephalic artery
Left sub-clavian artery
Right brachiocephalic vein
Mediastinal pleura
Right phrenic nerve
Left phrenic nerve
Superior vena cava
Thymus (right and left lobe)
Right lung
Anterior margin, Left lung
Parietal pericardium
Diaphragmatic pleura
Diaphragmatic lymph nodes (anterior inferior mediastinal)
Sternum
Diaphragm

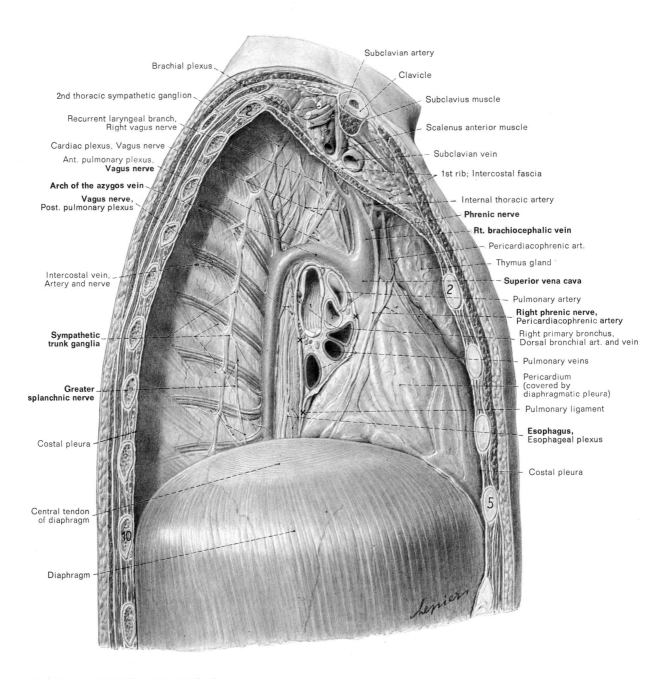

Fig. 129: The Right Side of the Mediastinum

Labels (clockwise from top):
Subclavian artery
Clavicle
Subclavius muscle
Scalenus anterior muscle
Subclavian vein
1st rib; Intercostal fascia
Internal thoracic artery
Phrenic nerve
Rt. brachiocephalic vein
Pericardiacophrenic art.
Thymus gland
Superior vena cava
Pulmonary artery
Right phrenic nerve, Pericardiacophrenic artery
Right primary bronchus, Dorsal bronchial art. and vein
Pulmonary veins
Pericardium (covered by diaphragmatic pleura)
Pulmonary ligament
Esophagus, Esophageal plexus
Costal pleura

Diaphragm
Central tendon of diaphragm
Costal pleura
Greater splanchnic nerve
Sympathetic trunk ganglia
Intercostal vein, Artery and nerve
Vagus nerve, Post. pulmonary plexus
Arch of the azygos vein
Ant. pulmonary plexus, Vagus nerve
Cardiac plexus, Vagus nerve
Recurrent laryngeal branch, Right vagus nerve
2nd thoracic sympathetic ganglion
Brachial plexus

NOTE: 1) with the right lung removed and the structures at its hilum transected, the organs of the mediastinum are exposed and their right lateral surface viewed.

2) the right side of the heart covered by the pericardium and the course of the phrenic nerve and pericardiacophrenic vessels.

3) the ascending course of the azygos vein, its arch and its junction with the superior vena cava.

4) that the right vagus nerve descends in the thorax behind the root of the right lung to form the posterior pulmonary plexus. It then helps form the esophageal plexus and leaves the thorax on the posterior aspect of the esophagus.

5) the dome of the diaphragm on the right side taking the rounded form of the underlying liver. The base of the heart rests on the diaphragm.

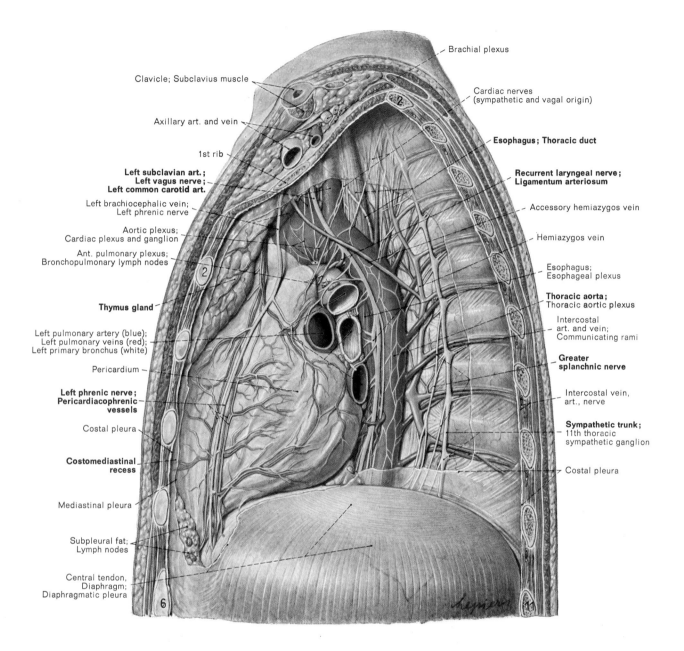

Brachial plexus

Clavicle; Subclavius muscle

Cardiac nerves
(sympathetic and vagal origin)

Axillary art. and vein

Esophagus; Thoracic duct

1st rib

**Recurrent laryngeal nerve;
Ligamentum arteriosum**

**Left subclavian art.;
Left vagus nerve;
Left common carotid art.**

Accessory hemiazygos vein

Left brachiocephalic vein;
Left phrenic nerve

Hemiazygos vein

Aortic plexus;
Cardiac plexus and ganglion

Esophagus;
Esophageal plexus

Ant. pulmonary plexus;
Bronchopulmonary lymph nodes

Thoracic aorta;
Thoracic aortic plexus

Thymus gland

Intercostal
art. and vein;
Communicating rami

Left pulmonary artery (blue);
Left pulmonary veins (red);
Left primary bronchus (white)

**Greater
splanchnic nerve**

Pericardium

Intercostal vein,
art., nerve

**Left phrenic nerve;
Pericardiacophrenic
vessels**

Sympathetic trunk;
11th thoracic
sympathetic ganglion

Costal pleura

Costal pleura

**Costomediastinal
recess**

Mediastinal pleura

Subpleural fat;
Lymph nodes

Central tendon,
Diaphragm;
Diaphragmatic pleura

Fig. 130: The Left Side of the Mediastinum

NOTE: 1) with the left lung removed along with most of the mediastinal pleura, the structures of the mediastinum are observed from their left side.

2) the left phrenic nerve and pericardiacophrenic vessels coursing to the diaphragm along the pericardium covering the left side of the heart.

3) the aorta ascends about two inches before it arches posteriorly and to the left of the vertebral column. The descending thoracic aorta commences at about the level of the 4th thoracic vertebra and as it descends, it comes to lie directly anterior to the vertebral column. The intercostal arteries branch directly from the thoracic aorta.

4) the left vagus nerve lies lateral to the aortic arch and gives off its recurrent laryngeal branch which passes inferior to the ligamentum arteriosum. The left vagus then continues to descend, contributes to the esophageal plexus, and enters the abdomen on the anterior aspect of the esophagus.

5) the position of the thymus gland anterior to the root of the great vessels at their attachments to the heart.

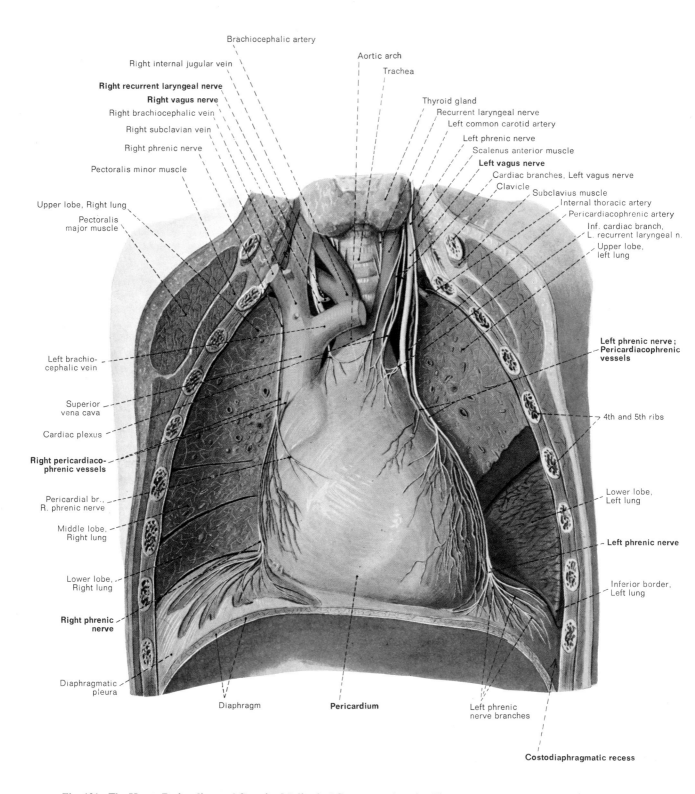

Brachiocephalic artery

Right internal jugular vein

Right recurrent laryngeal nerve

Right vagus nerve

Right brachiocephalic vein

Right subclavian vein

Right phrenic nerve

Pectoralis minor muscle

Upper lobe, Right lung

Pectoralis major muscle

Left brachio-cephalic vein

Superior vena cava

Cardiac plexus

Right pericardiaco-phrenic vessels

Pericardial br., R. phrenic nerve

Middle lobe, Right lung

Lower lobe, Right lung

Right phrenic nerve

Diaphragmatic pleura

Diaphragm

Pericardium

Aortic arch

Trachea

Thyroid gland

Recurrent laryngeal nerve

Left common carotid artery

Left phrenic nerve

Scalenus anterior muscle

Left vagus nerve

Cardiac branches, Left vagus nerve

Clavicle

Subclavius muscle

Internal thoracic artery

Pericardiacophrenic artery

Inf. cardiac branch, L. recurrent laryngeal n.

Upper lobe, left lung

Left phrenic nerve; Pericardiacophrenic vessels

4th and 5th ribs

Lower lobe, Left lung

Left phrenic nerve

Inferior border, Left lung

Left phrenic nerve branches

Costodiaphragmatic recess

Fig. 131: The Heart, Pericardium and Superior Mediastinal Structures, Anterior View

NOTE: 1) in this frontal section through the thorax, the anterior thoracic wall and the anterior aspect of the lungs and diaphragm have been removed leaving the pericardium, its contents and its associated vessels and nerves intact. The courses of the vagus nerves and their branches in the superior mediastinum are also demonstrated.

2) the phrenic nerves originate in the neck (C3, 4, 5) and descend almost vertically to innervate the diaphragm. In the superior mediastinum they join the pericardiacophrenic vessels, travel along the lateral surfaces of the pericardium and are distributed principally to the diaphragm, sending some sensory fibers to the pericardium as well.

3) the pericardium is formed by an outer fibrous layer which is lined by an inner serous sac. As the heart develops it invaginates into the inner serous sac, thereby being covered by a visceral layer of serous pericardium (epicardium) and a parietal layer of serous pericardium. The outer fibrous pericardium has only a parietal layer.

Fig. 132: The Coronary Vessels, Anterior View

NOTE: 1) both the left and right coronary arteries arise from the ascending aorta. The *left coronary* is directed toward the left and soon divides into a *descending anterior interventricular branch* which courses toward the apex and a circumflex branch which passes posteriorly as far as the posterior interventricular sulcus.

2) the right coronary artery is directed toward the right, passing to the posterior aspect of the heart within the coronary sulcus. In its course, branches from the right coronary supply the anterior surface of the right side (anterior cardiac artery). Its largest branch is the posterior interventricular artery which courses toward the apex on the posterior or diaphragmatic surface of the heart.

3) the principal veins of the heart drain into the coronary sinus which in turn flows into the right atrium. The distribution and course of the veins is generally similar to the arteries.

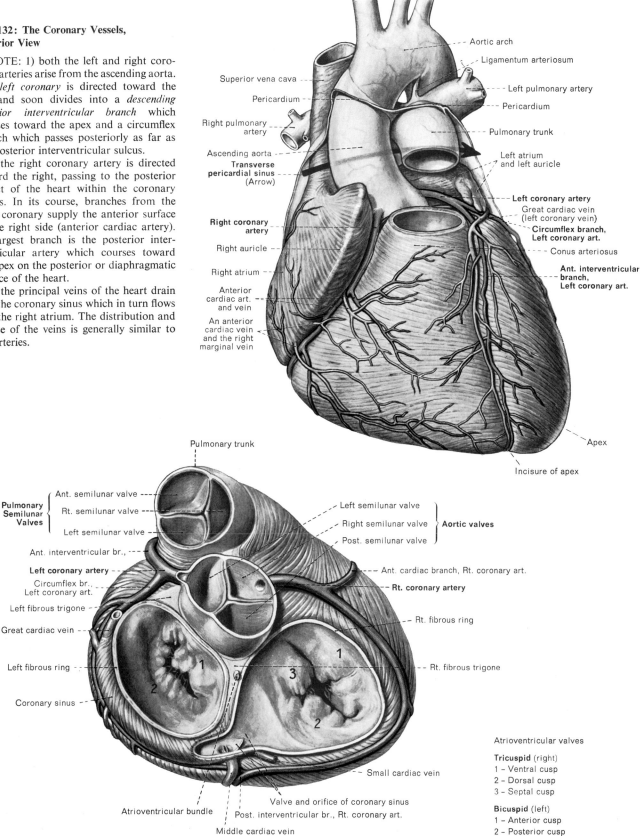

Fig. 132 labels:
Aortic arch
Ligamentum arteriosum
Superior vena cava
Left pulmonary artery
Pericardium
Pericardium
Right pulmonary artery
Pulmonary trunk
Ascending aorta
Left atrium and left auricle
Transverse pericardial sinus (Arrow)
Left coronary artery
Great cardiac vein (left coronary vein)
Right coronary artery
Circumflex branch, Left coronary art.
Conus arteriosus
Right auricle
Ant. interventricular branch, Left coronary art.
Right atrium
Anterior cardiac art. and vein
An anterior cardiac vein and the right marginal vein
Apex
Incisure of apex

Fig. 133 labels:
Pulmonary trunk
Pulmonary Semilunar Valves
Ant. semilunar valve
Rt. semilunar valve
Left semilunar valve
Left semilunar valve
Right semilunar valve
Post. semilunar valve
Aortic valves
Ant. interventricular br.,
Ant. cardiac branch, Rt. coronary art.
Left coronary artery
Rt. coronary artery
Circumflex br., Left coronary art.
Left fibrous trigone
Rt. fibrous ring
Great cardiac vein
Left fibrous ring
Rt. fibrous trigone
Coronary sinus
Small cardiac vein
Atrioventricular bundle
Valve and orifice of coronary sinus
Post. interventricular br., Rt. coronary art.
Middle cardiac vein

Atrioventricular valves

Tricuspid (right)
1 – Ventral cusp
2 – Dorsal cusp
3 – Septal cusp

Bicuspid (left)
1 – Anterior cusp
2 – Posterior cusp

Fig. 133: The Valves of the Heart and the Origin of the Coronary Vessels, Superior View

Note that the left coronary artery arises from the aortic sinus behind the left semilunar valve and the right coronary artery stems from the aortic sinus behind the right semilunar valve.

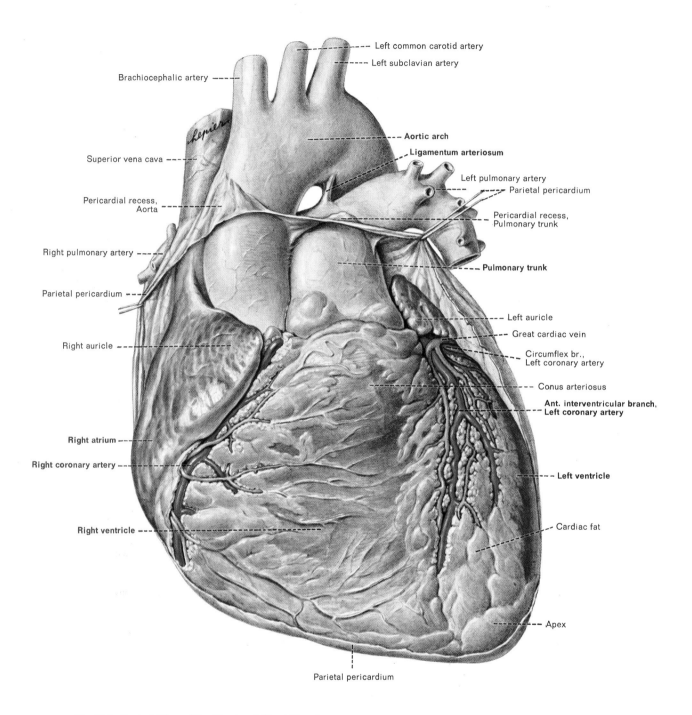

Left common carotid artery

Left subclavian artery

Brachiocephalic artery

Aortic arch

Ligamentum arteriosum

Superior vena cava

Left pulmonary artery

Parietal pericardium

Pericardial recess,
Aorta

Pericardial recess,
Pulmonary trunk

Right pulmonary artery

Pulmonary trunk

Parietal pericardium

Left auricle

Great cardiac vein

Right auricle

Circumflex br.,
Left coronary artery

Conus arteriosus

**Ant. interventricular branch,
Left coronary artery**

Right atrium

Right coronary artery

Left ventricle

Cardiac fat

Right ventricle

Apex

Parietal pericardium

Fig. 134: Ventral View of the Heart and Great Vessels

NOTE: 1) the heart is a muscular organ with its apex pointed inferiorly, toward the left and slightly anteriorly. The base of the heart is opposite to the apex and is, therefore, directed superiorly and toward the right. The great vessels attach to the heart at its base, and the pericardium is reflected over these vessels at their origin.

2) the anterior surface of the heart is its sternocostal surface. The auricular portion of the right atrium and especially the right ventricle is seen from this anterior view; also a small part of the left ventricle is visible on the left side.

3) the pulmonary trunk originates from the right ventricle. To its right and slightly behind can be seen the aorta which arises from the left ventricle. The superior vena cava can be seen opening into the upper aspect of the right atrium.

4) the ligamentum arteriosum. This fibrous structure, attaching the left pulmonary artery to the arch of the aorta, is the postnatal remnant of the fetal ductus arteriosus which, before birth, acted as a shunt diverting some of the blood directed for the lungs back into the aorta for general systemic distribution.

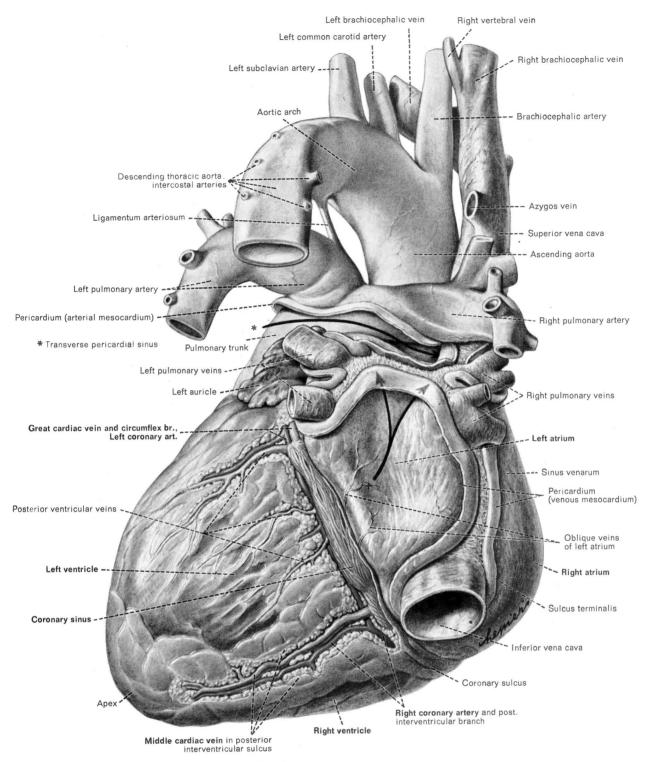

Left brachiocephalic vein

Left common carotid artery

Right vertebral vein

Left subclavian artery

Right brachiocephalic vein

Aortic arch

Brachiocephalic artery

Descending thoracic aorta,
intercostal arteries

Ligamentum arteriosum

Azygos vein

Superior vena cava

Ascending aorta

Left pulmonary artery

Pericardium (arterial mesocardium)

Right pulmonary artery

* Transverse pericardial sinus

Pulmonary trunk

Left pulmonary veins

Right pulmonary veins

Left auricle

Great cardiac vein and circumflex br.,
Left coronary art.

Left atrium

Sinus venarum

Pericardium
(venous mesocardium)

Posterior ventricular veins

Oblique veins
of left atrium

Right atrium

Left ventricle

Sulcus terminalis

Coronary sinus

Inferior vena cava

Coronary sulcus

Apex

Right coronary artery and post.
interventricular branch

Middle cardiac vein in posterior
interventricular sulcus

Right ventricle

Fig. 135: Posterior View of the Heart and Great Vessels

NOTE: 1) the two pericardial sinuses. The long transverse arrow indicates the *transverse pericardial sinus* which lies between the arterial mesocardium and the venus mesocardium. The double arrows lie in the *oblique pericardial sinus,* the boundaries of which are actually demarcated by the pericardial reflections around the pulmonary veins.

2) the transverse sinus can be identified by placing your index finger behind the pulmonary artery and aorta with the heart *in situ*. The oblique sinus is open inferiorly, while superiorly it forms a closed sac. This sinus can also be felt by cupping your fingers behind the heart and pushing superiorly.

3) the coronary sinus separates the posterior surface regions of the atria (above and to the right) and the ventricles (below and to the left). The posterior atrial surface principally consists of the left atrium, into which flow the pulmonary veins, although below and to the right can be seen the right atrium and its inferior vena cava. The posterior atrial surface lies anterior to the vertebral column. The posterior ventricular surface is formed principally by the left ventricle and this surface lies over the diaphragm.

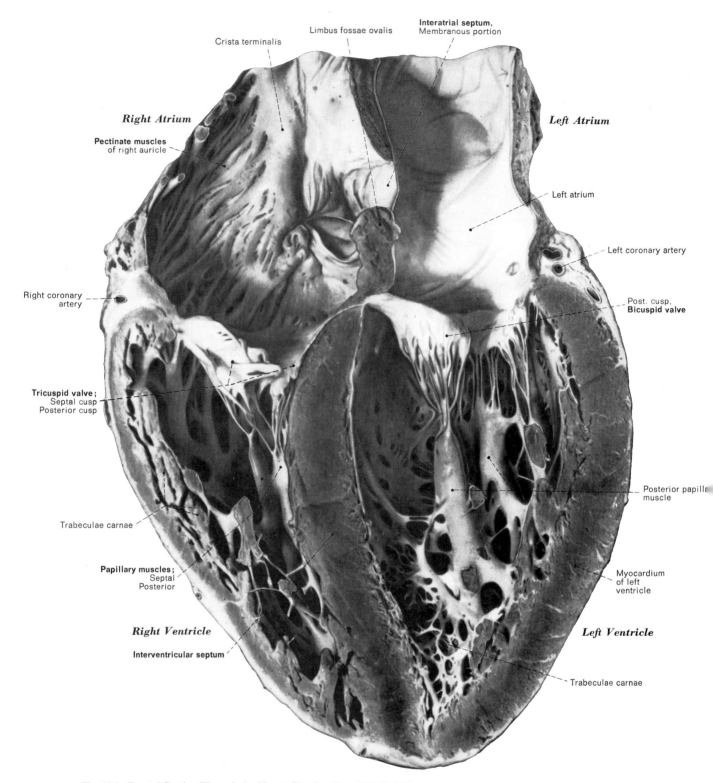

Labels on the figure:

Crista terminalis
Limbus fossae ovalis
Interatrial septum, Membranous portion

Right Atrium
Left Atrium

Pectinate muscles of right auricle

Left atrium

Left coronary artery

Right coronary artery

Post. cusp, **Bicuspid valve**

Tricuspid valve; Septal cusp Posterior cusp

Posterior papilla muscle

Trabeculae carnae

Myocardium of left ventricle

Papillary muscles; Septal Posterior

Right Ventricle
Left Ventricle

Interventricular septum

Trabeculae carnae

Fig. 136: Frontal Section Through the Heart, Showing Dorsal Half of Heart

NOTE: 1) the human heart is a four-chambered muscular organ consisting of an atrium and a ventricle on each side. The walls of the ventricles are thicker than those of the atria. The atrial chambers are separated by an interatrial septum, and this is continuous with the interventricular septum dividing the two ventricles. Blood passes simultaneously from the two atria into their respective ventricles through the atrioventricular valves.

2) on the right side the atrioventricular valve (AV valve) consists of three cusps and is called the tricuspid valve. On the left side the AV valve has two cusps and is called the bicuspid or mitral valve.

3) the inner surfaces of the atria are relatively smooth, whereas muscular projections, the papillary muscles, protrude from the inner walls of the ventricles to attach to the cusps of the AV valves by way of fibrous, thin cords, the chordae tendineae. (These cords are shown but not labelled.)

4) other elevated muscular bundles on the inner heart wall do not attach to the valves. In the ventricles these are called the trabeculae carnae, while in the right auricle they are named the pectinate muscles.

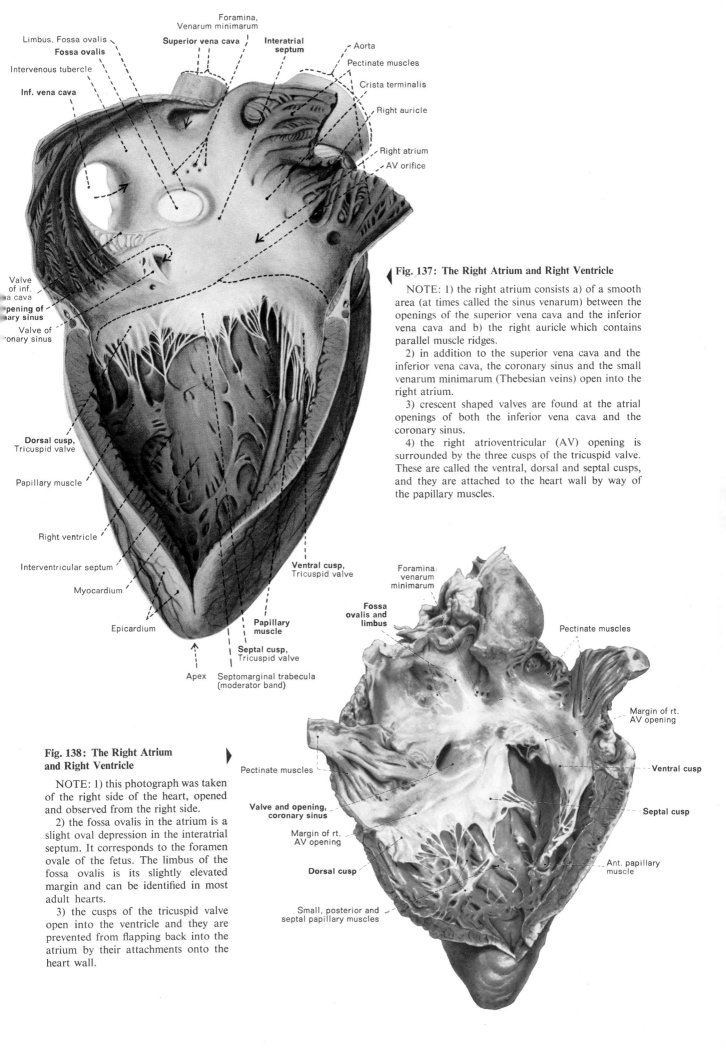

Foramina, Venarum minimarum

Limbus, Fossa ovalis
Fossa ovalis
Intervenous tubercle
Inf. vena cava
Superior vena cava
Interatrial septum
Aorta
Pectinate muscles
Crista terminalis
Right auricle
Right atrium
AV orifice

Valve of inf. vena cava
Opening of coronary sinus
Valve of coronary sinus

Dorsal cusp, Tricuspid valve
Papillary muscle
Right ventricle
Interventricular septum
Myocardium
Epicardium
Apex

Ventral cusp, Tricuspid valve
Papillary muscle
Septal cusp, Tricuspid valve
Septomarginal trabecula (moderator band)

Fig. 137: The Right Atrium and Right Ventricle

NOTE: 1) the right atrium consists a) of a smooth area (at times called the sinus venarum) between the openings of the superior vena cava and the inferior vena cava and b) the right auricle which contains parallel muscle ridges.

2) in addition to the superior vena cava and the inferior vena cava, the coronary sinus and the small venarum minimarum (Thebesian veins) open into the right atrium.

3) crescent shaped valves are found at the atrial openings of both the inferior vena cava and the coronary sinus.

4) the right atrioventricular (AV) opening is surrounded by the three cusps of the tricuspid valve. These are called the ventral, dorsal and septal cusps, and they are attached to the heart wall by way of the papillary muscles.

Foramina venarum minimarum
Fossa ovalis and limbus
Pectinate muscles
Pectinate muscles
Margin of rt. AV opening
Ventral cusp
Valve and opening, coronary sinus
Septal cusp
Margin of rt. AV opening
Dorsal cusp
Ant. papillary muscle
Small, posterior and septal papillary muscles

Fig. 138: The Right Atrium and Right Ventricle

NOTE: 1) this photograph was taken of the right side of the heart, opened and observed from the right side.

2) the fossa ovalis in the atrium is a slight oval depression in the interatrial septum. It corresponds to the foramen ovale of the fetus. The limbus of the fossa ovalis is its slightly elevated margin and can be identified in most adult hearts.

3) the cusps of the tricuspid valve open into the ventricle and they are prevented from flapping back into the atrium by their attachments onto the heart wall.

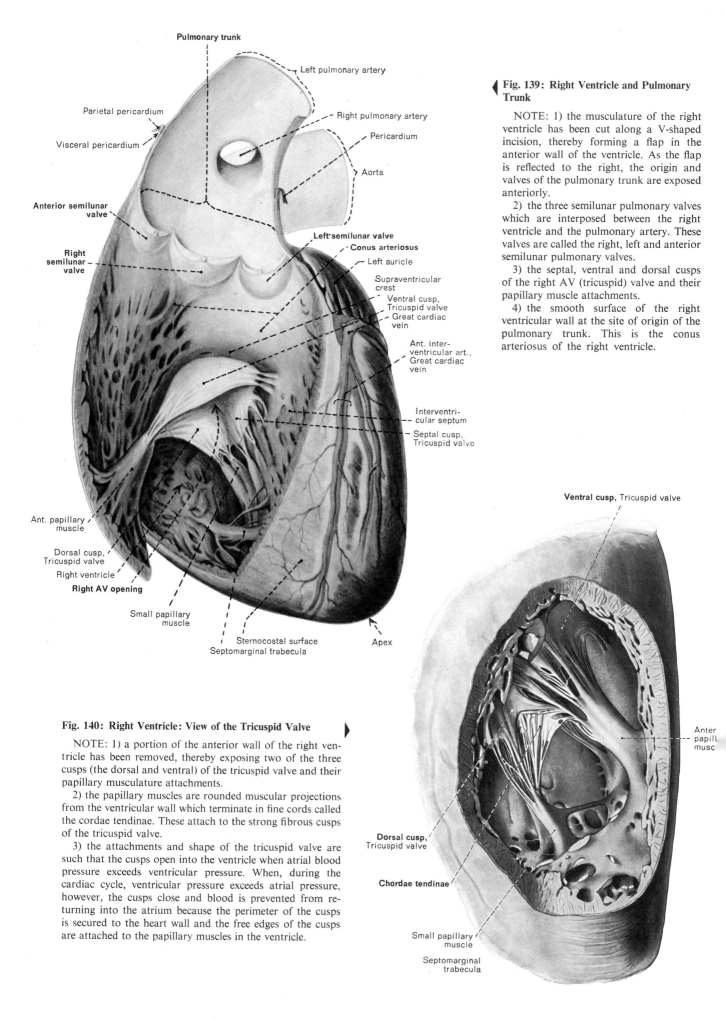

Pulmonary trunk

Left pulmonary artery

Parietal pericardium

Right pulmonary artery

Visceral pericardium

Pericardium

Aorta

Anterior semilunar valve

Left semilunar valve

Conus arteriosus

Right semilunar valve

Left auricle

Supraventricular crest

Ventral cusp, Tricuspid valve

Great cardiac vein

Ant. interventricular art., Great cardiac vein

Interventricular septum

Septal cusp, Tricuspid valve

Ant. papillary muscle

Dorsal cusp, Tricuspid valve

Right ventricle

Right AV opening

Small papillary muscle

Sternocostal surface
Septomarginal trabecula

Apex

Fig. 139: Right Ventricle and Pulmonary Trunk

NOTE: 1) the musculature of the right ventricle has been cut along a V-shaped incision, thereby forming a flap in the anterior wall of the ventricle. As the flap is reflected to the right, the origin and valves of the pulmonary trunk are exposed anteriorly.

2) the three semilunar pulmonary valves which are interposed between the right ventricle and the pulmonary artery. These valves are called the right, left and anterior semilunar pulmonary valves.

3) the septal, ventral and dorsal cusps of the right AV (tricuspid) valve and their papillary muscle attachments.

4) the smooth surface of the right ventricular wall at the site of origin of the pulmonary trunk. This is the conus arteriosus of the right ventricle.

Ventral cusp, Tricuspid valve

Anter papill musc

Dorsal cusp, Tricuspid valve

Chordae tendinae

Small papillary muscle

Septomarginal trabecula

Fig. 140: Right Ventricle: View of the Tricuspid Valve

NOTE: 1) a portion of the anterior wall of the right ventricle has been removed, thereby exposing two of the three cusps (the dorsal and ventral) of the tricuspid valve and their papillary musculature attachments.

2) the papillary muscles are rounded muscular projections from the ventricular wall which terminate in fine cords called the cordae tendinae. These attach to the strong fibrous cusps of the tricuspid valve.

3) the attachments and shape of the tricuspid valve are such that the cusps open into the ventricle when atrial blood pressure exceeds ventricular pressure. When, during the cardiac cycle, ventricular pressure exceeds atrial pressure, however, the cusps close and blood is prevented from returning into the atrium because the perimeter of the cusps is secured to the heart wall and the free edges of the cusps are attached to the papillary muscles in the ventricle.

Fig. 141: The Left Atrium and Left Ventricle

NOTE: 1) in this specimen a longitudinal section has been made through the left side of the heart, thereby exposing the smooth-walled left atrium above and the thickened, muscular-walled left ventricle below. The left atrium opens into the left ventricle through the left atrioventricular (AV) orifice at which is located the left AV valve. This valve is also called the mitral or bicuspid valve.

2) the mitral valve consists of two cusps, an anterior cusp and a posterior cusp, and these are attached to the left ventricular wall by means of papillary muscles in a manner similar to that seen on the right side of the heart. Observe the chordae tendineae interposed between the cusps and the papillary muscles.

3) the interatrial septum is marked by the valve of the foramen ovale (falx septi), which represents the remnant of the septum primum during the development of the interatrial septum.

4) the left atrium receives the four pulmonary veins (two from each lung) while the left ventricle leads into (indicated by arrow) the aorta.

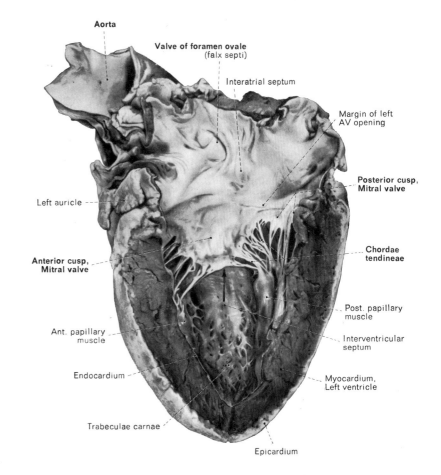

Fig. 142: The Left Ventricle and Ascending Aorta

NOTE: 1) the heart has been cut longitudinally in such a manner that the left ventricular cavity is exposed along with the origin of the ascending aorta.

2) the aortic opening is guarded by three semilunar valves. These are named the posterior, left and right semilunar aortic valves. Behind each valve a small *cul de sac* is formed by the cusp and the wall of the aorta. These small dilated pockets are called the aortic sinuses (sinuses of Valsalva) and from the aortic sinuses behind the left and right semilunar aortic valves, the left and right coronary arteries arise.

3) during ventricular contraction the blood pressure in the left ventricle is elevated over that in the aorta, thereby causing the aortic valves to open and blood to pass into the aorta. Soon, however, the aortic pressure exceeds ventricular pressure and blood then tends to rush back into the ventricle. In the normal heart, the aortic sinuses trap the regurgitating blood and thereby force the aortic valves to close.

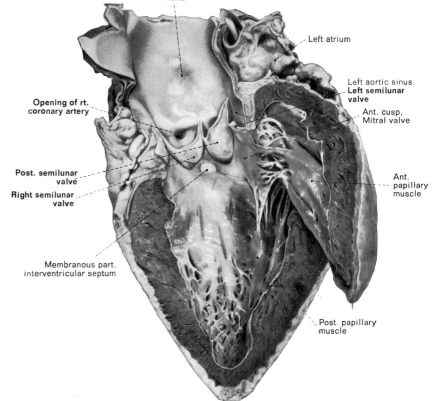

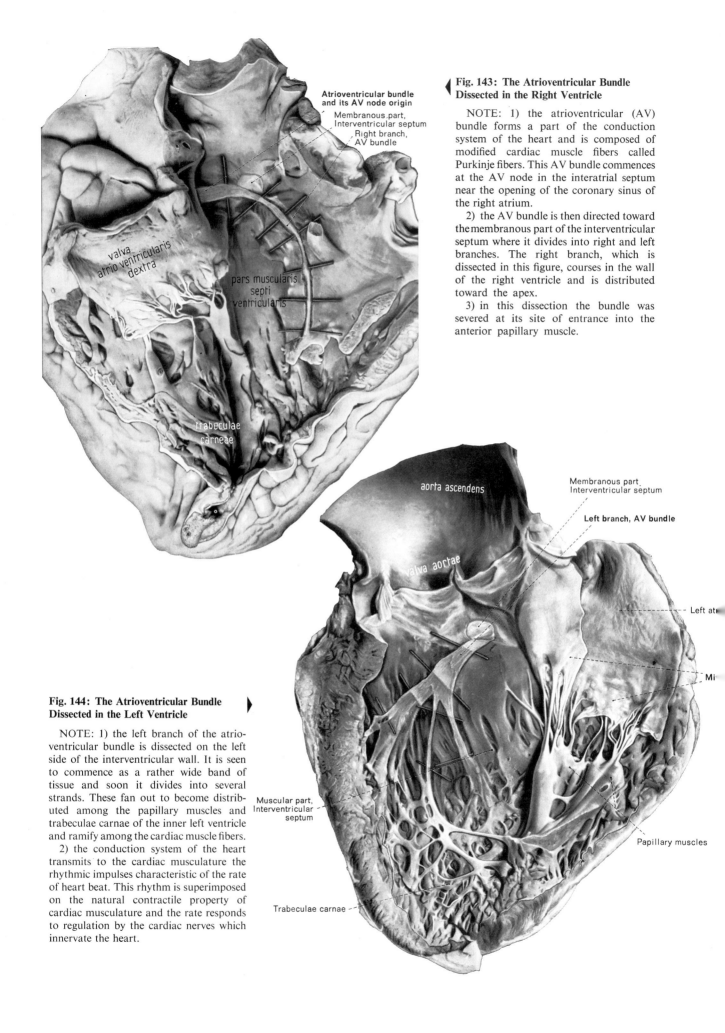

Atrioventricular bundle
and its AV node origin

Membranous part,
Interventricular septum

Right branch,
AV bundle

valva
atrio ventricularis
dextra

pars muscularis
septi
ventricularis

trabeculae
carneae

Fig. 143: The Atrioventricular Bundle Dissected in the Right Ventricle

NOTE: 1) the atrioventricular (AV) bundle forms a part of the conduction system of the heart and is composed of modified cardiac muscle fibers called Purkinje fibers. This AV bundle commences at the AV node in the interatrial septum near the opening of the coronary sinus of the right atrium.

2) the AV bundle is then directed toward the membranous part of the interventricular septum where it divides into right and left branches. The right branch, which is dissected in this figure, courses in the wall of the right ventricle and is distributed toward the apex.

3) in this dissection the bundle was severed at its site of entrance into the anterior papillary muscle.

aorta ascendens

Membranous part
Interventricular septum

Left branch, AV bundle

valva aortae

Left at

Mi

Muscular part,
Interventricular
septum

Papillary muscles

Trabeculae carneae

Fig. 144: The Atrioventricular Bundle Dissected in the Left Ventricle

NOTE: 1) the left branch of the atrioventricular bundle is dissected on the left side of the interventricular wall. It is seen to commence as a rather wide band of tissue and soon it divides into several strands. These fan out to become distributed among the papillary muscles and trabeculae carnae of the inner left ventricle and ramify among the cardiac muscle fibers.

2) the conduction system of the heart transmits to the cardiac musculature the rhythmic impulses characteristic of the rate of heart beat. This rhythm is superimposed on the natural contractile property of cardiac musculature and the rate responds to regulation by the cardiac nerves which innervate the heart.

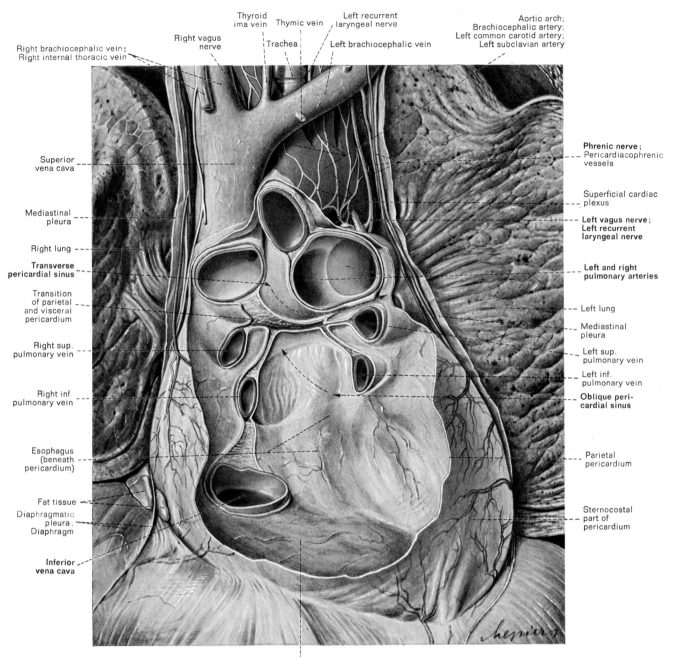

Right brachiocephalic vein;
Right internal thoracic vein

Right vagus
nerve

Thyroid
ima vein   Thymic vein

Trachea

Left recurrent
laryngeal nerve

Left brachiocephalic vein

Aortic arch;
Brachiocephalic artery;
Left common carotid artery;
Left subclavian artery

Phrenic nerve;
Pericardiacophrenic
vessels

Superior
vena cava

Superficial cardiac
plexus

Left vagus nerve;
Left recurrent
laryngeal nerve

Mediastinal
pleura

Right lung

Transverse
pericardial sinus

Left and right
pulmonary arteries

Transition
of parietal
and visceral
pericardium

Left lung

Mediastinal
pleura

Right sup.
pulmonary vein

Left sup.
pulmonary vein

Left inf.
pulmonary vein

Right inf
pulmonary vein

Oblique peri-
cardial sinus

Esophagus
(beneath
pericardium)

Parietal
pericardium

Fat tissue
Diaphragmatic
pleura;
Diaphragm

Sternocostal
part of
pericardium

Inferior
vena cava

Diaphragmatic part of pericardium

Fig. 145: Interior of the Pericardium, Anterior View

NOTE: 1) the pericardium has been opened anteriorly and the heart has been severed from the great vessels and removed. Eight vessels have been cut: the superior and inferior venae cavae, the four pulmonary veins, the pulmonary artery and the aorta.

2) the oblique pericardial sinus is located in the central portion of this posterior wall and is bounded by the pericardial reflections over the pulmonary veins and the venae cavae (venous mesocardium). With the heart in place, the oblique pericardial sinus may be palpated by inserting several fingers behind the heart and probing superiorly until the blind pouch of the sinus is felt.

3) the transverse pericardial sinus lies behind the pericardial reflection surrounding the aorta and pulmonary artery (arterial mesocardium). It may be located by probing from right to left with the index finger immediately posterior to the pulmonary artery.

4) the site of bifurcation of the pulmonary artery beneath the arch of the aorta and the course of the left recurrent laryngeal nerve beneath the ligamentum arteriosum (not labeled).

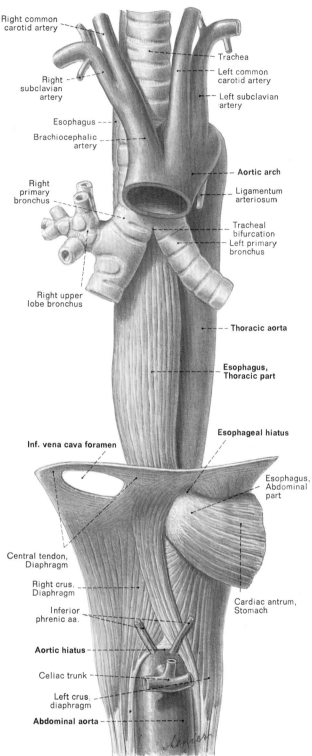

Fig. 146: (Above) the Aorta and Lower Esophagus at the Tracheal Bifurcation and Diaphragm

NOTE: 1) at the level of the bifurcation of the trachea (T-4), the esophagus lies between the trachea and the thoracic aorta. The esophagus then descends into the thorax with the aorta somewhat to its left. In the lower thorax the esophagus bends to the left and thus crosses over the aorta anteriorly from right to left.

2) the esophagus enters the abdomen through the esophageal hiatus of the diaphragm, while the aorta passes through the aortic hiatus.

Fig. 147: (Below) the Relationship of the Esophagus to the Aorta and Trachea, Viewed from Right Side

NOTE: the esophagus commences above as an inferior extension of the pharynx. Superiorly, the esophagus is in relationship with the larynx and thyroid gland. Its middle third courses in relation to the trachea, bronchi and the arch of the aorta, while its lower third descends with the thoracic aorta.

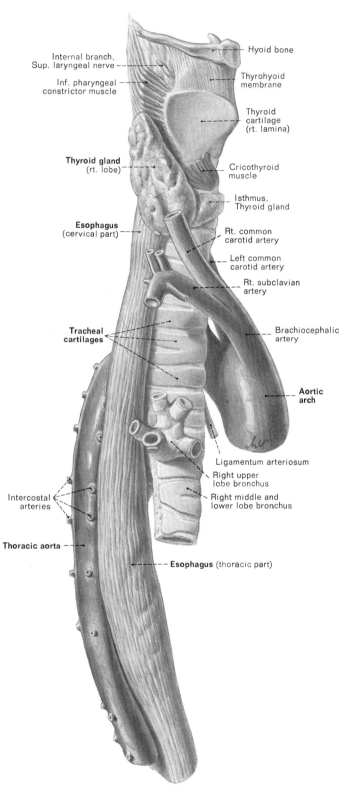

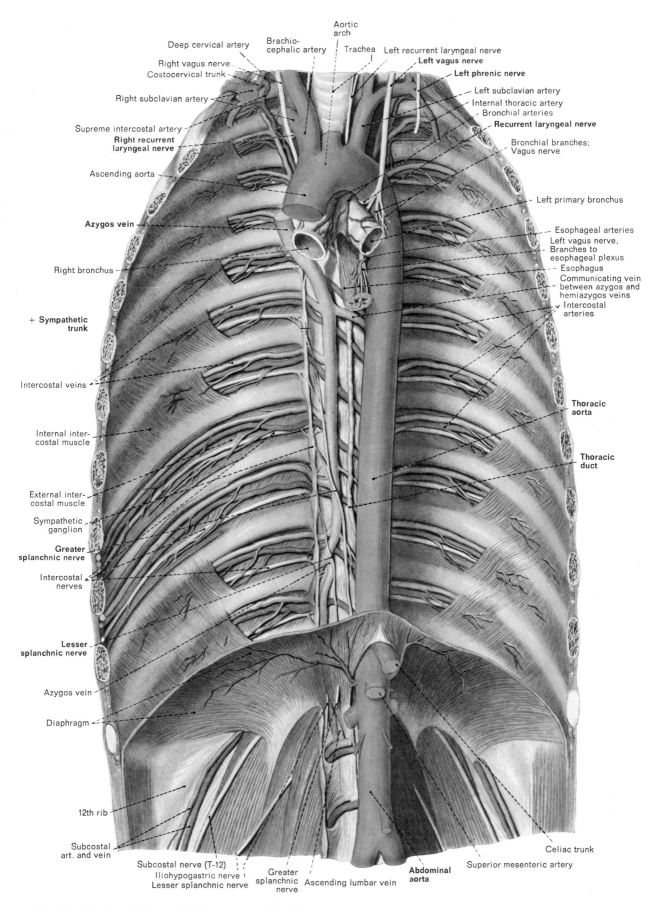

Fig. 148: **Vessels and Nerves of the Dorsal Thoracic Wall**

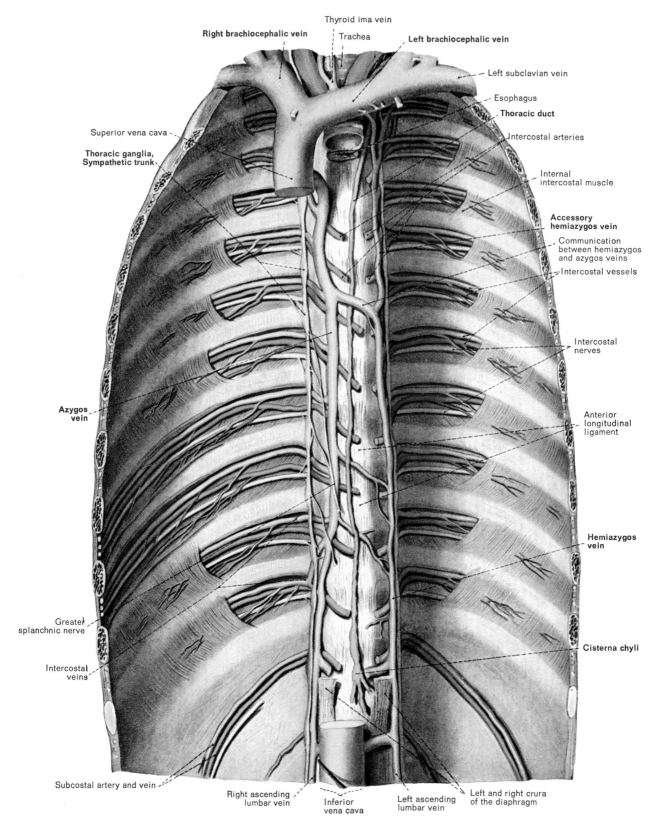

Fig. 149: The Azygos System of Veins, the Thoracic Duct and Other Posterior Thoracic Wall Structures

NOTE: 1) with all the organs of the thorax and mediastinum removed or cut, the hemiazygos and accessory hemiazygos veins to the left of the vertebral column are seen communicating across the midline with the larger azygos vein. This latter vessel also ascends in the thorax to flow into the superior vena cava.

2) the thoracic duct as it arises from the cisterna chyli at the 1st lumbar level.

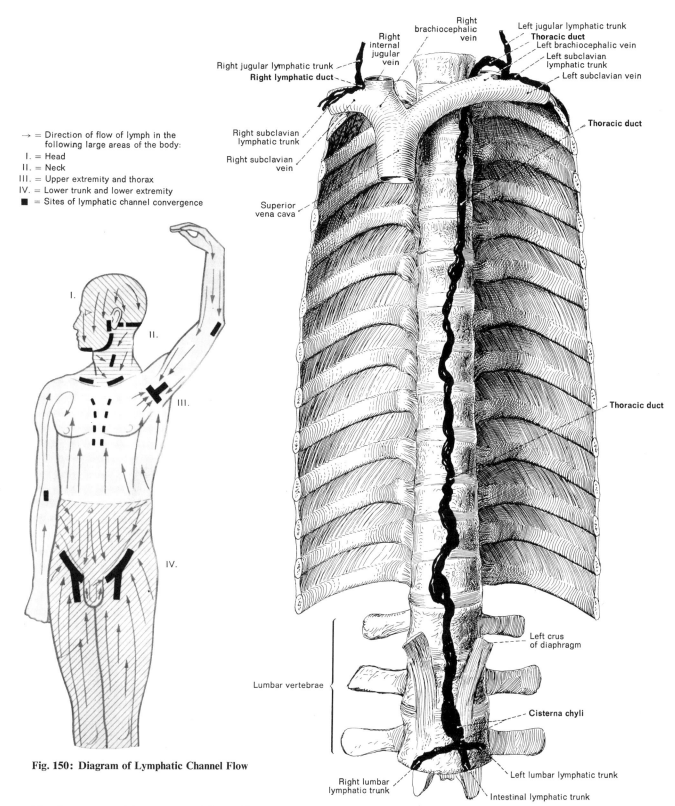

→ = Direction of flow of lymph in the
    following large areas of the body:
I. = Head
II. = Neck
III. = Upper extremity and thorax
IV. = Lower trunk and lower extremity
■ = Sites of lymphatic channel convergence

Fig. 150: Diagram of Lymphatic Channel Flow

Fig. 151: The Thoracic Duct: Its Origin and Course

NOTE: 1) the thoracic duct collects the lymph from most of the body tissues and transmits it back into the blood stream. It originates in the abdomen anterior to the 2nd lumbar vertebra at the cisterna chyli. The duct then ascends into the thorax through the aortic hiatus of the diaphragm slightly to the right of the midline. Within the posterior mediastinum of the thorax and still coursing just ventral to the vertebral column, it gradually crosses the midline to the left. The duct then ascends into the root of the neck on the left side and opens into the left subclavian vein near the junction of the right internal jugular vein.

2) the right lymphatic duct receives lymph from the right side of the head, neck and trunk and from the right upper extremity. It empties into the right subclavian vein.

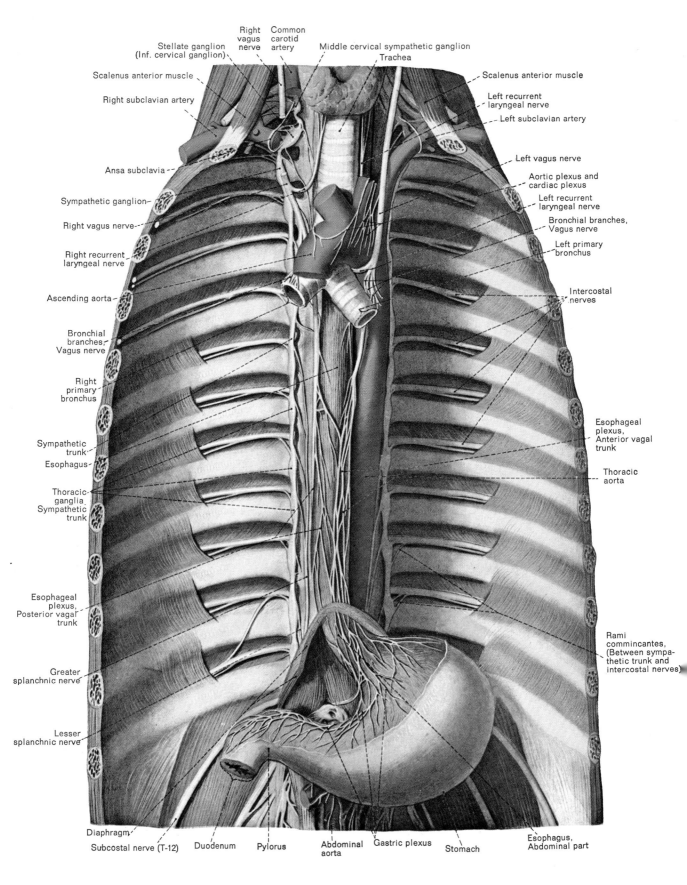

Right vagus nerve
Common carotid artery
Right vagus nerve
Common carotid artery

Stellate ganglion (Inf. cervical ganglion)
Middle cervical sympathetic ganglion
Trachea

Scalenus anterior muscle
Scalenus anterior muscle

Right subclavian artery
Left recurrent laryngeal nerve

Left subclavian artery

Ansa subclavia
Left vagus nerve

Aortic plexus and cardiac plexus

Sympathetic ganglion
Left recurrent laryngeal nerve

Right vagus nerve
Bronchial branches, Vagus nerve

Left primary bronchus

Right recurrent laryngeal nerve

Ascending aorta
Intercostal nerves

Bronchial branches, Vagus nerve

Right primary bronchus

Esophageal plexus, Anterior vagal trunk

Sympathetic trunk
Thoracic aorta

Esophagus

Thoracic ganglia, Sympathetic trunk

Esophageal plexus, Posterior vagal trunk
Rami commincantes, (Between sympathetic trunk and intercostal nerves)

Greater splanchnic nerve

Lesser splanchnic nerve

Diaphragm
Subcostal nerve (T-12)
Duodenum
Pylorus
Abdominal aorta
Gastric plexus
Stomach
Esophagus, Abdominal part

Fig. 152: The Sympathetic Trunks and Vagus Nerves in the Thorax and Upper Abdomen

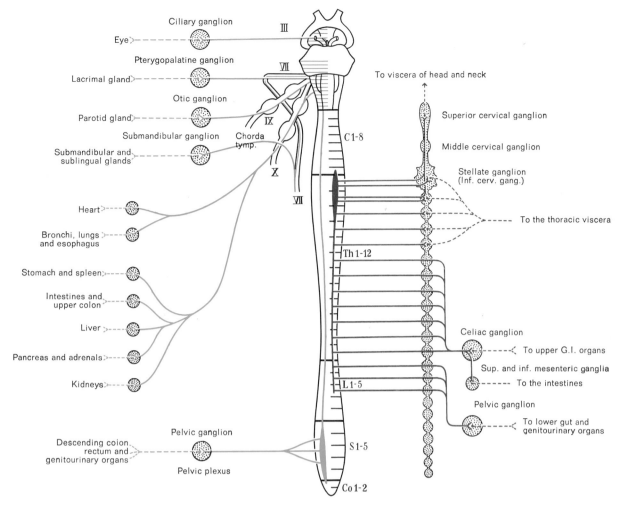

Fig. 153: Diagram of the Autonomic Nervous System. Blue = parasympathetic; red = sympathetic; solid lines = presynaptic neurons; broken lines = postsynaptic neurons.

NOTE: 1) the autonomic nervous system, by definition, is a two motor neuron system with the neuron cell bodies of the *presynaptic neurons* (solid lines) somewhere within the central nervous system, and the cell bodies of the *postsynaptic neurons* (broken lines) located in ganglia distributed peripherally in the body.

2) the autonomic nervous system is comprised of the nerve fibers which supply all the glands and blood vessels of the body including the heart. In so doing, all the smooth and cardiac muscle tissues (sometimes called involuntary muscles) are thereby innervated.

3) the autonomic nervous system is composed of two major divisions called the parasympathetic (in blue) and sympathetic (in red) divisions. The autonomic regulation of visceral function is, therefore, a dualistic control, i.e., most organs receive postganglionic fibers of both parasympathetic and sympathetic source.

4) the *parasympathetic division* is sometimes called a craniosacral outflow because the preganglionic cell bodies of this division lie in the brainstem and in the sacral segments of the spinal cord. Parasympathetic preganglionic fibers are found in four cranial nerves, III (oculomotor), VII (facial), IX (glossopharyngeal) and X (vagus) and in the 2nd, 3rd and 4th sacral nerves.

5) these *pre*ganglionic parasympathetic fibers then synapse with *post*ganglionic parasympathetic cell bodies in peripheral ganglia. From these ganglia the *post*ganglionic nerve fibers innervate the various organs.

6) the *sympathetic division* is sometimes called the thoracolumbar outflow because the *pre*ganglionic sympathetic neuron cell bodies are located in the lateral horn of the spinal cord between the 1st thoracic spinal segment and the 2nd or 3rd lumbar spinal segment, (i.e., from T-1 to L-3).

7) these *pre*ganglionic fibers emerge from the cord with their corresponding spinal roots and communicate with the sympathetic trunk and its ganglia where some *pre*synaptic sympathetic fibers synapse with *post*ganglionic sympathetic neurons. Other presynaptic fibers (especially those of the upper thoracic segments) ascend in the sympathetic chain and synapse with *post*ganglionic neurons in the inferior, middle and superior cervical ganglia. *Post*ganglionic fibers from these latter ganglia are then distributed to the viscera of the head and neck. Still other *pre*synaptic sympathetic fibers do not synapse in the sympathetic chain of ganglia at all, but collect to form the splanchnic nerves. These nerves course to the collateral sympathetic ganglia (celiac, superior and inferior mesenteric and pelvic ganglia) where synapse with the *post*ganglionic neuron occurs. The *post*ganglionic neurons of the sympathetic division then course to the viscera to supply sympathetic innervation.

8) the functions of the parasympathetic and sympathetic divisions of the autonomic nervous system are antagonistic to each other. The parasympathetic division constricts the pupil, decelerates the heart, lowers blood pressure, relaxes the sphincters of the gut and contracts the longitudinal musculature of the hollow organs. It is the division which is active during periods of calm and tranquility and aids in digestion and absorption. In contrast, the *sympathetic division* dilates the pupil, accelerates the heart, increases blood pressure, contracts the sphincters of the gut and relaxes the longitudinal musculature of hollow organs. It is active when the organism is challenged. It prepares for fight and flight and generally comes to the individual's defense during periods of stress and adversity.

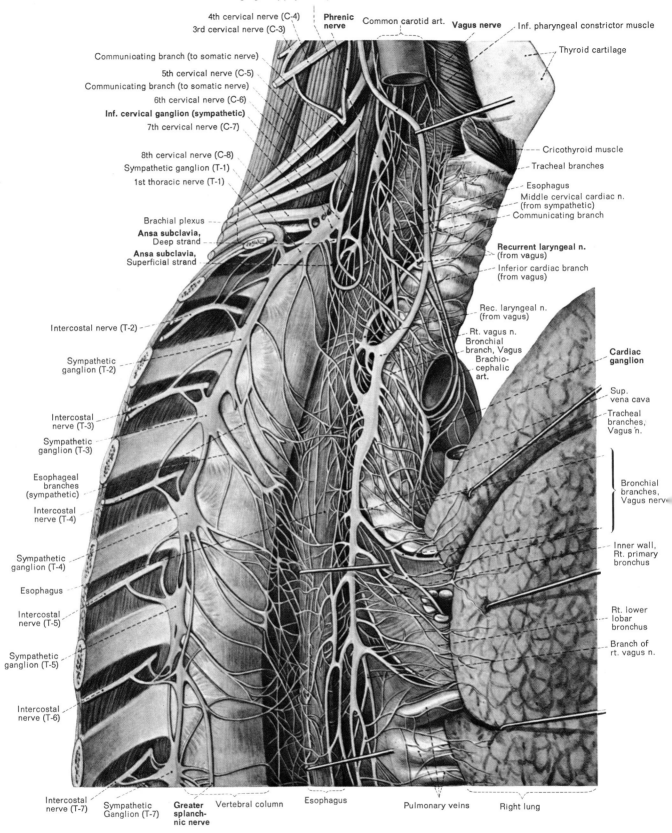

Middle cervical ganglion (sympathetic)

4th cervical nerve (C-4) — **Phrenic** — Common carotid art. — **Vagus nerve** — Inf. pharyngeal constrictor muscle
3rd cervical nerve (C-3) — **nerve**

Communicating branch (to somatic nerve) — Thyroid cartilage

5th cervical nerve (C-5)
Communicating branch (to somatic nerve)
6th cervical nerve (C-6)
Inf. cervical ganglion (sympathetic)
7th cervical nerve (C-7)

Cricothyroid muscle
Tracheal branches

8th cervical nerve (C-8)
Sympathetic ganglion (T-1)
1st thoracic nerve (T-1)

Esophagus
Middle cervical cardiac n. (from sympathetic)
Communicating branch

Brachial plexus
Ansa subclavia, Deep strand
Ansa subclavia, Superficial strand

Recurrent laryngeal n. (from vagus)
Inferior cardiac branch (from vagus)

Rec. laryngeal n. (from vagus)

Intercostal nerve (T-2)

Rt. vagus n. Bronchial branch, Vagus Brachio-cephalic art.

Cardiac ganglion

Sympathetic ganglion (T-2)

Sup. vena cava
Tracheal branches, Vagus n.

Intercostal nerve (T-3)

Sympathetic ganglion (T-3)

Bronchial branches, Vagus nerve

Esophageal branches (sympathetic)

Intercostal nerve (T-4)

Inner wall, Rt. primary bronchus

Sympathetic ganglion (T-4)

Esophagus

Rt. lower lobar bronchus

Intercostal nerve (T-5)

Branch of rt. vagus n.

Sympathetic ganglion (T-5)

Intercostal nerve (T-6)

Intercostal nerve (T-7)   Sympathetic Ganglion (T-7)   **Greater splanch-nic nerve**   Vertebral column   Esophagus   Pulmonary veins   Right lung

Fig. 154: The Cervical and Upper Thoracic Distribution of Autonomic Nerves

NOTE: the organs of the posterior mediastinum are viewed from the right side by pulling the lungs forward and removing certain of the organs. Observe the two major descending nerve trunks and their associated complexes: the right vagus nerve situated more anteriorly and the right sympathetic trunk descending more posteriorly in the thorax adjacent to the costo-vertebral joints.

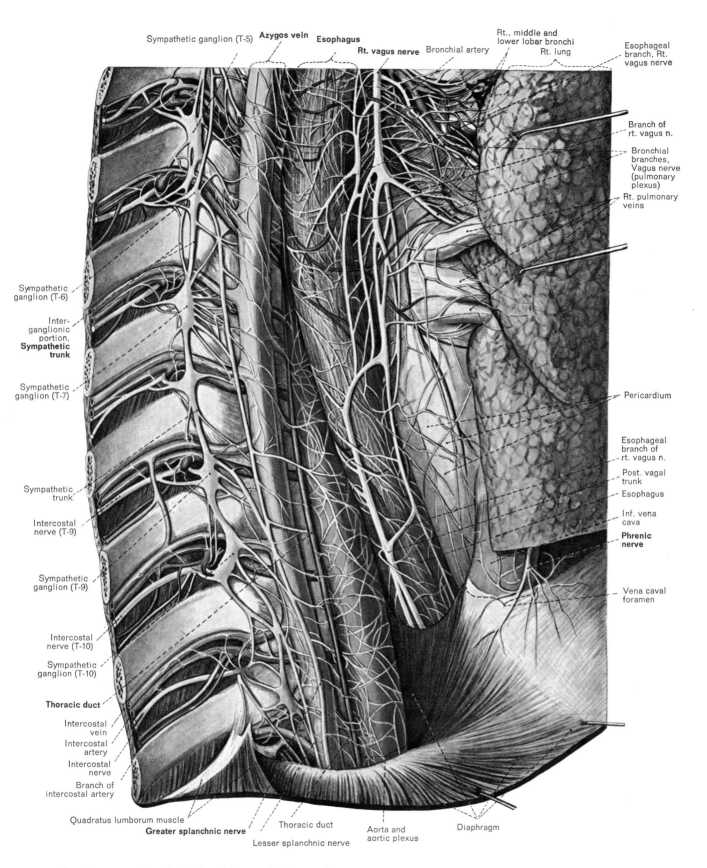

Esophageal branch, Rt. vagus nerve

Sympathetic ganglion (T-5)   Azygos vein   Esophagus
Rt. vagus nerve   Bronchial artery   Rt., middle and lower lobar bronchi   Rt. lung

Branch of rt. vagus n.

Bronchial branches, Vagus nerve (pulmonary plexus)

Rt. pulmonary veins

Sympathetic ganglion (T-6)

Inter-ganglionic portion, **Sympathetic trunk**

Sympathetic ganglion (T-7)

Pericardium

Esophageal branch of rt. vagus n.

Post. vagal trunk

Sympathetic trunk

Esophagus

Intercostal nerve (T-9)

Inf. vena cava

Phrenic nerve

Sympathetic ganglion (T-9)

Intercostal nerve (T-10)

Vena caval foramen

Sympathetic ganglion (T-10)

Thoracic duct

Intercostal vein

Intercostal artery

Intercostal nerve

Branch of intercostal artery

Quadratus lumborum muscle   **Greater splanchnic nerve**   Thoracic duct   Aorta and aortic plexus   Diaphragm
Lesser splanchnic nerve

Fig. 155: Lower Thoracic Portion of Autonomic Nervous System

NOTE: 1) the formation of the greater and lesser splanchnic nerves. The greater splanchnic nerve is derived from preganglionic sympathetic fibers which emerge from sympathetic ganglia T-6 to T-9 or T-10, whereas the lesser splanchnic nerve is derived from ganglia T-10 and T-11.

2) the right vagus nerve after contributing parasympathetic fibers to the esophageal plexus becomes the posterior vagal trunk dorsal to the esophagus as that organ passes through the diaphragm.

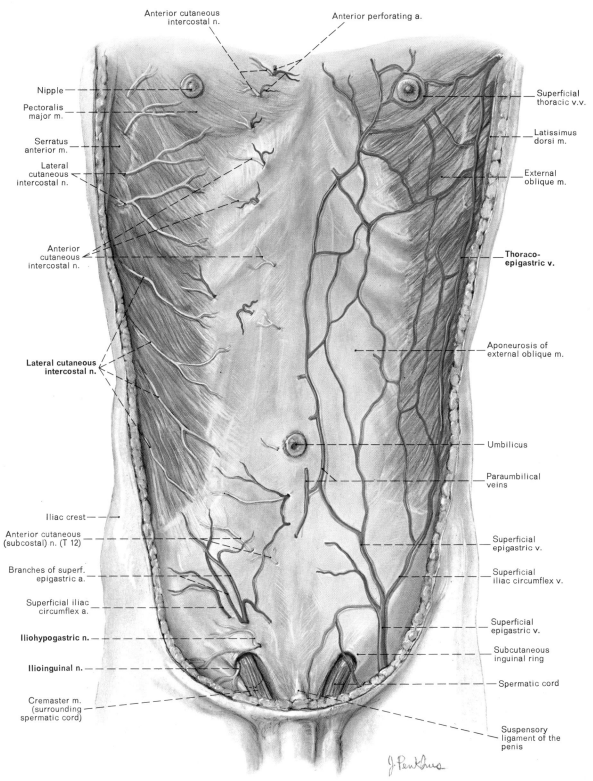

Anterior cutaneous
intercostal n.

Anterior perforating a.

Nipple

Pectoralis
major m.

Serratus
anterior m.

Lateral
cutaneous
intercostal n.

Anterior
cutaneous
intercostal n.

Lateral cutaneous
intercostal n.

Iliac crest

Anterior cutaneous
(subcostal) n. (T 12)

Branches of superf.
epigastric a.

Superficial iliac
circumflex a.

Iliohypogastric n.

Ilioinguinal n.

Cremaster m.
(surrounding
spermatic cord)

Superficial
thoracic v.v.

Latissimus
dorsi m.

External
oblique m.

Thoraco-
epigastric v.

Aponeurosis of
external oblique m.

Umbilicus

Paraumbilical
veins

Superficial
epigastric v.

Superficial
iliac circumflex v.

Superficial
epigastric v.

Subcutaneous
inguinal ring

Spermatic cord

Suspensory
ligament of the
penis

J. Penkhus

Fig. 156: Superficial Nerves and Vessels of the Anterior Abdominal Wall

NOTE: 1) the distribution of the superficial vessels and cutaneous nerves is demonstrated upon the removal of the skin and superficial fatty layers over the lower thoracic and anterior abdominal wall.

2) the thoracic intercostal nerves supply the abdominal surface with lateral and anterior cutaneous branches.

3) in the inguinal region, the ilioinguinal and iliohypogastric branches of the 1st lumbar nerve become superficial in the region of the superficial inguinal ring.

4) the branches of superficial epigastric artery (which arises from the femoral artery) as they ascend in the inguinal region toward the umbilicus. Note also the superficial branches of the intercostal arteries.

5) the thoracoepigastric vein which serves as a means of communication between the femoral vein and the axillary vein. In cases of obstruction of the portal vein, these superficial veins become greatly enlarged forming varicose veins over the abdominal wall (sometimes this condition is called *caput medusae*).

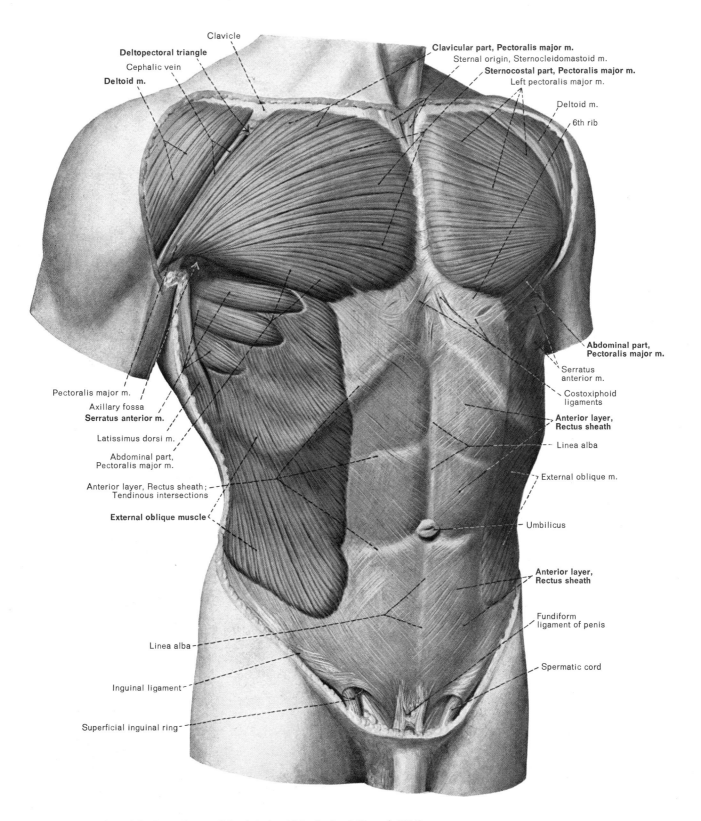

Fig. 157: Superficial Musculature of the Anterior Abdominal and Thoracic Wall

NOTE: 1) the first layer of abdominal musculature consists principally of the external oblique muscle and its broad, flat aponeurosis which extends medially to the midline (forming the anterior layer of the sheath of the rectus abdominis muscle) and inferiorly as the inguinal ligament.

2) the external oblique arises by means of 7 or 8 fleshy slips from the outer surfaces of the lower ribs (ribs 5 to 12), thereby interdigitating with the fleshy origin of the serratus anterior muscle.

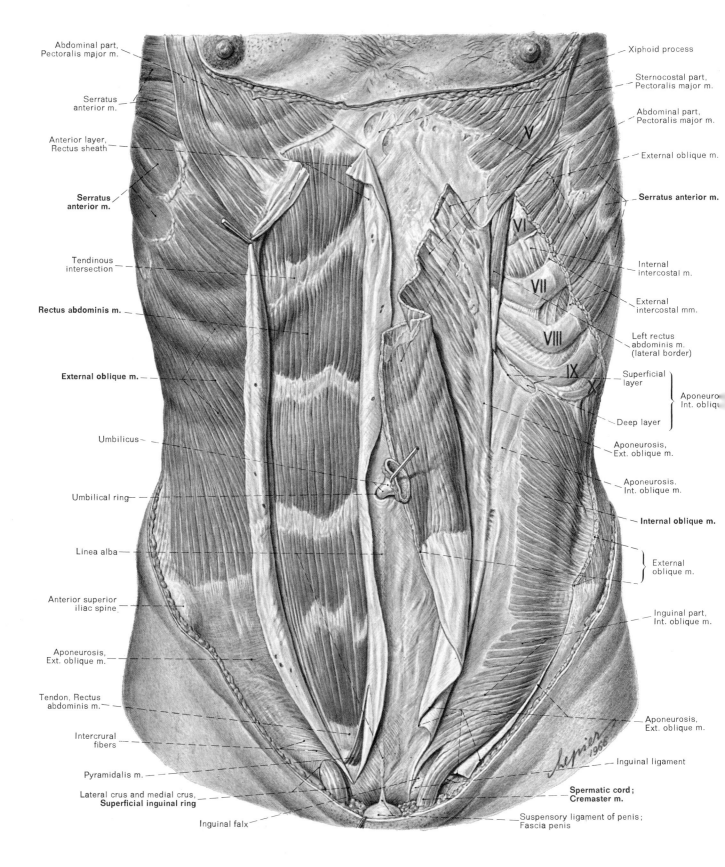

Abdominal part,
Pectoralis major m.

Serratus
anterior m.

Anterior layer,
Rectus sheath

**Serratus
anterior m.**

Tendinous
intersection

Rectus abdominis m.

External oblique m.

Umbilicus

Umbilical ring

Linea alba

Anterior superior
iliac spine

Aponeurosis,
Ext. oblique m.

Tendon, Rectus
abdominis m.

Intercrural
fibers

Pyramidalis m.

Lateral crus and medial crus,
Superficial inguinal ring

Inguinal falx

Xiphoid process

Sternocostal part,
Pectoralis major m.

Abdominal part,
Pectoralis major m.

External oblique m.

Serratus anterior m.

Internal
intercostal m.

External
intercostal mm.

Left rectus
abdominis m.
(lateral border)

Superficial
layer

Aponeuro
Int. obliqu

Deep layer

Aponeurosis,
Ext. oblique m.

Aponeurosis.
Int. oblique m.

Internal oblique m.

External
oblique m.

Inguinal part,
Int. oblique m.

Aponeurosis,
Ext. oblique m.

Inguinal ligament

**Spermatic cord;
Cremaster m.**

Suspensory ligament of penis;
Fascia penis

V

VI

VII

VIII

IX

X

Fig. 158: Anterior Abdominal Wall: Rectus Abdominis and Internal Oblique Muscles

NOTE: 1) the specimen's right rectus sheath has been opened (reader's left) to reveal the right rectus abdominis muscle which is marked by transversely oriented tendinous intersections. On the specimen's left side, the external oblique muscle has been severed to reveal the second muscular layer, the internal oblique muscle. This also reveals ribs 6 through 10.

2) the muscle fibers of the external oblique course inferomedially (or in the same direction as you would put your hands in your side pockets), whereas most of the fibers of the internal oblique course in the opposite direction.

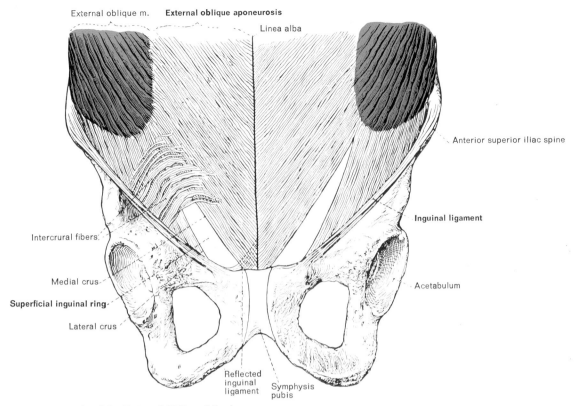

Fig. 159: The Aponeurosis of the External Oblique Muscle

NOTE: 1) the superficial inguinal ring is a triangular slit-like opening in the aponeurosis of the external oblique muscle. Observe how the intercrural fibers would strengthen the lateral aspect of the superficial ring by extending between the medial crus and lateral crus.

2) the inguinal ligament which extends between the anterior superior iliac spine and the pubic tubercle. This ligament is formed by the lowermost fibers of the external oblique aponeurosis and lends support to the inferior portion of the anterior abdominal wall.

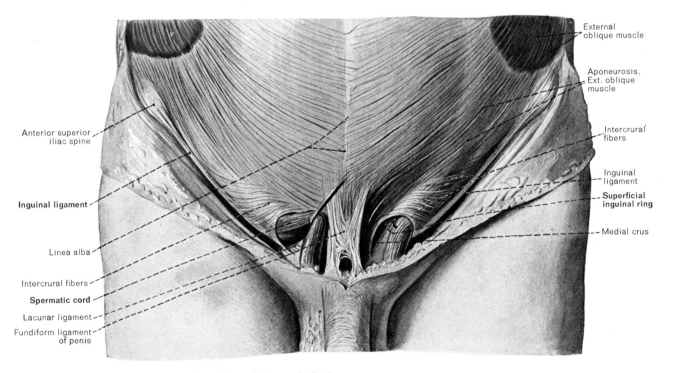

Fig. 160: The Superficial Inguinal Ring and Spermatic Cord

NOTE: 1) the superficial inguinal ring transmits the spermatic cord in the male and the round ligament of the uterus in the female. In this dissection, the right spermatic cord has been lifted in order to show the lateral crus of the inguinal ring.

2) the tendinous fibers of the aponeurosis are continuous with the fleshy fibers of the external oblique. They are directed inferiorly and medially and either decussate or insert into the linea alba.

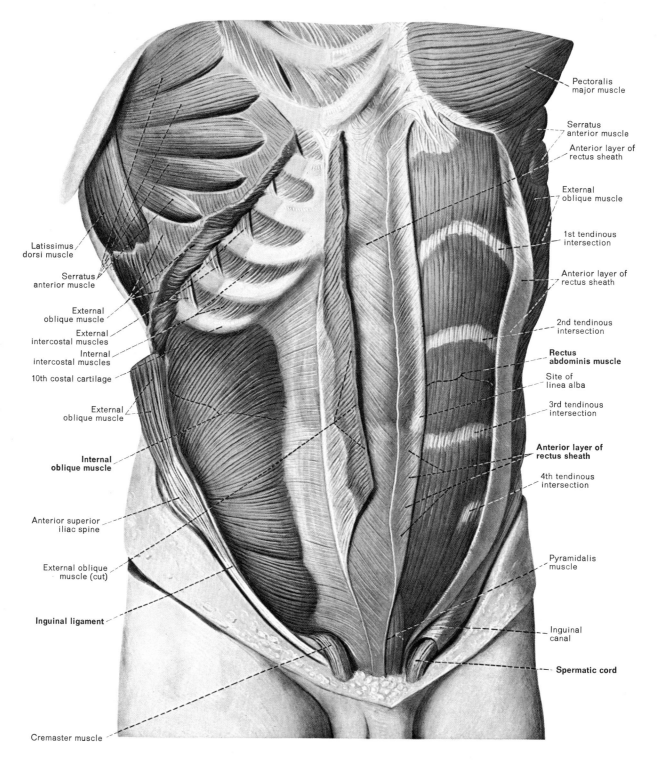

Pectoralis
major muscle

Serratus
anterior muscle

Anterior layer of
rectus sheath

External
oblique muscle

1st tendinous
intersection

Anterior layer of
rectus sheath

2nd tendinous
intersection

**Rectus
abdominis muscle**

Site of
linea alba

3rd tendinous
intersection

**Anterior layer of
rectus sheath**

4th tendinous
intersection

Pyramidalis
muscle

Inguinal
canal

Spermatic cord

Latissimus
dorsi muscle

Serratus
anterior muscle

External
oblique muscle

External
intercostal muscles

Internal
intercostal muscles

10th costal cartilage

External
oblique muscle

**Internal
oblique muscle**

Anterior superior
iliac spine

External oblique
muscle (cut)

Inguinal ligament

Cremaster muscle

Fig. 161: Middle Layer of Abdominal Musculature: Internal Oblique Muscle

NOTE: 1) on the right side, the external oblique muscle has been severed and reflected to expose the right internal oblique muscle. On the left side, the anterior layer of the rectus sheath has been incised longitudinally to expose the left rectus abdominis muscle with its tendinous intersections and the small pyramidalis muscle.

2) the muscle fibers of the internal oblique muscle arise from the inguinal ligament, the iliac crest and the lumbar aponeurosis. They insert into the lower ribs above, and into an aponeurosis which contributes to the formation of the rectus sheath medially. Inferiorly, the aponeurosis of the internal oblique along with the aponeurosis of the transversus abdominis muscle forms the conjoint tendon, which is also known as the inguinal falx (shown, but not labelled). The conjoint tendon inserts into the pubic crest along with the lower end of the rectus sheath, thereby helping to provide strength to the inherently weak inguinal-pubic region.

3) the cremaster muscle. This muscular covering over the outer surface of the spermatic cord in the male represents an extension of the internal oblique (also possibly the transversus abdominis). It originates on the inguinal ligament and, after its fibers loop around the spermatic cord, inserts onto the pubis. Upon contraction this muscle lifts the testis within the scrotum toward the subcutaneous inguinal ring.

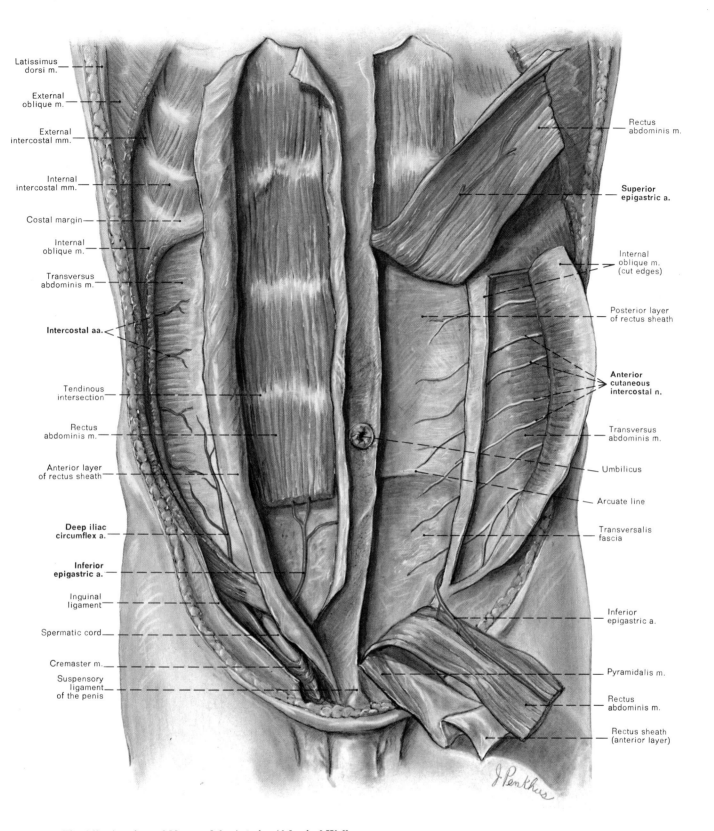

Fig. 162: Arteries and Nerves of the Anterior Abdominal Wall

NOTE: 1) on each side the first two layers of muscle (external oblique and internal oblique muscles) have been removed, since the vessels and nerves supplying the musculature of the anterior abdominal wall course between the internal oblique and transversus abdominis muscles.

2) thoracic nerves T7 to T12 and the 1st lumbar nerve (ilioinguinal and iliohypogastric nn.) supply the anterior abdominal musculature in their segmental course around the body.

3) in addition to segmental branches of the intercostal arteries, deep circumflex iliac artery and the inferior epigastric artery supply the abdominal muscles. This latter artery anastomoses with the superior epigastric artery within the rectus abdominis muscle.

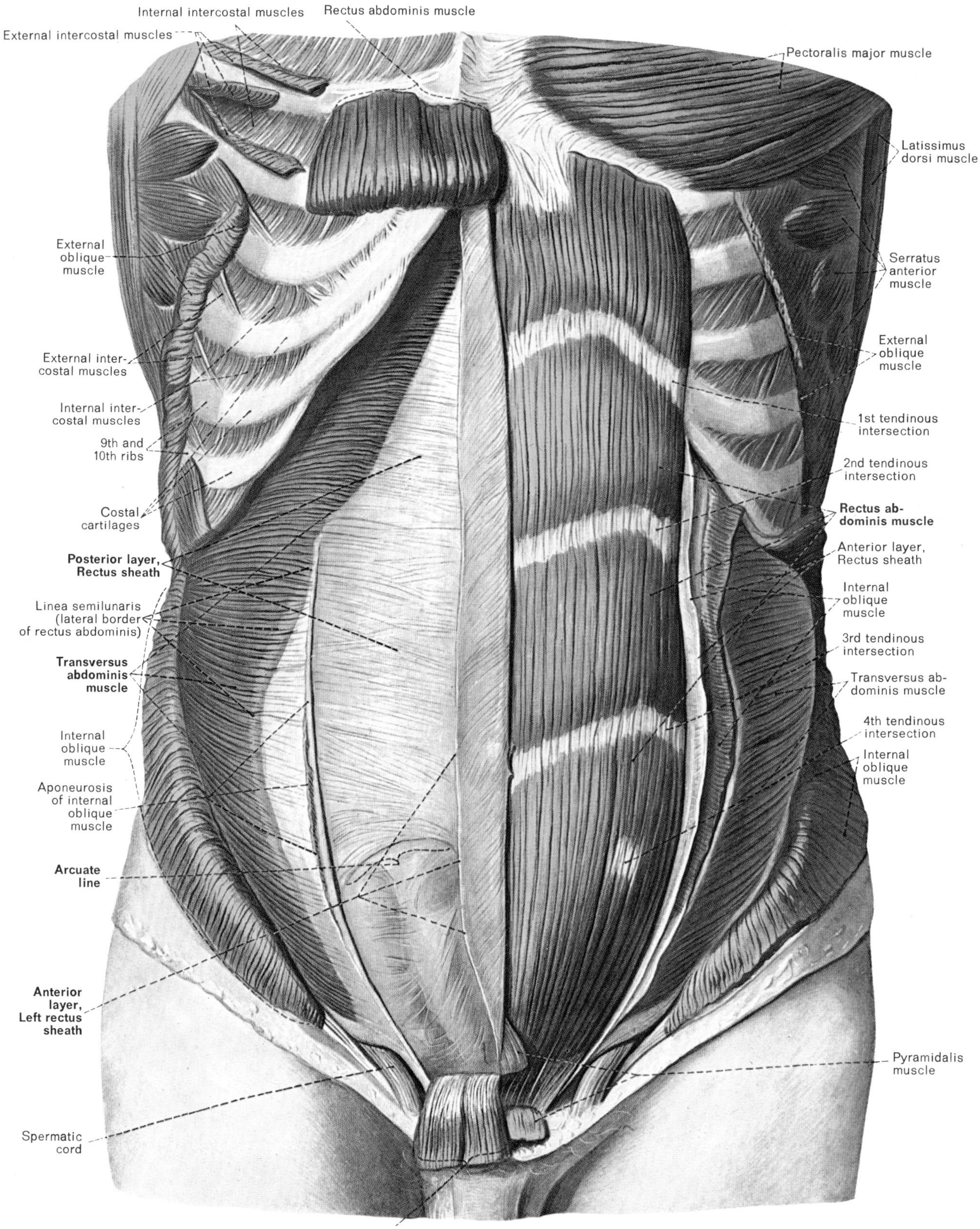

Fig. 163: Deep Layer of Abdominal Musculature: The Transversus Abdominis Muscle

NOTE: 1) on the right, the external and internal oblique and rectus abdominis muscles have been resected demonstrating the transversus abdominis muscle. On the left, the rectus abdominis muscle remains intact but the small pyramidalis muscle was severed to show the insertion of the left rectus.

2) on the right, the posterior layer of the rectus sheath is exposed while on the left, the anterior layer of the sheath has been opened to demonstrate the rectus muscle. Below the arcuate line, the posterior sheath of the rectus abdominis is wanting and the overlying rectus muscle lies directly anterior to the transversalis fascia.

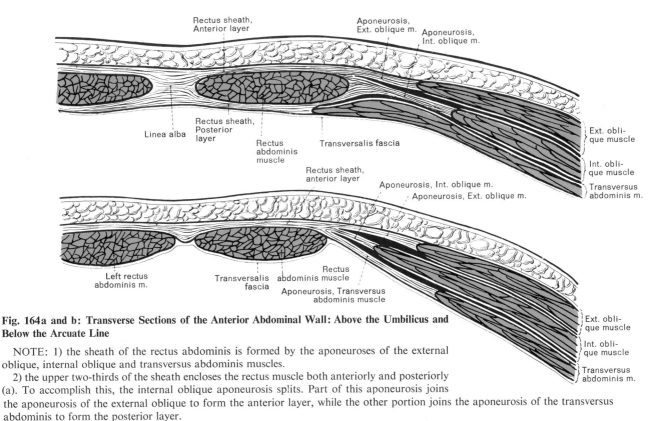

Fig. 164a and b: Transverse Sections of the Anterior Abdominal Wall: Above the Umbilicus and Below the Arcuate Line

NOTE: 1) the sheath of the rectus abdominis is formed by the aponeuroses of the external oblique, internal oblique and transversus abdominis muscles.

2) the upper two-thirds of the sheath encloses the rectus muscle both anteriorly and posteriorly (a). To accomplish this, the internal oblique aponeurosis splits. Part of this aponeurosis joins the aponeurosis of the external oblique to form the anterior layer, while the other portion joins the aponeurosis of the transversus abdominis to form the posterior layer.

3) the lower one-third of the sheath (b), below the arcuate line, is deficient posteriorly since the aponeuroses of all three muscles pass anterior to the rectus abdominis muscle.

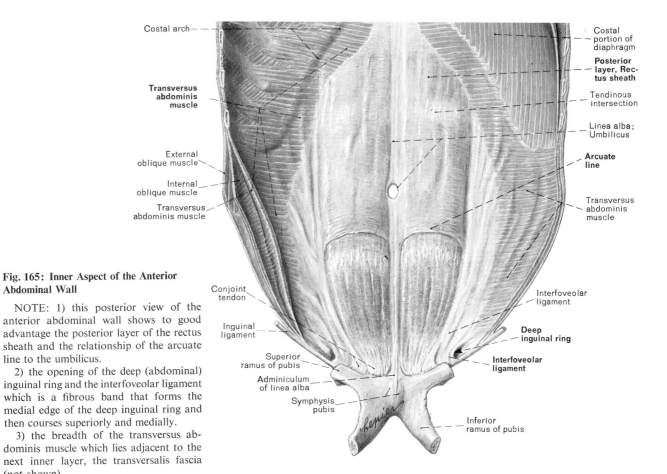

Fig. 165: Inner Aspect of the Anterior Abdominal Wall

NOTE: 1) this posterior view of the anterior abdominal wall shows to good advantage the posterior layer of the rectus sheath and the relationship of the arcuate line to the umbilicus.

2) the opening of the deep (abdominal) inguinal ring and the interfoveolar ligament which is a fibrous band that forms the medial edge of the deep inguinal ring and then courses superiorly and medially.

3) the breadth of the transversus abdominis muscle which lies adjacent to the next inner layer, the transversalis fascia (not shown).

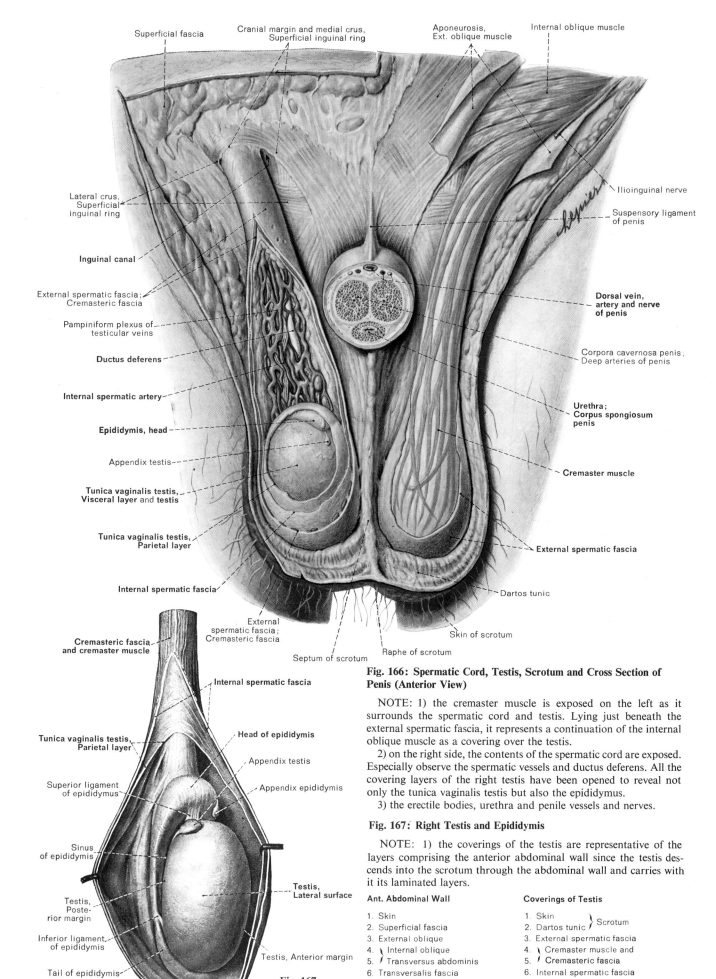

Superficial fascia

Cranial margin and medial crus, Superficial inguinal ring

Aponeurosis, Ext. oblique muscle

Internal oblique muscle

Lateral crus, Superficial inguinal ring

Inguinal canal

External spermatic fascia; Cremasteric fascia

Pampiniform plexus of testicular veins

Ductus deferens

Internal spermatic artery

Epididymis, head

Appendix testis

Tunica vaginalis testis, Visceral layer and testis

Tunica vaginalis testis, Parietal layer

Internal spermatic fascia

Ilioinguinal nerve

Suspensory ligament of penis

Dorsal vein, artery and nerve of penis

Corpora cavernosa penis; Deep arteries of penis

Urethra; Corpus spongiosum penis

Cremaster muscle

External spermatic fascia

Dartos tunic

Skin of scrotum

External spermatic fascia; Cremasteric fascia

Septum of scrotum

Raphe of scrotum

Cremasteric fascia and cremaster muscle

Internal spermatic fascia

Tunica vaginalis testis, Parietal layer

Head of epididymis

Appendix testis

Superior ligament of epididymus

Appendix epididymis

Sinus of epididymis

Testis, Lateral surface

Testis, Posterior margin

Inferior ligament of epididymis

Tail of epididymis

Testis, Anterior margin

Fig. 167

Fig. 166: Spermatic Cord, Testis, Scrotum and Cross Section of Penis (Anterior View)

NOTE: 1) the cremaster muscle is exposed on the left as it surrounds the spermatic cord and testis. Lying just beneath the external spermatic fascia, it represents a continuation of the internal oblique muscle as a covering over the testis.

2) on the right side, the contents of the spermatic cord are exposed. Especially observe the spermatic vessels and ductus deferens. All the covering layers of the right testis have been opened to reveal not only the tunica vaginalis testis but also the epididymus.

3) the erectile bodies, urethra and penile vessels and nerves.

Fig. 167: Right Testis and Epididymis

NOTE: 1) the coverings of the testis are representative of the layers comprising the anterior abdominal wall since the testis descends into the scrotum through the abdominal wall and carries with it its laminated layers.

Ant. Abdominal Wall	Coverings of Testis
1. Skin	1. Skin
2. Superficial fascia	2. Dartos tunic } Scrotum
3. External oblique	3. External spermatic fascia
4. \ Internal oblique	4. \ Cremaster muscle and
5. / Transversus abdominis	5. / Cremasteric fascia
6. Transversalis fascia	6. Internal spermatic fascia
7. Extraperitoneal fat	7. Fatty layer
8. Peritoneum	8. Processus vaginalis

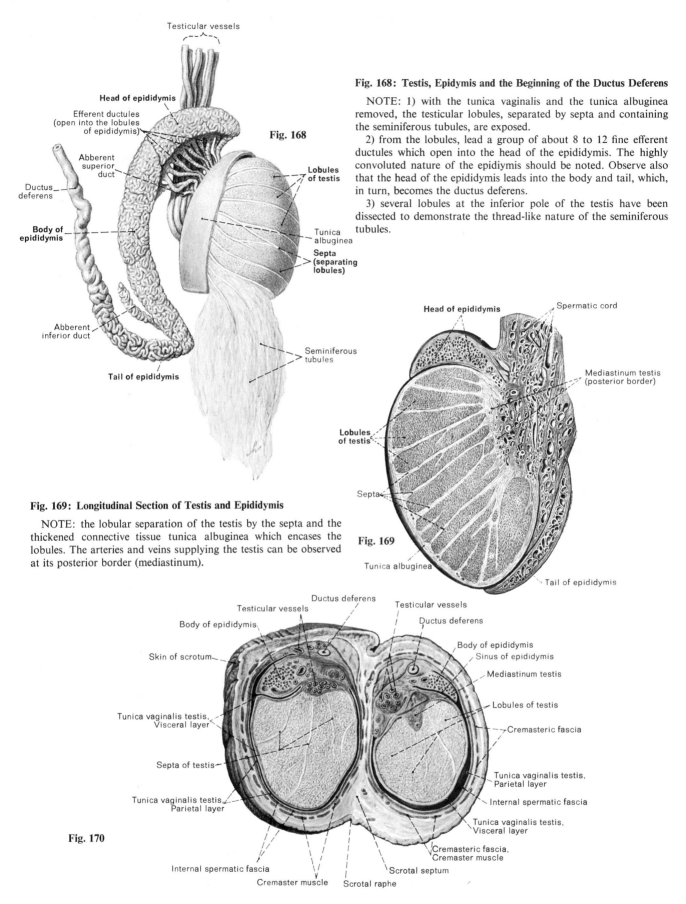

Fig. 168: Testis, Epidymis and the Beginning of the Ductus Deferens

NOTE: 1) with the tunica vaginalis and the tunica albuginea removed, the testicular lobules, separated by septa and containing the seminiferous tubules, are exposed.

2) from the lobules, lead a group of about 8 to 12 fine efferent ductules which open into the head of the epididymis. The highly convoluted nature of the epidiymis should be noted. Observe also that the head of the epididymis leads into the body and tail, which, in turn, becomes the ductus deferens.

3) several lobules at the inferior pole of the testis have been dissected to demonstrate the thread-like nature of the seminiferous tubules.

Fig. 169: Longitudinal Section of Testis and Epididymis

NOTE: the lobular separation of the testis by the septa and the thickened connective tissue tunica albuginea which encases the lobules. The arteries and veins supplying the testis can be observed at its posterior border (mediastinum).

Fig. 170: Cross Section of Testis and Scrotum

NOTE: the scrotum is divided by the median raphe and septum into two lateral compartments, each surrounding an ovoid-shaped testis which is suspended in the scrotal sac by the spermatic cord.

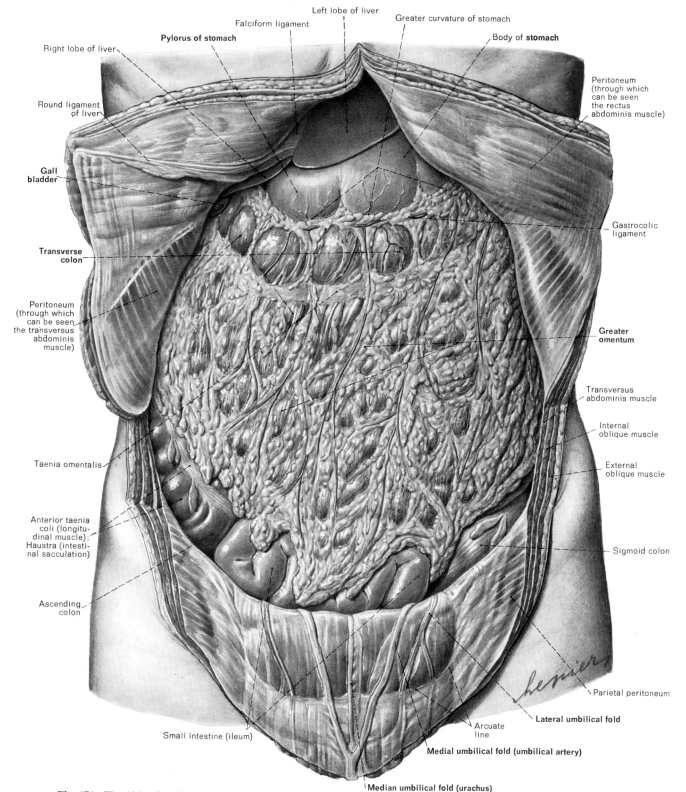

Right lobe of liver

Round ligament
of liver

**Gall
bladder**

**Transverse
colon**

Peritoneum
(through which
can be seen
the transversus
abdominis
muscle)

Taenia omentalis

Anterior taenia
coli (longitu-
dinal muscle);
Haustra (intesti-
nal sacculation)

Ascending
colon

Small intestine (ileum)

Pylorus of stomach

Falciform ligament

Left lobe of liver

Greater curvature of stomach

Body of **stomach**

Peritoneum
(through which
can be seen
the rectus
abdominis muscle)

Gastrocolic
ligament

**Greater
omentum**

Transversus
abdominis muscle

Internal
oblique muscle

External
oblique muscle

Sigmoid colon

Parietal peritoneum

Lateral umbilical fold

Arcuate
line

Medial umbilical fold (umbilical artery)

Median umbilical fold (urachus)

Fig. 171: The Abdominal Cavity (1), the Viscera Left Intact

NOTE: 1) the greater omentum which attaches along the greater curvature of the stomach, covers most of the intestines like an apron, and extends inferiorly almost as far as the pelvis.

2) the falciform ligament and round ligament of the liver (ligamentum teres). The falciform ligament is a remnant of the ventral mesogastrium. It extends between the liver and the anterior wall and separates the left and right lobes of the liver. The round ligament is the remains of the obliterated umbilical vein.

3) on the inner surface of the anterior wall identify

a) *the median umbilical fold* = the remains of the urachus, which in the fetus extends between the bladder and the umbilicus.

b) *the medial umbilical folds* = the obliterated umbilical arteries, which, before birth, coursed from the common iliac arteries to the umbilicus.

c) *the lateral umbilical folds* = which represent a reflection of peritoneum over the inferior epigastric vessels.

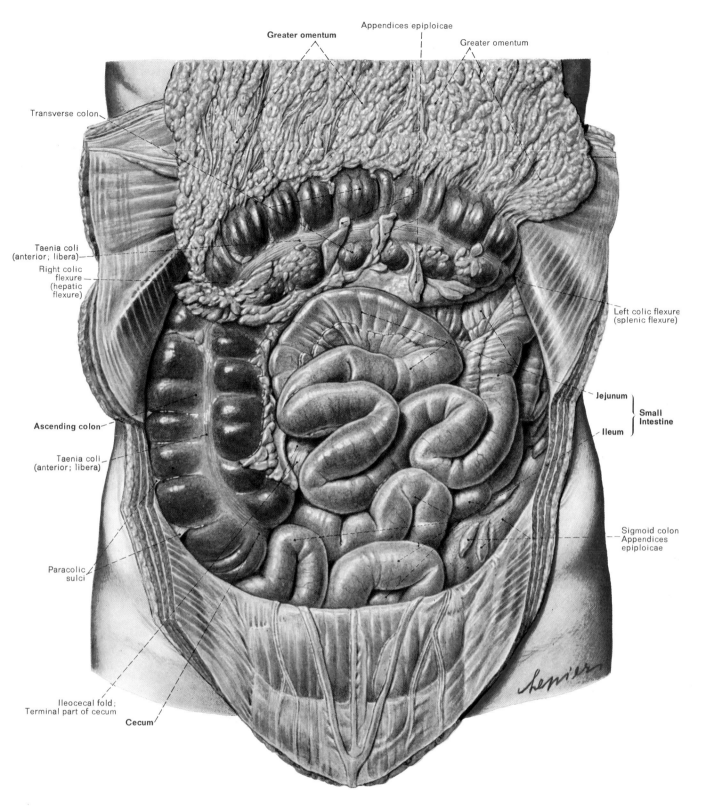

Greater omentum

Appendices epiploicae

Greater omentum

Transverse colon

Taenia coli
(anterior; libera)

Right colic
flexure
(hepatic
flexure)

Left colic flexure
(splenic flexure)

Jejunum

Small
Intestine

Ileum

Ascending colon

Taenia coli
(anterior; libera)

Sigmoid colon
Appendices
epiploicae

Paracolic
sulci

Ileocecal fold;
Terminal part of cecum

Cecum

Fig. 172: The Abdominal Cavity (2), the Ascending Colon and the Transverse Colon and its Mesocolon

NOTE: 1) with the greater omentum reflected superiorly, the transverse colon comes into view as it crosses the abdominal cavity from right to left in continuity with the ascending colon on the right and the descending colon (not shown in this figure; see Figs. 206 and 207) on the left. Observe the longitudinal muscles (taeniae) along the outer surface of the colon. Since these muscles are shorter than the other coats of the large intestine, they cause sacculations which are called haustrae.

2) that small, smooth irregular fatty masses called appendices epiploicae are suspended from the large intestine, thereby assisting in its identification.

3) below the mesocolon (inframesocolic) can be seen the small intestine which consists of three portions, the duodenum (see Figs. 195–197), jejunum and ileum. The outer walls of the small intestine are smooth and glistening and are not sacculated.

4) the small intestine measures about 22 feet in length, commencing at the pyloric end of the stomach and terminating at the ileocecal junction which marks the commencement of the large intestine.

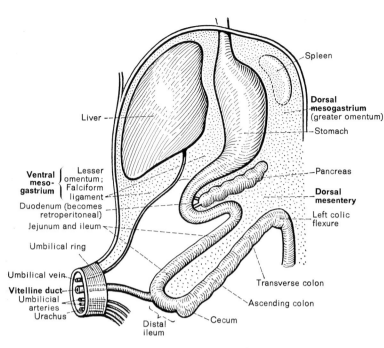

Liver

Ventral meso-gastrium { Lesser omentum; Falciform ligament

Duodenum (becomes retroperitoneal)

Jejunum and ileum

Umbilical ring

Umbilical vein

Vitelline duct
Umbilical arteries
Urachus

Distal ileum

Cecum

Spleen

Dorsal mesogastrium (greater omentum)

Stomach

Pancreas

Dorsal mesentery

Left colic flexure

Transverse colon

Ascending colon

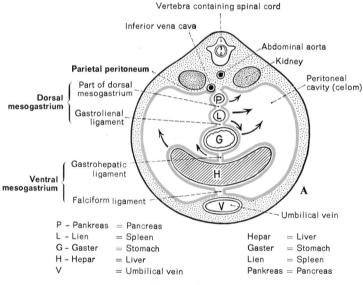

Vertebra containing spinal cord

Inferior vena cava

Parietal peritoneum

Dorsal mesogastrium { Part of dorsal mesogastrium | Gastrolienal ligament

Ventral mesogastrium { Gastrohepatic ligament | Falciform ligament

Abdominal aorta

Kidney

Peritoneal cavity (celom)

Umbilical vein

A

P – Pankreas = Pancreas
L – Lien = Spleen
G – Gaster = Stomach
H – Hepar = Liver
V = Umbilical vein

Hepar = Liver
Gaster = Stomach
Lien = Spleen
Pankreas = Pancreas

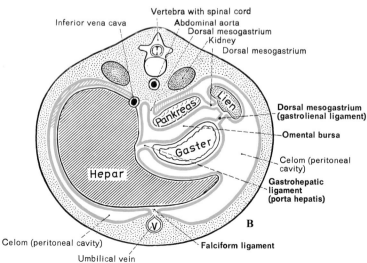

Vertebra with spinal cord

Inferior vena cava

Abdominal aorta
Dorsal mesogastrium
Kidney
Dorsal mesogastrium

Pankreas

Lien

Gaster

Hepar

Dorsal mesogastrium (gastrolienal ligament)

Omental bursa

Celom (peritoneal cavity)

Gastrohepatic ligament (porta hepatis)

B

Celom (peritoneal cavity)

Falciform ligament

Umbilical vein

Fig. 173: The Developing Gastrointestinal Organs and their Mesenteries

NOTE: 1) as the primitive gastrointestinal tube develops within the abdominal celom, it is suspended to the body wall by primitive peritoneal reflections, both ventrally and dorsally. The early peritoneal attachments to the expanding stomach are called the ventral mesogastrium and dorsal mesogastrium, while the dorsal mesentery develops on the posterior aspect of the primitive small and large intestine.

2) the embryonic liver develops into the ventral mesogastrium, thereby dividing this ventral peritoneal attachment into:

a) a portion between the anterior body wall and the liver which eventually becomes the falciform ligament, and

b) a portion between the liver and the stomach which becomes the lesser omentum.

3) on the dorsal aspect:

a) the pancreas develops in relation to the primitive duodenum, both of which lose their mesenteries during gut rotation to become retroperitoneal;

b) the dorsal mesogastrium, attaching along the greater curvature of the stomach and rotating with the stomach, becomes the greater omentum. This eventually encases the transverse colon;

c) the dorsal mesentery remains attached to the small intestine while the ascending and descending colon become displaced to the right and left side respectively, becoming adherent to the posterior body wall;

d) the sigmoid colon usually retains its mesentery while that of the rectum becomes obliterated.

4) near the cecal end of the small intestine the developing G.I. canal communicates with the vitelline duct. After birth, this duct usually becomes resorbed; when it persists (2% of cases), it results in a diverticulum of the ileum called Meckel's diverticulum.

Cross Sectional Diagram of Development of Mesogastria
Fig. 174A: Early Stage (about six weeks)

NOTE: 1) the primitive peritoneal reflections are indicated in red. The arrows show the direction of growth and, therefore, of movement by the various organs to achieve the positions shown in Fig. 174B.

2) at this early stage, the peritoneum completely surrounds the organs in the upper abdominal region (visceral petitoneum) and attaches peripherally to the body wall (parietal peritoneum). Attaching along the posterior border of the stomach, the dorsal mesogastrium then surrounds the spleen and pancreas. Anterior to the stomach, the liver becomes interposed between the stomach and the anterior body wall. This forms the gastrohepatic ligament (also called lesser omentum) between the lesser curvature of the stomach and the liver, and the falciform ligament between the liver and the anterior body wall.

Cross Sectional Diagram of Development of Mesogastria
Fig. 174B: Late Fetal Stage

NOTE: 1) with the rotation of the organs (in the direction of the arrows in Fig. 174A), the liver grows into the celomic cavity toward the right and contacts the inferior vena cava while the stomach rotates such that its dorsal mesogastrium (greater curvature) is shifted to the left. The pancreas and spleen still retain their position posterior to the stomach.

2) the reflection of dorsal mesogastrium between the stomach and spleen becomes established as the gastrolienal ligament while one layer of mesogastrium surrounding the pancreas (and duodenum) fuses to the posterior body wall. This latter development fixates these two organs with a layer of peritoneum on their anterior surface, causing them to become retroperitoneal. The omental bursa also develops posterior to the stomach and anterior to the pancreas.

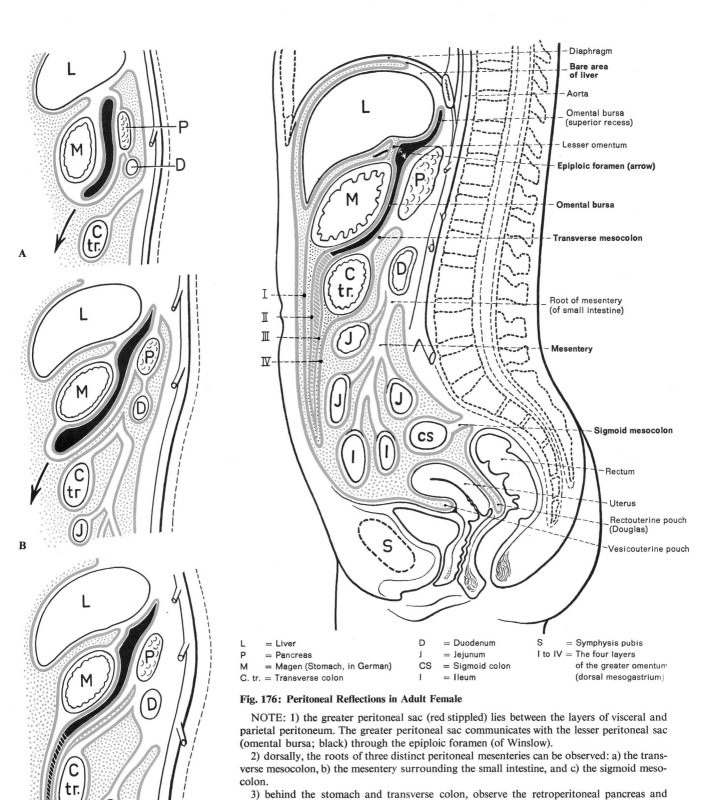

Fig. 176: Peritoneal Reflections in Adult Female

L	= Liver	D	= Duodenum	S	= Symphysis pubis
P	= Pancreas	J	= Jejunum	I to IV	= The four layers
M	= Magen (Stomach, in German)	CS	= Sigmoid colon		of the greater omentum
C. tr.	= Transverse colon	I	= Ileum		(dorsal mesogastrium)

NOTE: 1) the greater peritoneal sac (red stippled) lies between the layers of visceral and parietal peritoneum. The greater peritoneal sac communicates with the lesser peritoneal sac (omental bursa; black) through the epiploic foramen (of Winslow).

2) dorsally, the roots of three distinct peritoneal mesenteries can be observed: a) the transverse mesocolon, b) the mesentery surrounding the small intestine, and c) the sigmoid mesocolon.

3) behind the stomach and transverse colon, observe the retroperitoneal pancreas and duodenum. Note also that a portion of the liver is not surrounded by peritoneum (bare area of the liver) and lies adjacent to the diaphragm.

Fig. 175 A, B, & C: Stages in the Development of the Omental Bursa (Sagittal Diagrams)

NOTE: 1) at four weeks the dorsal border of the stomach (Magen, M) grows faster than the ventral border assisting in rotation of the stomach on its long axis. The greater curvature and its dorsal mesogastrium becomes directed to the left while the lesser curvature and the ventral mesogastrium is directed to the right.

2) by eight weeks (Fig. 175 A) the omental bursa (black) forms behind the stomach between the two leaves of dorsal mesogastrium. The pancreas and duodenum are still surrounded by dorsal mesentery. As gut rotation continues the dorsal mesogastrium extends inferiorly (Fig. 175 B, arrow) to form the greater omentum which becomes a double reflection (4 leaves) of the dorsal mesogastrium "trapping" the cavity of the omental bursa between the 2nd and 3rd leaves.

3) continued development (Fig. 175 C) results in a further descent of the greater omentum over the abdominal viscera and a fusion (cross-hatched) of the 2nd and 3rd leaves inferiorly.

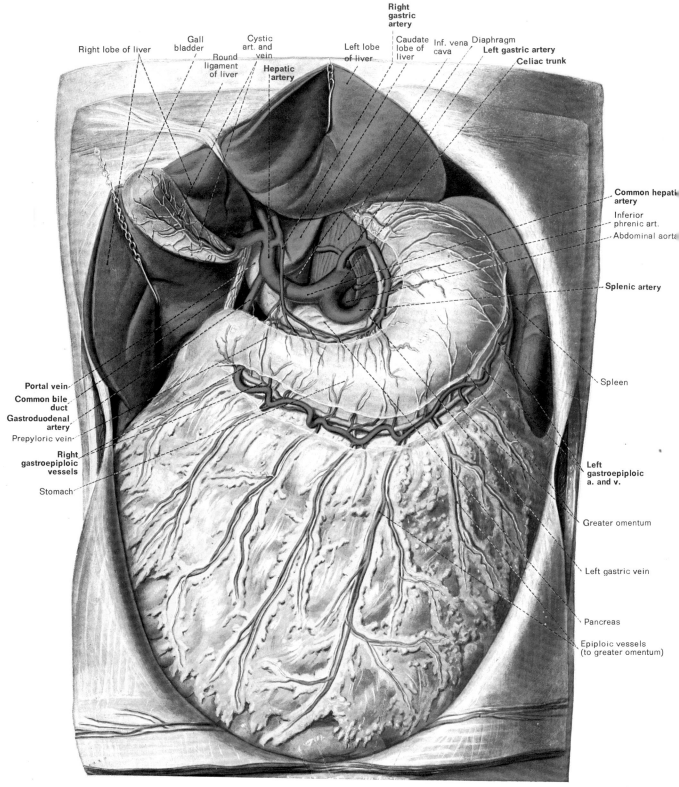

Right lobe of liver — Gall bladder — Cystic art. and vein — Round ligament of liver — Hepatic artery — Left lobe of liver — Right gastric artery — Caudate lobe of liver — Inf. vena cava — Diaphragm — Left gastric artery — Celiac trunk

Common hepatic artery
Inferior phrenic art.
Abdominal aorta

Splenic artery

Spleen

Portal vein
Common bile duct
Gastroduodenal artery
Prepyloric vein
Right gastroepiploic vessels
Stomach

Left gastroepiploic a. and v.

Greater omentum

Left gastric vein

Pancreas

Epiploic vessels (to greater omentum)

Fig. 177: The Abdominal Cavity (3): The Celiac Trunk and its Branches

NOTE: 1) the right and left lobes of the liver have been elevated and the lesser omentum has been removed between the lesser curvature of the stomach and the liver to reveal the celiac trunk and its branches and three major structures at the porta hepatis, the hepatic artery, portal vein and common bile duct.

2) the celiac trunk lies anterior to the 12th thoracic vertebra and almost immediately divides into the left gastric artery, and the hepatic and splenic arteries:

a) the left gastric artery courses along the lesser curvature of the stomach and anastomoses with the right gastric branch of the hepatic artery;

b) the hepatic artery courses to the right and gives off the gastroduodenal artery before dividing to enter the lobes of the liver;

c) the splenic artery courses to the left toward the hilum of the spleen;

d) the gastroduodenal artery gives rise to the right gastroepiploic artery which follows along the greater curvature of the stomach to anastomose with the left gastroepiploic branch of the splenic artery.

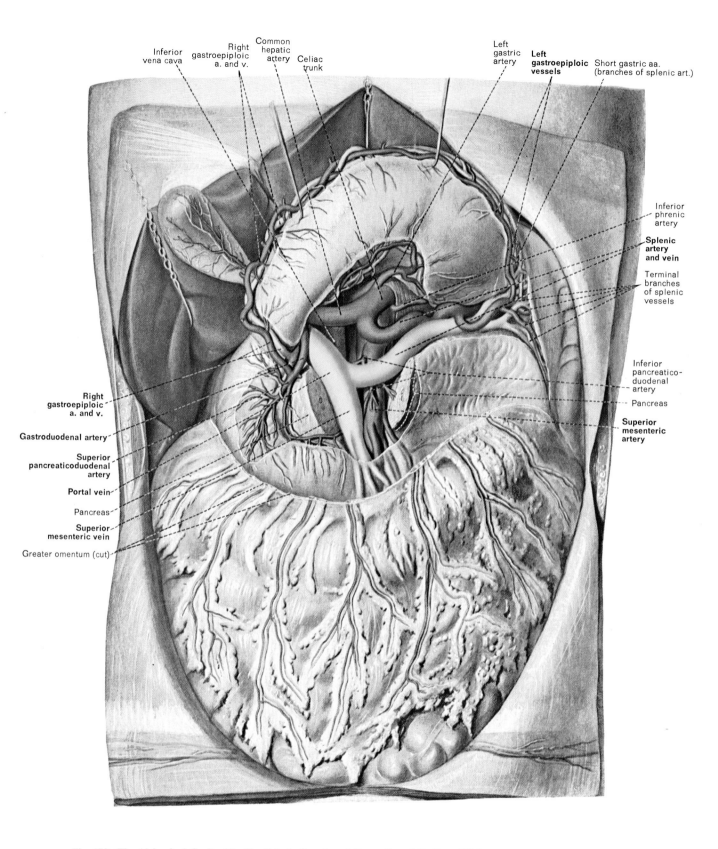

Fig. 178: The Abdominal Cavity (4): The Splenic Vessels and Formation of the Portal Vein

NOTE: 1) the attachment of the greater omentum has been cut along the greater curvature of the stomach. The stomach has been lifted to expose its posterior surface and the underlying pancreas, duodenum and blood vessels. A portion of the body of the pancreas has been removed to reveal the formation of the portal vein by the junction of the splenic and superior mesenteric veins.

2) the splenic artery in its tortuous course across the left upper abdomen to the hilum of the spleen. Observe also how the gastroduodenal artery lies posterior to the pyloric end of the stomach and divides into the right gastroepiploic artery and the superior pancreaticoduodenal artery. The origin of the left gastroepiploic artery from the splenic is also visible.

3) the root of the superior mesenteric artery as it branches from the abdominal aorta just below the celiac trunk.

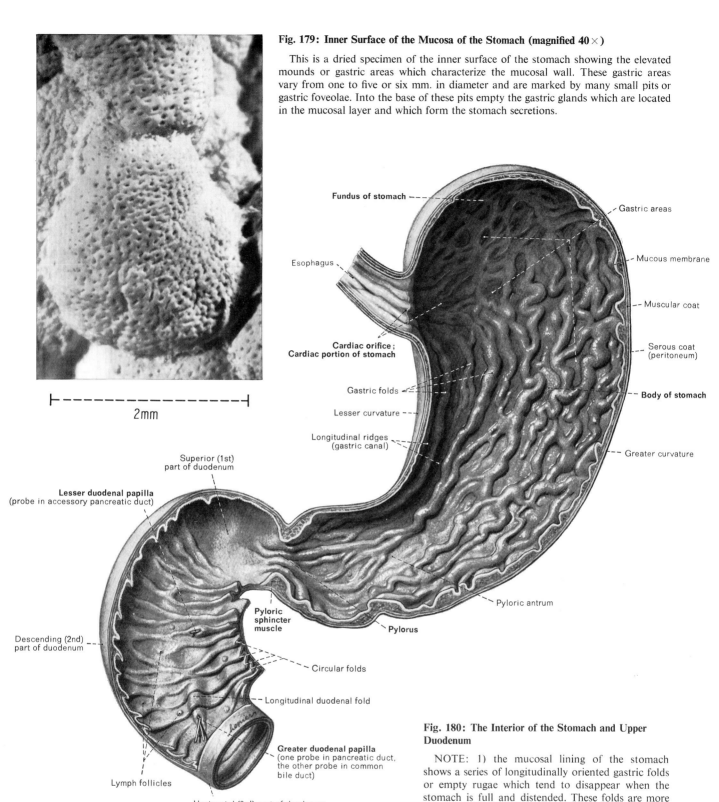

Fig. 179: Inner Surface of the Mucosa of the Stomach (magnified 40 ×)

This is a dried specimen of the inner surface of the stomach showing the elevated mounds or gastric areas which characterize the mucosal wall. These gastric areas vary from one to five or six mm. in diameter and are marked by many small pits or gastric foveolae. Into the base of these pits empty the gastric glands which are located in the mucosal layer and which form the stomach secretions.

2mm

Fundus of stomach

Gastric areas

Esophagus

Mucous membrane

Muscular coat

Cardiac orifice ;
Cardiac portion of stomach

Serous coat
(peritoneum)

Gastric folds

Body of stomach

Lesser curvature

Longitudinal ridges
(gastric canal)

Greater curvature

Superior (1st)
part of duodenum

Lesser duodenal papilla
(probe in accessory pancreatic duct)

Pyloric antrum

Pyloric
sphincter
muscle

Pylorus

Descending (2nd)
part of duodenum

Circular folds

Longitudinal duodenal fold

Fig. 180: The Interior of the Stomach and Upper Duodenum

Greater duodenal papilla
(one probe in pancreatic duct,
the other probe in common
bile duct)

Lymph follicles

Horizontal (3rd) part of duodenum

NOTE: 1) the mucosal lining of the stomach shows a series of longitudinally oriented gastric folds or empty rugae which tend to disappear when the stomach is full and distended. These folds are more regular along the lesser curvature and form the grooved gastric canal. The concept that food travels along this canal (magenstrasse) is not correct.

2) the surface of the first portion of the duodenum (superior) is smooth, whereas the circular ridges characteristic of the small intestine can be seen to commence in the second or descending portion of the duodenum.

3) the pyloric junction of the stomach with the duodenum. A circular muscle, the pyloric sphincter, guards this junction. It diminishes significantly in size the lumen of the gastrointestinal tract at this point. The pylorus is to the right of midline at the level of the 1st lumbar vertebra.

4) the openings in the wall of the duodenum. The greater duodenal papilla serves as the site of the openings of both the common bile duct and the main pancreatic duct. The accessory pancreatic duct opens two centimeters more proximally through the lesser duodenal papilla.

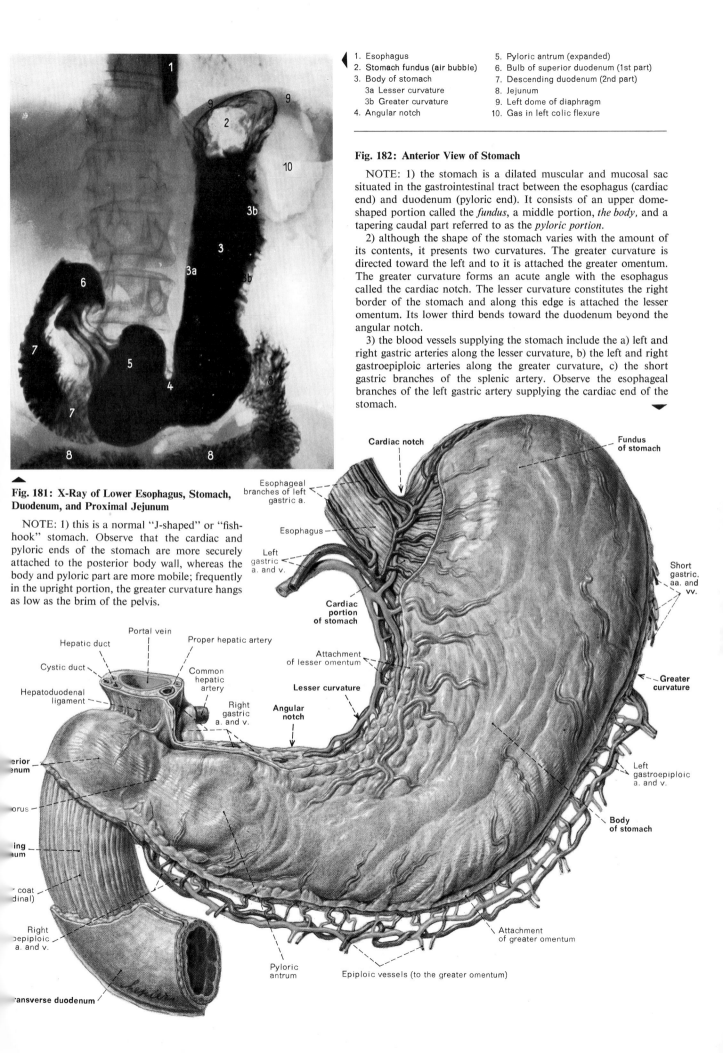

1. Esophagus
2. Stomach fundus (air bubble)
3. Body of stomach
  3a Lesser curvature
  3b Greater curvature
4. Angular notch
5. Pyloric antrum (expanded)
6. Bulb of superior duodenum (1st part)
7. Descending duodenum (2nd part)
8. Jejunum
9. Left dome of diaphragm
10. Gas in left colic flexure

Fig. 182: Anterior View of Stomach

NOTE: 1) the stomach is a dilated muscular and mucosal sac situated in the gastrointestinal tract between the esophagus (cardiac end) and duodenum (pyloric end). It consists of an upper dome-shaped portion called the *fundus*, a middle portion, *the body,* and a tapering caudal part referred to as the *pyloric portion.*

2) although the shape of the stomach varies with the amount of its contents, it presents two curvatures. The greater curvature is directed toward the left and to it is attached the greater omentum. The greater curvature forms an acute angle with the esophagus called the cardiac notch. The lesser curvature constitutes the right border of the stomach and along this edge is attached the lesser omentum. Its lower third bends toward the duodenum beyond the angular notch.

3) the blood vessels supplying the stomach include the a) left and right gastric arteries along the lesser curvature, b) the left and right gastroepiploic arteries along the greater curvature, c) the short gastric branches of the splenic artery. Observe the esophageal branches of the left gastric artery supplying the cardiac end of the stomach.

Fig. 181: X-Ray of Lower Esophagus, Stomach, Duodenum, and Proximal Jejunum

NOTE: 1) this is a normal "J-shaped" or "fish-hook" stomach. Observe that the cardiac and pyloric ends of the stomach are more securely attached to the posterior body wall, whereas the body and pyloric part are more mobile; frequently in the upright portion, the greater curvature hangs as low as the brim of the pelvis.

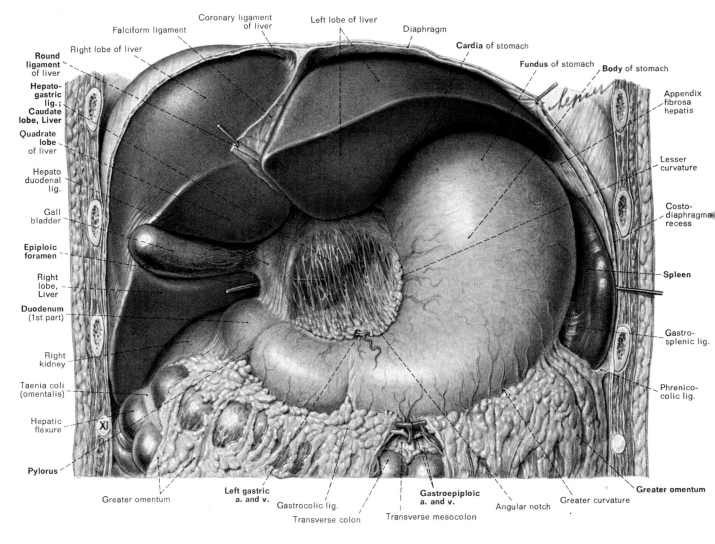

Fig. 183: The Lesser Omentum, Stomach, Liver and Spleen

NOTE: 1) with the liver elevated, a probe has been inserted through the epiploic foramen into the vestibule of the omental bursa. By way of this opening, the greater peritoneal sac communicates with the lesser peritoneal sac. Observe that the lesser omentum consists of the hepatogastric and hepatoduodenal ligaments.

2) the epiploic foramen is situated just caudal to the liver and readily admits two fingers. It is bound superiorly by the caudate lobe of the liver, inferiorly by the 1st part of the duodenum, posteriorly by the inferior vena cava, and anteriorly by the lesser omentum which ensheathes the structures of the porta hepatis (hepatic artery, portal vein and bile ducts).

3) the greater omentum extends along the greater curvature from the spleen to the duodenum. The gall bladder is situated between the right and quadrate lobes of the liver and projects just beyond the inferior border of the liver, thereby coming into contact directly with the anterior abdominal wall at this site.

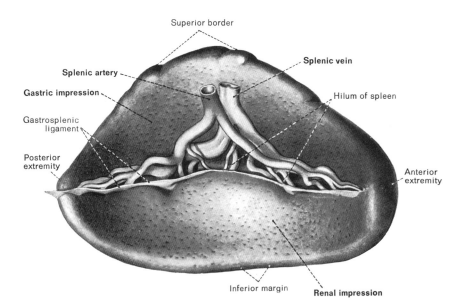

Fig. 184: The Spleen, Visceral Surface

Note that the spleen is situated in the left hypochondriac region between the fundus of the stomach and the diaphragm. Its visceral surface shows the contours of the organs related to it. A gastric impression and a renal impression conform to the shapes of the stomach and left kidney. Additionally, the left colic flexure, the tail of the pancreas and the left adrenal gland which overlies the left kidney are related to this visceral surface.

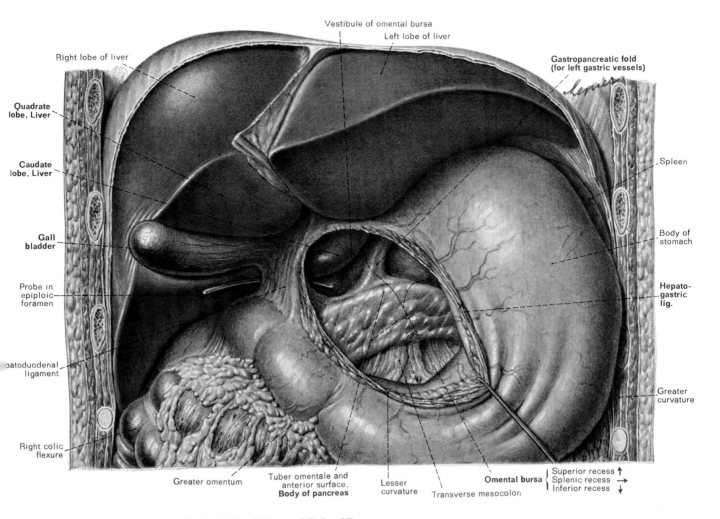

Fig. 185: The Omental Bursa, Caudate Lobe of Liver and Body of Pancreas

NOTE: 1) the liver has been elevated and the lesser curvature of the stomach has been pulled down and to the left in order to enlarge the exposure obtained by opening the omental bursa through the hepatogastric ligament (indicated by X and XX). The superior, splenic and inferior recesses of this bursa have been indicated by the arrows.

2) the portion of the omental bursa adjacent to the epiploic foramen is called the vestibule. Observe the gastropancreatic fold which crosses the dorsal wall of the bursa. This fold is formed by a reflection of peritoneum covering the left gastric artery which courses (from its origin on the celiac trunk) to the left of the superior recess of the omental bursa to achieve its destination, the lesser curvature of the stomach.

3) exposure of the omental bursa in this manner reveals the caudate lobe of the liver which can be seen situated on the dorsal surface of the liver's right lobe as well as the anterior surface of the body of the pancreas coursing transversely behind the stomach.

4) the left lobe of the liver overlies the lesser curvature, the fundus and part of the body of the stomach. While the caudate lobe is situated to the right of the esophagus (not visible in this figure), the quadrate lobe, which lies between the fossa of the gall bladder and the round ligament, comes into contact with the pylorus and the first part of the duodenum.

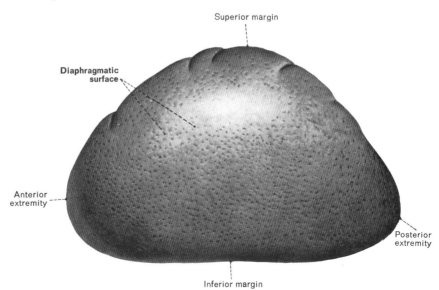

Fig. 186: The Spleen, Diaphragmatic Surface

NOTE: the diaphragmatic surface of the spleen is directed posterolaterally. It is smooth and convex and conforms to the concave abdominal surface of the adjacent diaphragm. Although the normal adult spleen may vary considerably in size from 100 grams to 400 grams, its proximity to the 9th, 10th and 11th ribs of the left side makes it vulnerable to costal fractures in this region.

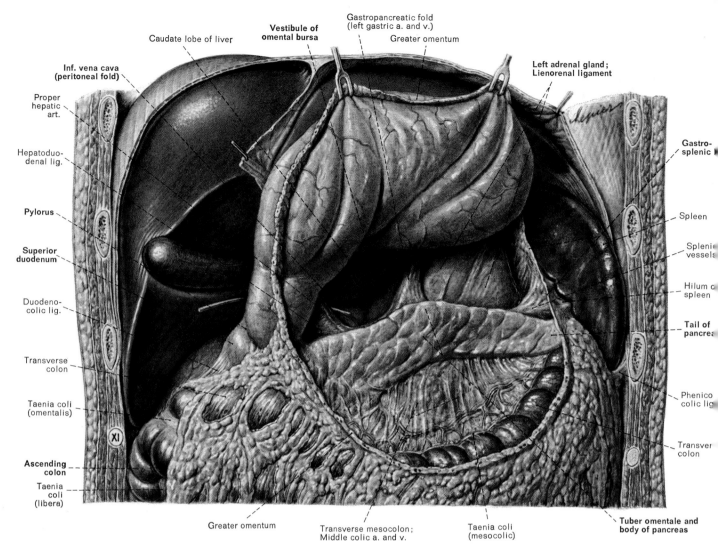

Caudate lobe of liver

Inf. vena cava (peritoneal fold)

Proper hepatic art.

Hepatoduo-denal lig.

Pylorus

Superior duodenum

Duodeno-colic lig.

Transverse colon

Taenia coli (omentalis)

Ascending colon

Taenia coli (libera)

Vestibule of omental bursa

Gastropancreatic fold (left gastric a. and v.)

Greater omentum

Left adrenal gland; Lienorenal ligament

Gastro-splenic

Spleen

Splenic vessels

Hilum of spleen

Tail of pancreas

Phenico-colic lig

Transverse colon

Greater omentum

Transverse mesocolon; Middle colic a. and v.

Taenia coli (mesocolic)

Tuber omentale and body of pancreas

Fig. 187: The Omental Bursa and Structures of the Stomach Bed

NOTE: 1) the attachment of the greater omentum has been cut along the entire greater curvature of the stomach and the stomach has been elevated to expose the dorsal wall of the omental bursa.

2) the transverse course of the pancreas across the posterior abdomen and the pointed direction of the tail of the pancreas toward the hilum of the spleen.

3) the severed peritoneal reflection between the stomach and the spleen, the gastrosplenic ligament and its continuation from the spleen to the kidney, the lienorenal ligament. Covering the upper pole of the left kidney, observe the adrenal gland.

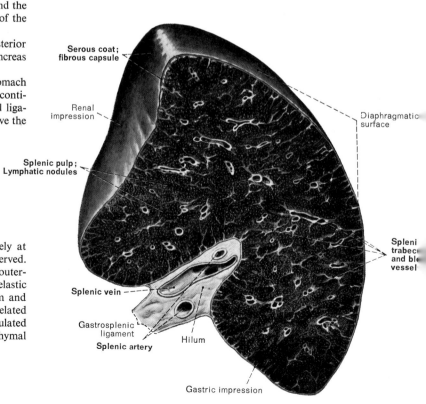

Serous coat; fibrous capsule

Renal impression

Splenic pulp; Lymphatic nodules

Diaphragmatic surface

Splenic trabeculae and blood vessel

Splenic vein

Gastrosplenic ligament

Hilum

Splenic artery

Gastric impression

Fig. 188: Spleen, Cross Section

NOTE: 1) the spleen has been sectioned transversely at the hilum where the severed splenic vessels can be observed.

2) covering the spleen are two external coats. The outermost is a serous coat and beneath this is the fibrous elastic capsule. The serous coat derives from the peritoneum and is continuous at the hilum with the peritoneal folds related to the spleen. The fibrous, elastic coat invests the trabeculated soft masses of splenic pulp which compose the parenchymal tissue of the organ.

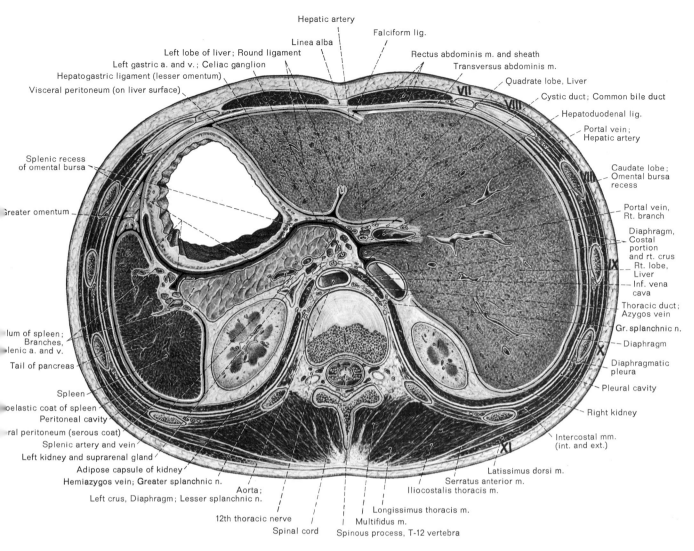

Hepatic artery

Linea alba

Falciform lig.

Left lobe of liver; Round ligament

Left gastric a. and v.; Celiac ganglion

Hepatogastric ligament (lesser omentum)

Visceral peritoneum (on liver surface)

Rectus abdominis m. and sheath

Transversus abdominis m.

Quadrate lobe, Liver

VII

VIII

Cystic duct; Common bile duct

Hepatoduodenal lig.

Portal vein; Hepatic artery

Splenic recess of omental bursa

Caudate lobe; Omental bursa recess

Greater omentum

VII

Portal vein, Rt. branch

Diaphragm, Costal portion and rt. crus

IX

Rt. lobe, Liver

Inf. vena cava

Thoracic duct; Azygos vein

Gr. splanchnic n.

lum of spleen; Branches, lenic a. and v.

Tail of pancreas

X

Diaphragm

Diaphragmatic pleura

Spleen

Pleural cavity

oelastic coat of spleen

Peritoneal cavity

Right kidney

ral peritoneum (serous coat)

Splenic artery and vein

Left kidney and suprarenal gland

Adipose capsule of kidney

Hemiazygos vein; Greater splanchnic n.

XI

Intercostal mm. (int. and ext.)

Latissimus dorsi m.

Serratus anterior m.

Iliocostalis thoracis m.

Aorta;

Left crus, Diaphragm; Lesser splanchnic n.

Longissimus thoracis m.

12th thoracic nerve

Multifidus m.

Spinal cord

Spinous process, T-12 vertebra

Fig. 189: Transverse Section Through the Upper Abdomen (between T-12 and L-1)

NOTE: 1) in light red is outlined the peritoneum of the greater peritoneal cavity while in dark red is the peritoneum of the omental bursa or lesser peritoneal cavity.

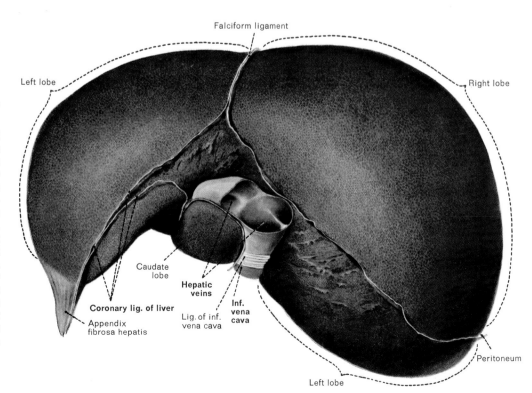

Falciform ligament

Left lobe

Right lobe

Fig. 190: Dorsocranial View of Liver

NOTE: 1) the visceral peritoneum closely adheres to the surface of the liver and is called the coronary ligament. Between the two leaves of the coronary ligament a portion of the liver is devoid of peritoneum. This is called the bare area of the liver and it is in direct contact with the diaphragm.

2) the hepatic veins as they converge superiorly from the liver lobes to empty into the inferior vena cava; this latter vessel lies in its sulcus on the posterior surface of the liver.

Caudate lobe

Hepatic veins

Inf. vena cava

Coronary lig. of liver

Lig. of inf. vena cava

Appendix fibrosa hepatis

Peritoneum

Left lobe

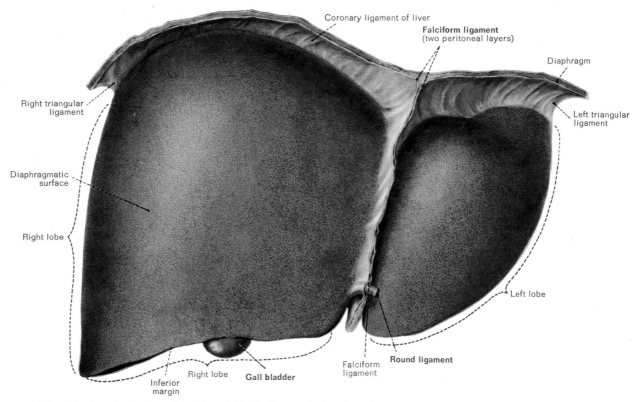

Fig. 191: Anterior Surface of the Liver (with Diaphragmatic Attachment)

NOTE: 1) the falciform ligament (derived from the ventral mesogastrium) separates the large right from the smaller left lobe of the liver. It contains the fibrous cord called the round ligament of the liver which is the resultant structure from the obliteration of the umbilical vein.

2) the fundus of the gall bladder extending below the sharply angled hepatic inferior margin.

Fig. 192: Posterior (Visceral) Surface of Liver and the Gall Bladder

NOTE: 1) the impressions made by the esophagus and stomach on the left lobe of the liver and the right kidney, right suprarenal gland, duodenum and transverse colon on the right lobe.

2) the sulcus formed by the inferior vena cava, which subdivides the caudate lobe from the right lobe. The gall bladder along with the portal vein, hepatic artery and common bile duct bound the quadrate lobe.

3) the continuity of the round ligament (umbilical vein) with the ligamentum venosum (ductus venosus).

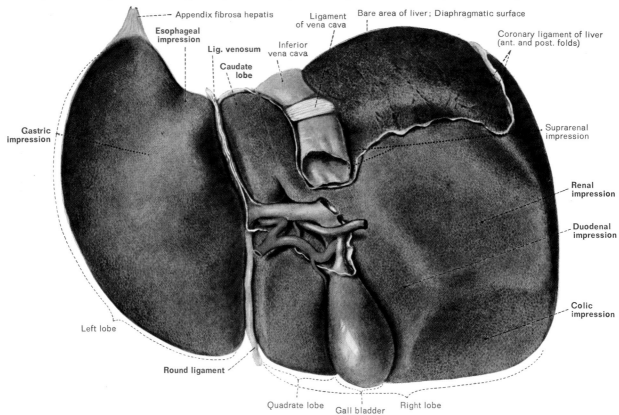

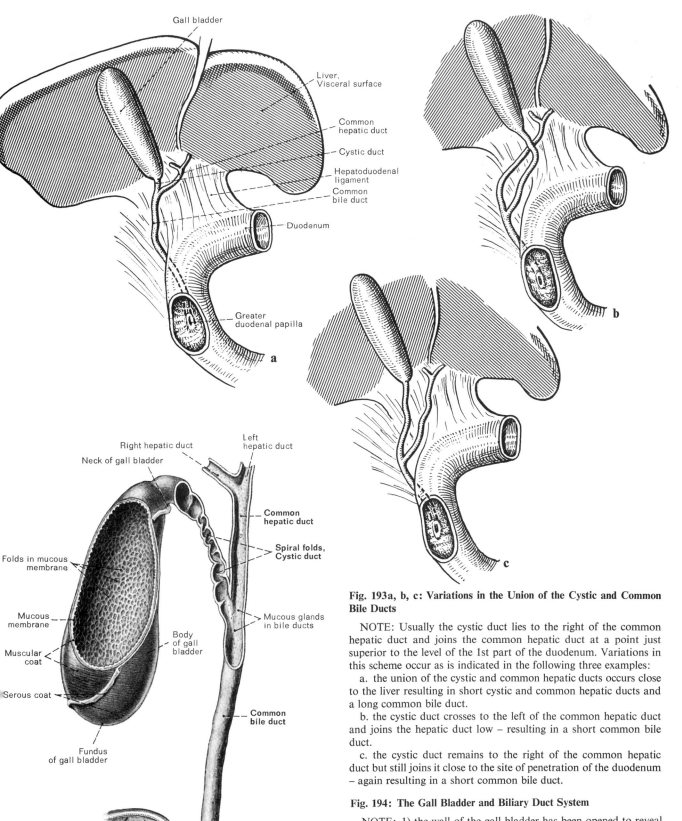

Fig. 193a, b, c: Variations in the Union of the Cystic and Common Bile Ducts

NOTE: Usually the cystic duct lies to the right of the common hepatic duct and joins the common hepatic duct at a point just superior to the level of the 1st part of the duodenum. Variations in this scheme occur as is indicated in the following three examples:

a. the union of the cystic and common hepatic ducts occurs close to the liver resulting in short cystic and common hepatic ducts and a long common bile duct.

b. the cystic duct crosses to the left of the common hepatic duct and joins the hepatic duct low – resulting in a short common bile duct.

c. the cystic duct remains to the right of the common hepatic duct but still joins it close to the site of penetration of the duodenum – again resulting in a short common bile duct.

Fig. 194: The Gall Bladder and Biliary Duct System

NOTE: 1) the wall of the gall bladder has been opened to reveal the meshwork characteristic of the surface of the mucosal layer. The pear-shaped gall bladder stores bile which reaches it from the liver. Its capacity is about 35 cc.

2) the spiral nature of the cystic duct which leads from the neck of the gall bladder. Normally the cystic duct measures about 1½ inches long and joins the common hepatic duct (which also is about 1½ inches long) to form the common bile duct. The common bile duct descends about 3 inches to open into the 2nd or descending portion of the duodenum.

3) at its point of entrance into the duodenum (the greater duodenal papilla), the common bile duct is joined by the main pancreatic duct (duct of Wirsung).

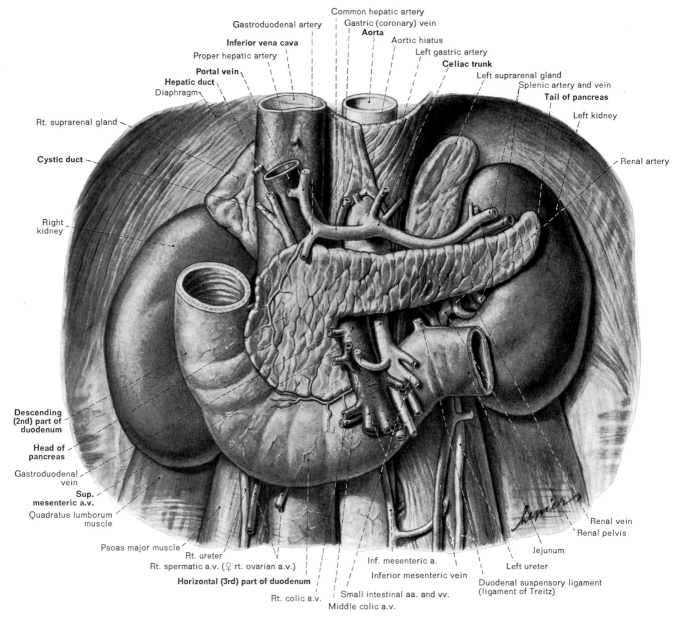

Fig. 195: Pancreas and Duodenum

NOTE: 1) the *head* of the pancreas lies to the right of midline and is in contact with the inferior vena cava and the common bile duct dorsally and the transverse colon ventrally.

2) the body of the pancreas crosses the midline at vertebral level L-1, just caudal to the origin of the celiac trunk. It is in contact posteriorly with the aorta, superior mesenteric vessels, left suprarenal gland and left kidney.

3) the tail of the pancreas is in contact with the spleen laterally, the left kidney posteriorly, and the splenic flexure of the colon anteriorly.

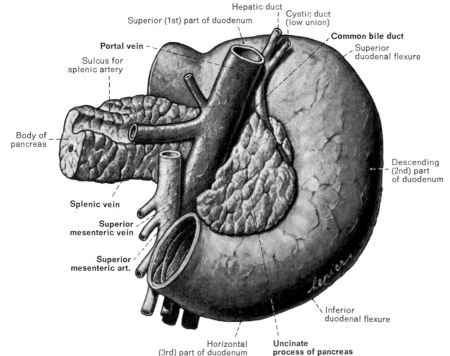

Fig. 196: Head of Pancreas and Duodenum (Dorsal View)

NOTE: that this posterior view of the head of the pancreas and its uncinate process shows how the common bile duct is actually embedded within the pancreas as the duct courses adjacent to the duodenum prior to penetration.

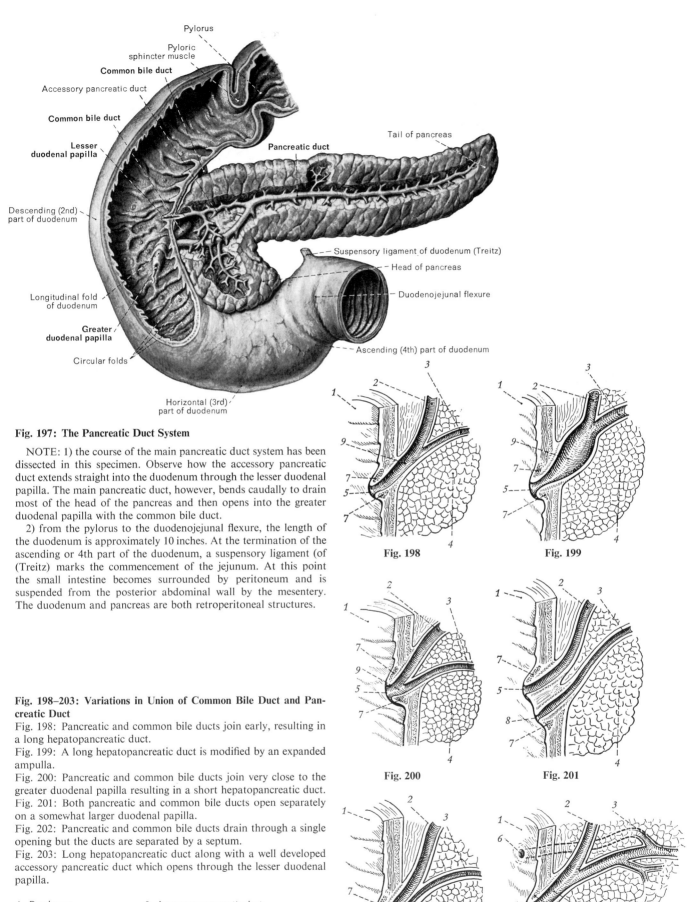

Fig. 197: The Pancreatic Duct System

NOTE: 1) the course of the main pancreatic duct system has been dissected in this specimen. Observe how the accessory pancreatic duct extends straight into the duodenum through the lesser duodenal papilla. The main pancreatic duct, however, bends caudally to drain most of the head of the pancreas and then opens into the greater duodenal papilla with the common bile duct.

2) from the pylorus to the duodenojejunal flexure, the length of the duodenum is approximately 10 inches. At the termination of the ascending or 4th part of the duodenum, a suspensory ligament (of (Treitz) marks the commencement of the jejunum. At this point the small intestine becomes surrounded by peritoneum and is suspended from the posterior abdominal wall by the mesentery. The duodenum and pancreas are both retroperitoneal structures.

Fig. 198–203: Variations in Union of Common Bile Duct and Pancreatic Duct

Fig. 198: Pancreatic and common bile ducts join early, resulting in a long hepatopancreatic duct.
Fig. 199: A long hepatopancreatic duct is modified by an expanded ampulla.
Fig. 200: Pancreatic and common bile ducts join very close to the greater duodenal papilla resulting in a short hepatopancreatic duct.
Fig. 201: Both pancreatic and common bile ducts open separately on a somewhat larger duodenal papilla.
Fig. 202: Pancreatic and common bile ducts drain through a single opening but the ducts are separated by a septum.
Fig. 203: Long hepatopancreatic duct along with a well developed accessory pancreatic duct which opens through the lesser duodenal papilla.

1	Duodenum	6	Accessory pancreatic duct (Santorini)
2	Common bile duct	7	Sphincter (Oddi) at duodenal papilla
3	Pancreatic duct (Wirsung)		
4	Pancreas	8	Pancreatic duct separate opening
5	Greater duodenal papilla	9	Hepatopancreatic duct

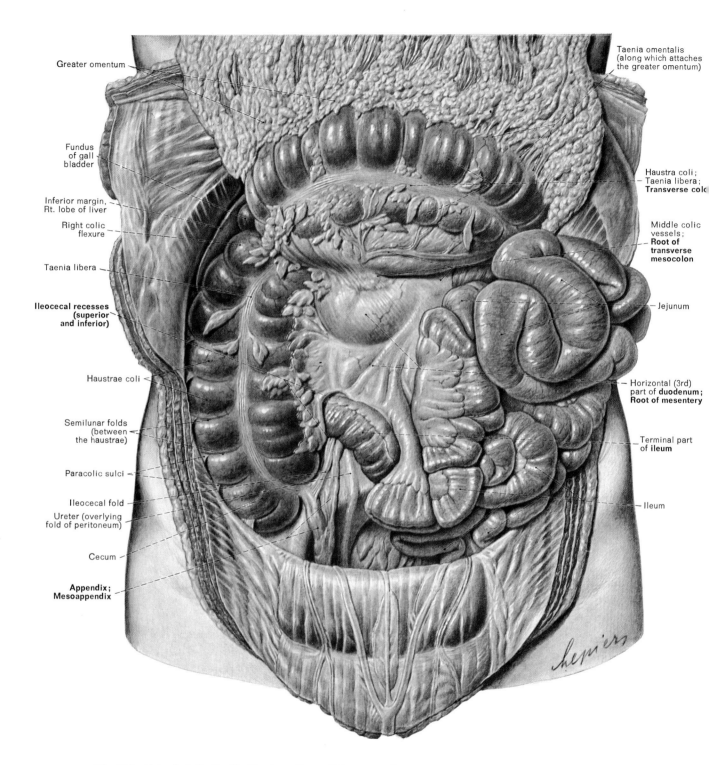

Greater omentum

Taenia omentalis
(along which attaches
the greater omentum)

Fundus
of gall
bladder

Haustra coli;
Taenia libera;
Transverse colc

Inferior margin,
Rt. lobe of liver

Middle colic
vessels;
**Root of
transverse
mesocolon**

Right colic
flexure

Taenia libera

Jejunum

**Ileocecal recesses
(superior
and inferior)**

Haustrae coli

Horizontal (3rd)
part of **duodenum;
Root of mesentery**

Semilunar folds
(between
the haustrae)

Terminal part
of **ileum**

Paracolic sulci

Ileocecal fold

Ileum

Ureter (overlying
fold of peritoneum)

Cecum

**Appendix;
Mesoappendix**

Fig. 204: Abdominal Cavity (5): The Ascending and Transverse Colon

NOTE: 1) the greater omentum has been reflected superiorly and the jejunum and ileum have been pulled to the left in order to expose the root of the mesentery of the small intestine on the right side.

2) the horizontal (3rd) part of the duodenum which is retroperitoneal and which is covered by the smooth and glistening peritoneum. Observe also the distal portion of the ileum at its junction with the cecum. At this ileocecal junction, identify the ileocecal fold, the appendix and the mesoappendix. The appendix may extend cranially behind the cecum, toward the left and behind the ileum, or as demonstrated here, inferiorly over the pelvic brim.

3) the transverse colon and the small intestine beyond the duodenal junction are more mobile than most other organs because they are attached to the transverse mesocolon and the mesentery.

4) the retroperitoneal position of the right ureter as it descends over the pelvic brim on its course toward the bladder in the pelvis.

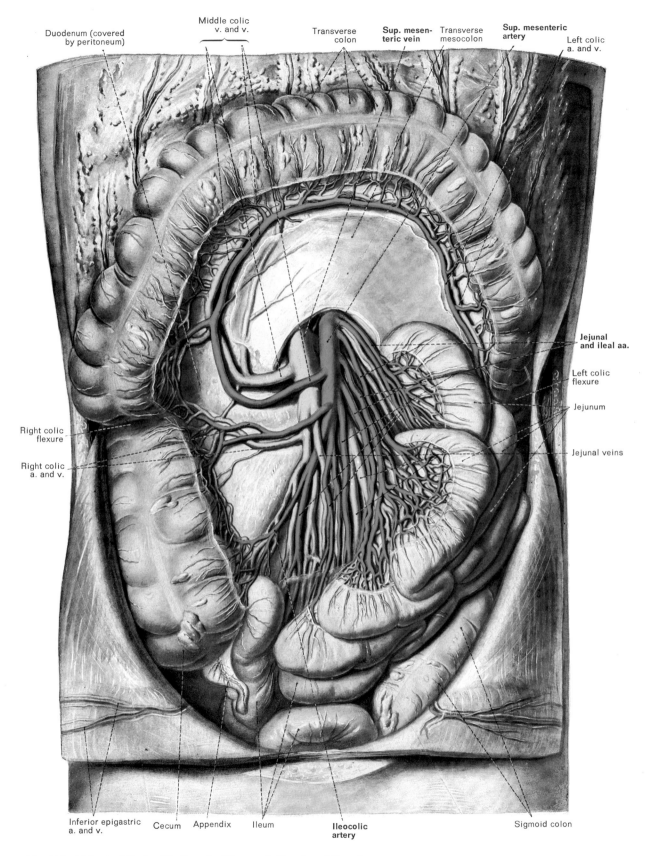

Duodenum (covered by peritoneum) — Middle colic v. and v. — Transverse colon — **Sup. mesenteric vein** — Transverse mesocolon — **Sup. mesenteric artery** — Left colic a. and v.

Jejunal and ileal aa.

Left colic flexure

Jejunum

Jejunal veins

Right colic flexure

Right colic a. and v.

Inferior epigastric a. and v. — Cecum — Appendix — Ileum — **Ileocolic artery** — Sigmoid colon

Fig. 205: Abdominal Cavity (6): Superior Mesenteric Vessels and Branches

NOTE: 1) the transverse colon has been turned upward and the small intestine was pushed to the left. The peritoneal attachment along the coils of small intestine and colon have been dissected to reveal the branches of the superior mesenteric vessels which supply the small intestine, ascending colon and transverse colon.

2) the intestinal arteries (jejunal and ileal) branch from the left side of the superior mesenteric artery. There are about 12 of these vessels and they are distributed to the jejunum and ileum.

3) branching from the right side of the superior mesenteric artery are the ileocolic (to the ileocecal region), right colic (to the ascending colon) and middle colic (transverse colon) arteries. Observe the elaborate branching of these vessels and the rich anastomoses which exist among them.

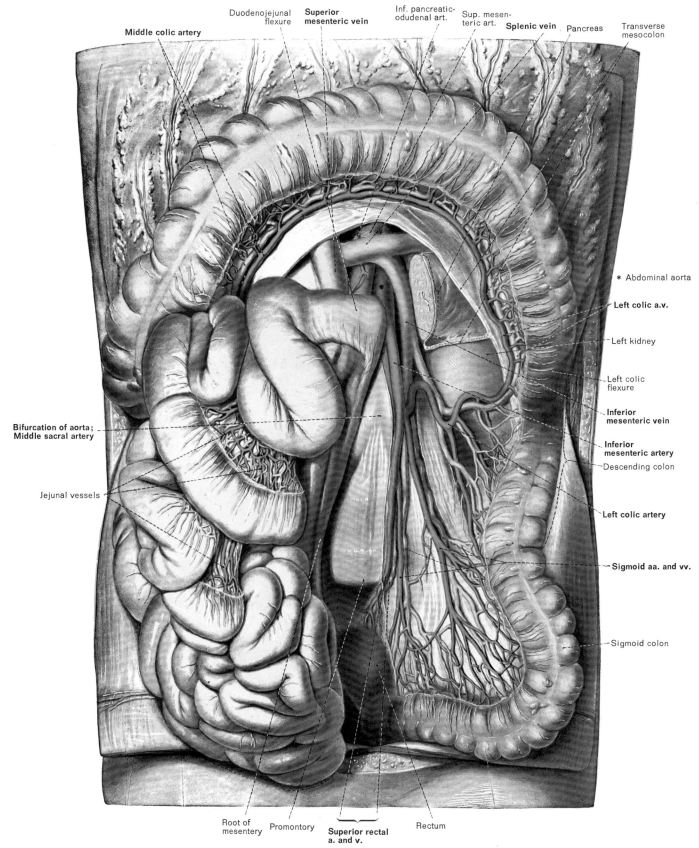

Middle colic artery

Duodenojejunal flexure

Superior mesenteric vein

Inf. pancreatic-odudenal art.

Sup. mesenteric art.

Splenic vein

Pancreas

Transverse mesocolon

* Abdominal aorta

Left colic a.v.

Left kidney

Left colic flexure

Inferior mesenteric vein

Inferior mesenteric artery

Descending colon

Left colic artery

Bifurcation of aorta; Middle sacral artery

Sigmoid aa. and vv.

Sigmoid colon

Jejunal vessels

Root of mesentery

Promontory

Superior rectal a. and v.

Rectum

Fig. 206: Abdominal Cavity (7): The Inferior Mesenteric Vessels and Branches

NOTE: 1) the small intestine has been pushed to the right side of the abdomen to reveal origin of the inferior mesenteric artery from the aorta and the drainage of the inferior mesenteric vein into the splenic vein. Also a portion of the body of the pancreas and transverse mesocolon was removed to show these relationships more clearly.

2) the inferior mesenteric artery supplies the descending colon via the left colic artery. Observe the anastomosis around the margin of the large bowel between the left colic artery and the middle colic artery. Somewhat lower, the inferior mesenteric gives rise to the sigmoid arteries and the superior rectal vessels.

3) the bifurcation of the abdominal aorta retroperitoneally and the middle sacral artery descending in the midline.

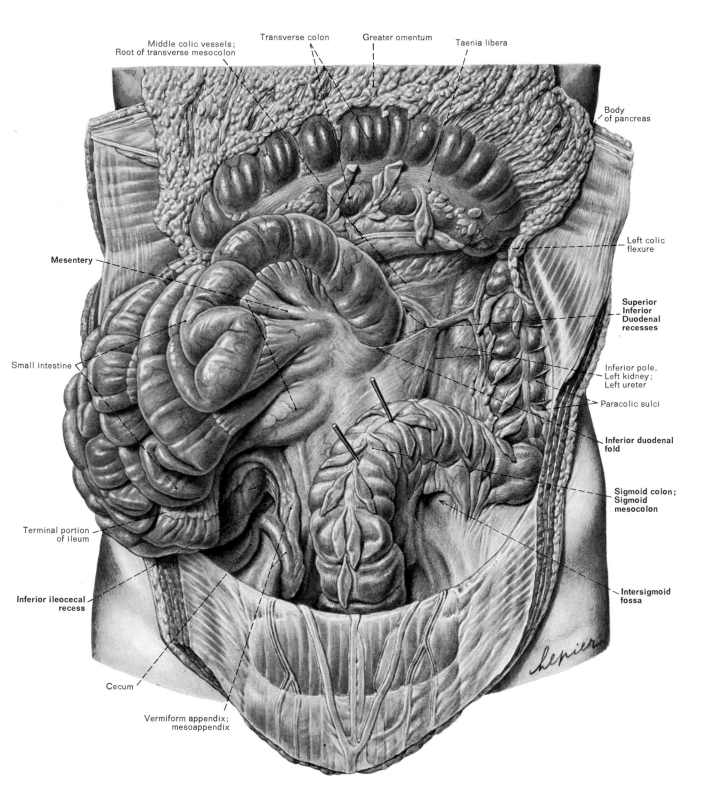

Fig. 207: Abdominal Cavity (8): Duodenojejunal Junction: Descending and Sigmoid Colon

NOTE: 1) the transverse colon and greater omentum have been reflected superiorly and the jejunum and ileum have been pulled to the right to reveal the duodenojejunal junction and the descending and sigmoid colon.

2) as the ascending (4th) part of the duodenum becomes jejunum, and the small intestine acquires a mesentery at that site, there frequently are found duodenal fossae or recesses situated in relation to the junction. Look for the inferior and superior duodenal recesses (present in over 50% of the cases). These are of importance because they represent possible sites of introtinal herniae within the abdomen.

3) the mobility of the sigmoid colon because of its mesocolic attachment in contrast to the descending colon which is more fixed to the posterior wall of the abdomen. Observe the intersigmoid fossa located behind the sigmoid mesocolon and between it and the peritoneum reflected over the external iliac vessels.

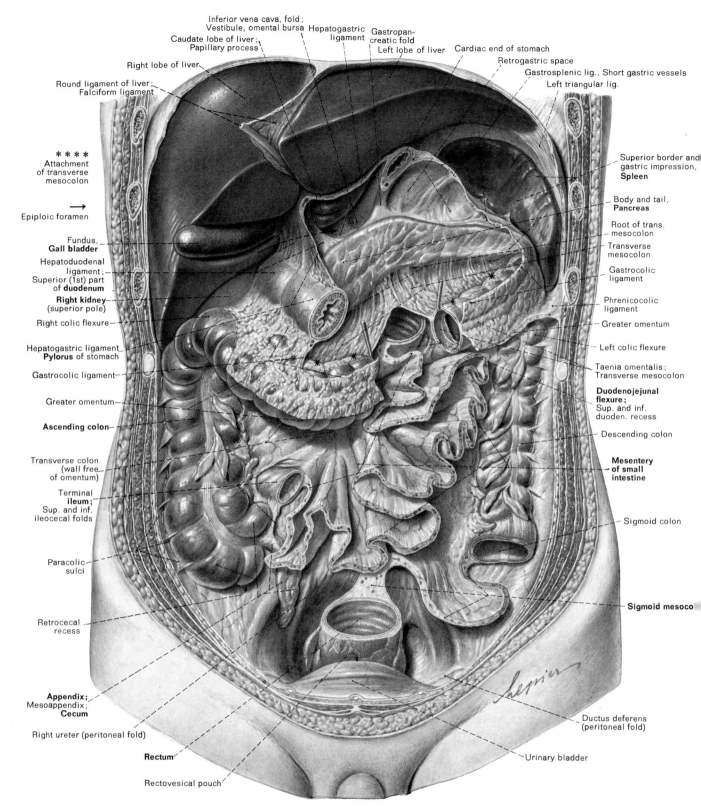

Inferior vena cava, fold;
Vestibule, omental bursa
Caudate lobe of liver;
Papillary process
Right lobe of liver
Round ligament of liver;
Falciform ligament

Hepatogastric ligament
Gastropancreatic fold
Left lobe of liver
Cardiac end of stomach
Retrogastric space
Gastrosplenic lig., Short gastric vessels
Left triangular lig.

**** Attachment of transverse mesocolon

→ Epiploic foramen

Fundus, **Gall bladder**

Hepatoduodenal ligament; Superior (1st) part of **duodenum**

Right kidney (superior pole)

Right colic flexure

Hepatogastric ligament **Pylorus** of stomach

Gastrocolic ligament

Greater omentum

Ascending colon

Transverse colon (wall free of omentum)

Terminal **ileum**; Sup. and inf. ileocecal folds

Paracolic sulci

Retrocecal recess

Appendix; Mesoappendix; **Cecum**

Right ureter (peritoneal fold)

Rectum

Rectovesical pouch

Superior border and gastric impression, **Spleen**

Body and tail, **Pancreas**

Root of trans. mesocolon

Transverse mesocolon

Gastrocolic ligament

Phrenicocolic ligament

Greater omentum

Left colic flexure

Taenia omentalis; Transverse mesocolon

Duodenojejunal flexure; Sup. and inf. duoden. recess

Descending colon

Mesentery of small intestine

Sigmoid colon

Sigmoid mesoco

Ductus deferens (peritoneal fold)

Urinary bladder

Fig. 208: Abdominal Cavity (9): The Large Intestine and the Mesenteries

NOTE: 1) the stomach was cut just proximal to the pylorus and the small intestine was severed at the duodenojejunal junction and at the distal ileum and then removed by cutting the mesentery. A portion of the transverse colon was removed along with the greater omentum and the sigmoid colon was resected to reveal its mesocolon.

2) the mesentery of the small intestine extends obliquely across the posterior abdominal wall from the duodenojejunal flexure to the ilocecal junction. In this distance of about 6 to 7 inches, the mesentery is thrown into many folds to accommodate all the loops of jejunum and ileum.

3) the ascending and descending colon is fused to the posterior abdominal wall while the transverse and sigmoid colon are suspended by their respective mesocolons.

Fig. 209: The Ileocecal Junction

NOTE: 1) the terminal ileum, cecum and lower ascending colon have been opened anteriorly to reveal the ileocecal junction and the opening of the vermiform appendix.

2) the leaves of the ileocecal valve have been separated. Observe that this valve is formed by two reflected folds of the wall of the large intestine. These folds unite and then project further around the large intestine as the frenulum.

3) the orifice of the appendix opens into the cecum, although the position and the direction of the appendix are quite variable. Observe the semilunar folds, the sacculations (haustrae) and longitudinal muscle bands (taeniae) which characterize the large intestine.

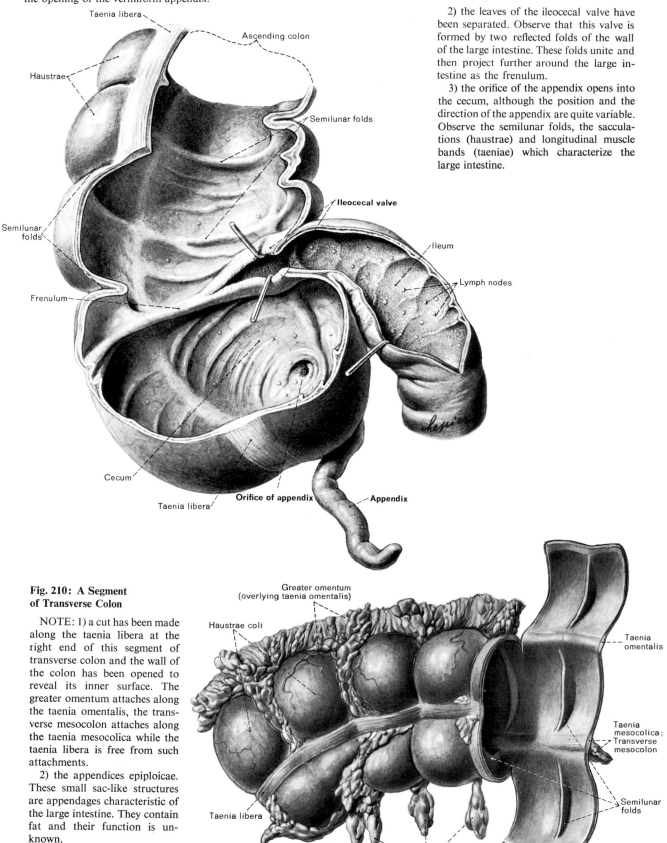

Fig. 210: A Segment of Transverse Colon

NOTE: 1) a cut has been made along the taenia libera at the right end of this segment of transverse colon and the wall of the colon has been opened to reveal its inner surface. The greater omentum attaches along the taenia omentalis, the transverse mesocolon attaches along the taenia mesocolica while the taenia libera is free from such attachments.

2) the appendices epiploicae. These small sac-like structures are appendages characteristic of the large intestine. They contain fat and their function is unknown.

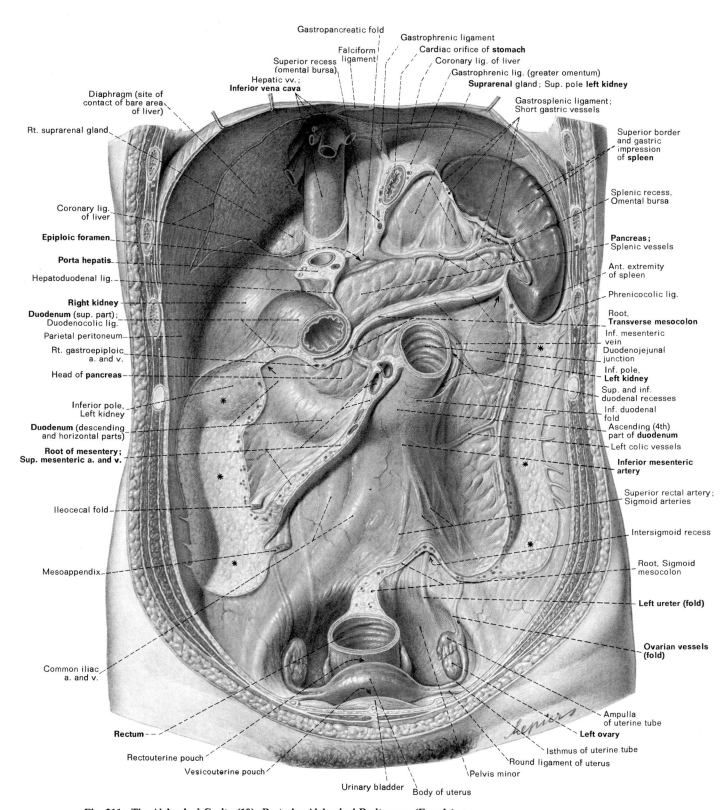

Gastropancreatic fold

Falciform ligament

Gastrophrenic ligament

Cardiac orifice of **stomach**

Coronary lig. of liver

Gastrophrenic lig. (greater omentum)

Superior recess (omental bursa)

Hepatic vv.; **Inferior vena cava**

Suprarenal gland; Sup. pole **left kidney**

Gastrosplenic ligament; Short gastric vessels

Diaphragm (site of contact of bare area of liver)

Rt. suprarenal gland

Superior border and gastric impression of **spleen**

Splenic recess, Omental bursa

Coronary lig. of liver

Pancreas; Splenic vessels

Epiploic foramen

Ant. extremity of spleen

Porta hepatis

Phrenicocolic lig.

Hepatoduodenal lig.

Root, **Transverse mesocolon**

Right kidney

Duodenum (sup. part); Duodenocolic lig.

Inf. mesenteric vein

Duodenojejunal junction

Parietal peritoneum

Rt. gastroepiploic a. and v.

Inf. pole, **Left kidney**

Head of **pancreas**

Sup. and inf. duodenal recesses

Inferior pole, Left kidney

Inf. duodenal fold

Ascending (4th) part of **duodenum**

Duodenum (descending and horizontal parts)

Left colic vessels

Root of mesentery; Sup. mesenteric a. and v.

Inferior mesenteric artery

Superior rectal artery; Sigmoid arteries

Ileocecal fold

Intersigmoid recess

Mesoappendix

Root, Sigmoid mesocolon

Left ureter (fold)

Ovarian vessels (fold)

Common iliac a. and v.

Ampulla of uterine tube

Rectum

Left ovary

Rectouterine pouch

Isthmus of uterine tube

Round ligament of uterus

Vesicouterine pouch

Pelvis minor

Urinary bladder

Body of uterus

Fig. 211: The Abdominal Cavity (10): Posterior Abdominal Peritoneum (Female)

NOTE: 1) the stomach and intestine (except duodenum and rectum) have been removed and their associated mesenteries have been cut close to their roots on the posterior abdominal wall. The liver and its attachments and the gall bladder were removed, leaving intact the spleen and the retroperitoneal organs (duodenum, pancreas, adrenal glands, kidneys and ureters, aorta and inferior vena cava).

2) ascending and descending portions of the large intestine are fused to the posterior abdominal wall (sites marked by *) with a peritoneal layer covering their anterior surfaces. Observe the small black arrows at the right and left colic flexures.

3) the course of the ureters and ovarian vessels as they descend over the pelvic brim. Notice the ovary, uterine tubes and uterus located in the pelvis and their relationship to the rectum and bladder.

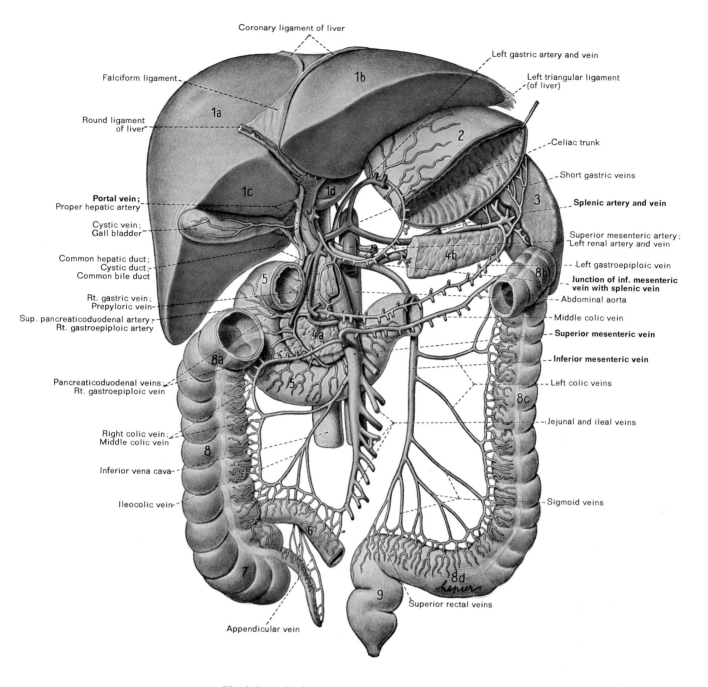

Coronary ligament of liver

Falciform ligament

Round ligament of liver

1b

Left gastric artery and vein

Left triangular ligament (of liver)

2

Celiac trunk

Short gastric veins

1a

1c

1d

Portal vein;
Proper hepatic artery

Cystic vein;
Gall bladder

Common hepatic duct;
Cystic duct;
Common bile duct

Rt. gastric vein;
Prepyloric vein

Sup. pancreaticoduodenal artery;
Rt. gastroepiploic artery

Pancreaticoduodenal veins;
Rt. gastroepiploic vein

Right colic vein;
Middle colic vein

Inferior vena cava

Ileocolic vein

3

Splenic artery and vein

Superior mesenteric artery;
Left renal artery and vein

4b

Left gastroepiploic vein

Junction of inf. mesenteric vein with splenic vein

Abdominal aorta

Middle colic vein

Superior mesenteric vein

Inferior mesenteric vein

Left colic veins

8c

Jejunal and ileal veins

Sigmoid veins

5

4a

8a

8

7

6

9

8d

Superior rectal veins

Appendicular vein

Fig. 212: Abdominal Portal System of Veins

NOTE: 1) the abdominal portal system of veins drains venous blood from the gastro-intestinal tract, the gall bladder, pancreas and spleen through the liver via the large portal vein. This is done in order to subject this venous blood to the various functions of the liver before it is returned to the general systemic circulation by way of the hepatic veins into the inferior vena cava.

2) the portal vein is formed by the union of the superior mesenteric vein and the splenic vein. The inferior mesenteric vein drains into the splenic vein. At the esophageal end of the stomach (esophageal veins) and at the distal end of the rectum (inferior rectal veins), the portal system of veins anastomoses with the systemic veins. Certain disease states which may cause a reduction of blood flow through the liver result in greater use of these anastomotic channels in the return of blood in the portal system.

3) the functions of the liver are numerous, varied and vital to life. The liver secretes bile which is then stored in the gall bladder and released when food appears in the duodenum. Bile aids in the digestion and absorption of fats. The liver converts glucose to glycogen, stores the glycogen and then reconverts it to glucose again when needed. Further, the liver is involved in the synthesis of Vitamin A, heparin, prothrombin, fibrinogen and other substances. It functions also in detoxification of substances in the blood. It is involved in the breakdown of hemoglobin and stores both iron and copper.

1a Right lobe of liver
1b Left lobe of liver
1c Quadrate lobe of liver
1d Caudate lobe of liver
2 Stomach
3 Spleen
4a Head of pancreas
4b Tail of pancreas
5 Duodenum
6 Ileum
7 Cecum
8 Ascending colon
8a Right colic flexure
8b Left colic flexure
8c Descending colon
8d Sigmoid colon
9 Rectum
↑ = Junction of sup. mesenteric v. and splenic vein to form portal vein

Fig. 213: The Inner Surface of the Rectum and Anal Canal

NOTE: 1) at about the level of the 3rd sacral vertebra, the sigmoid colon becomes the rectum. Measuring about 5 inches in length, the rectum then becomes the anal canal which is the terminal 1½ inches of the intestinal tract. The rectum is dilated near its junction with the anal canal, giving rise to the rectal ampulla.

2) the internal mucosa of the rectum is thrown into transverse folds of which there are usually three in number. They are also known as the valves of Houston.

3) below the rectal ampulla, the mucosa of the anal canal shows a series of longitudinal folds called the anal columns (columns of Morgagni). Each of these folds usually posseses an artery and vein and between the anal columns are small fossae called the anal sinuses. The veins in this region are dilated and tortuous and can become varicosed, giving rise to a condition called hemorrhoids or piles.

4) distal to the anal column is an abrupt zone of epithelial transition. The stratified squamous of the distalmost part of the anal canal becomes the simple columnar of the rectum. This transition line can be identified in a living person and is referred to as Hilton's line.

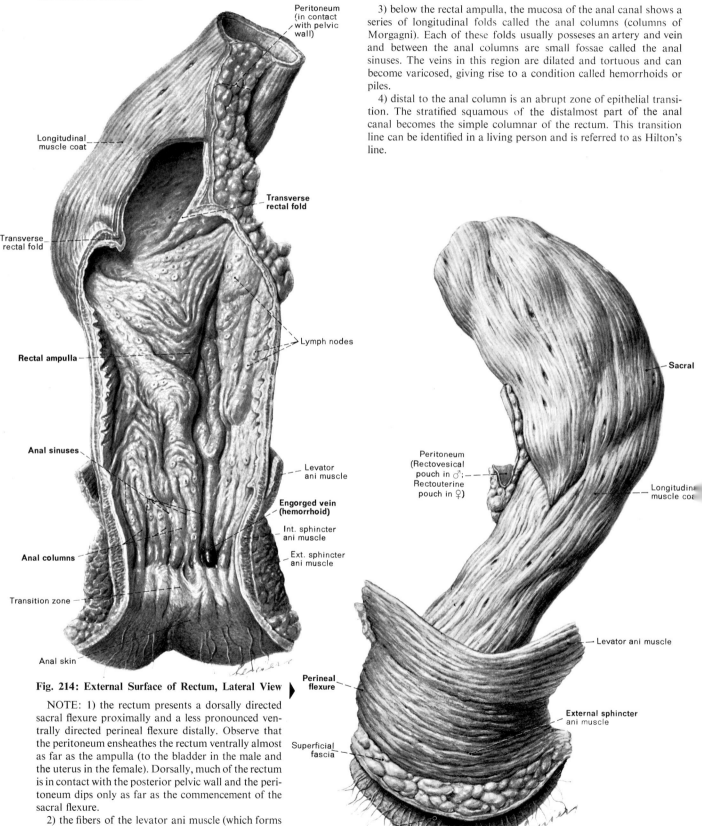

Fig. 214: External Surface of Rectum, Lateral View

NOTE: 1) the rectum presents a dorsally directed sacral flexure proximally and a less pronounced ventrally directed perineal flexure distally. Observe that the peritoneum ensheathes the rectum ventrally almost as far as the ampulla (to the bladder in the male and the uterus in the female). Dorsally, much of the rectum is in contact with the posterior pelvic wall and the peritoneum dips only as far as the commencement of the sacral flexure.

2) the fibers of the levator ani muscle (which forms the floor of the pelvis) surround the rectum and are

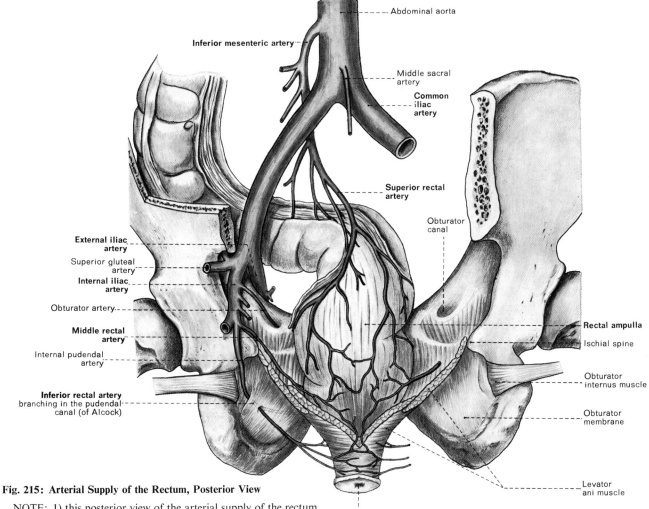

Fig. 215: **Arterial Supply of the Rectum, Posterior View**

NOTE: 1) this posterior view of the arterial supply of the rectum shows the superior rectal artery which branches from the inferior mesenteric artery and distributes to the rectum as far as the ampulla. The middle rectal artery coming off the internal iliac artery and the inferior rectal artery branching from the internal pudendal artery supply the more caudal parts of the rectum.

2) from the bifurcation of the aorta, the middle sacral artery descends down the midline of the sacrum. The common iliac arteries branch into external and internal iliac vessels. From the internal iliac (hypogastric), many of the pelvic organs derive their blood supply.

3) the internal pudendal artery coursing within the pudendal canal (of Alcock). The inferior rectal artery branches from the internal pudendal within this canal.

Fig. 216: **Distribution Pattern of the Rectal Arteries**
This figure shows the distribution of the superior, middle and inferior rectal arteries as they supply the rectum and the anal canal. Observe that the region of distribution of the superior rectal artery is much greater than either the middle or inferior rectal arteries. Note the rich anastomoses among these three vessels.

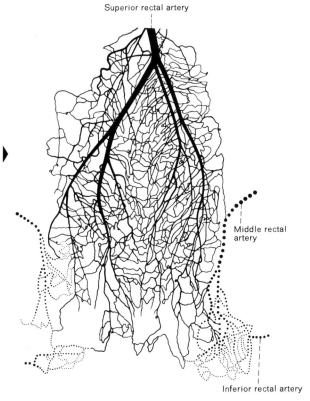

continued distally as the external sphincter ani muscle. The internal sphincter ani muscle (seen in Figure 213) is composed of smooth muscle and really represents a thickening of inner circular muscle layer of the wall of the rectum. Observe also the outer longitudinal (smooth) muscle layer.

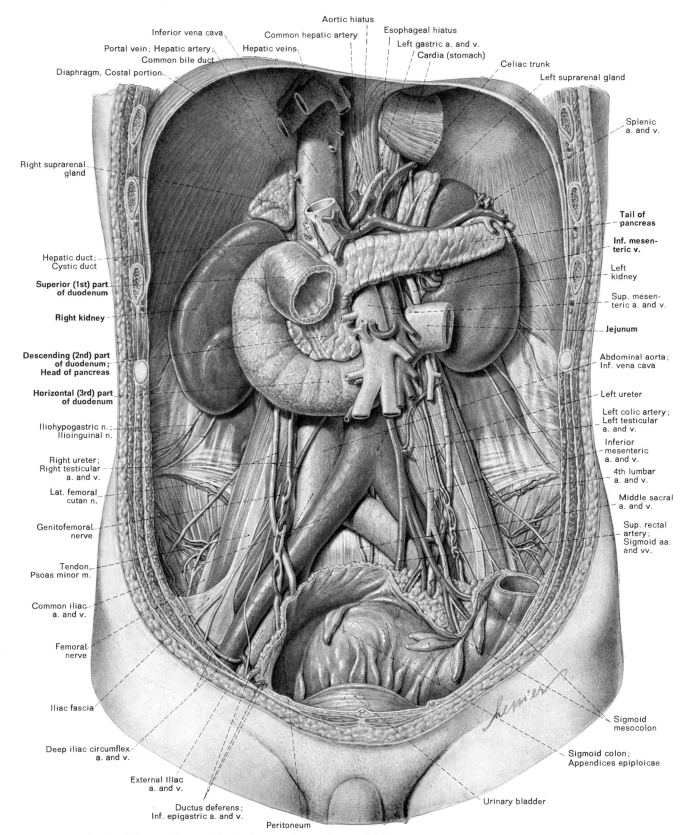

Inferior vena cava
Portal vein; Hepatic artery;
Common bile duct
Diaphragm, Costal portion

Common hepatic artery
Hepatic veins

Aortic hiatus
Esophageal hiatus
Left gastric a. and v.
Cardia (stomach)
Celiac trunk
Left suprarenal gland

Right suprarenal gland

Splenic a. and v.

Hepatic duct; Cystic duct
Superior (1st) part of duodenum
Right kidney
Descending (2nd) part of duodenum; Head of pancreas
Horizontal (3rd) part of duodenum
Iliohypogastric n.; Ilioinguinal n.
Right ureter; Right testicular a. and v.
Lat. femoral cutan n.
Genitofemoral nerve
Tendon, Psoas minor m.
Common iliac a. and v.
Femoral nerve
Iliac fascia
Deep iliac circumflex a. and v.
External Iliac a. and v.
Ductus deferens; Inf. epigastric a. and v.
Peritoneum

Tail of pancreas
Inf. mesenteric v.
Left kidney
Sup. mesenteric a. and v.
Jejunum
Abdominal aorta; Inf. vena cava
Left ureter
Left colic artery; Left testicular a. and v.
Inferior mesenteric a. and v.
4th lumbar a. and v.
Middle sacral a. and v.
Sup. rectal artery; Sigmoid aa. and vv.
Sigmoid mesocolon
Sigmoid colon; Appendices epiploicae
Urinary bladder

Fig. 217: The Abdominal Cavity (11): The Retroperitoneal Organs (Male)

NOTE: 1) that the curvature of the duodenum lies ventral to the hilum of the right kidney while the duodenojejunal junction is situated ventral to the lower medial border of the left kidney. Observe that the right kidney is slightly lower than the left.

2) the head of the pancreas lies ventral to the inferior vena cava and within the curve of the duodenum. A small extension of the head of the pancreas, the uncinate process, projects posterior to the superior mesenteric vessels. Upon crossing the midline at the level of the 1st lumbar vertebra, the posterior surface of the body and tail of the pancreas is in contact with the middle third of the left kidney.

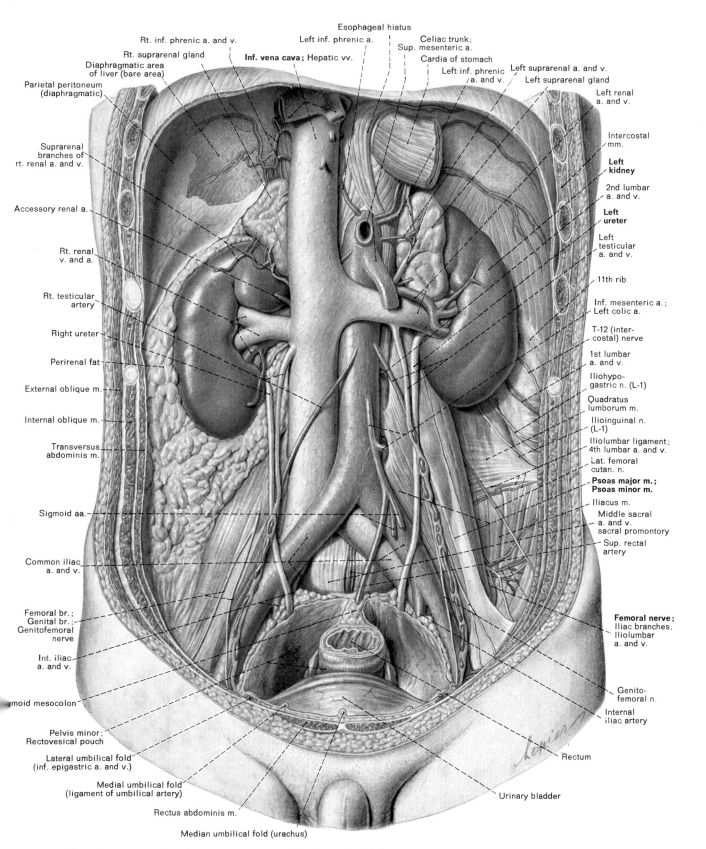

Rt. inf. phrenic a. and v.
Rt. suprarenal gland
Diaphragmatic area
of liver (bare area)
Parietal peritoneum
(diaphragmatic)

Suprarenal
branches of
rt. renal a. and v.

Accessory renal a.

Rt. renal
v. and a.

Rt. testicular
artery

Right ureter

Perirenal fat

External oblique m.

Internal oblique m.

Transversus
abdominis m.

Sigmoid aa.

Common iliac
a. and v.

Femoral br.;
Genital br.;
Genitofemoral
nerve

Int. iliac
a. and v.

ʃmoid mesocolon

Pelvis minor;
Rectovesical pouch

Lateral umbilical fold
(inf. epigastric a. and v.)

Medial umbilical fold
(ligament of umbilical artery)

Rectus abdominis m.

Median umbilical fold (urachus)

Esophageal hiatus
Left inf. phrenic a.
Inf. vena cava; Hepatic vv.

Celiac trunk;
Sup. mesenteric a.
Cardia of stomach
Left inf. phrenic
a. and v.
Left suprarenal a. and v.
Left suprarenal gland

Left renal
a. and v.

Intercostal
mm.

Left
kidney

2nd lumbar
a. and v.

Left
ureter

Left
testicular
a. and v.

11th rib

Inf. mesenteric a.;
Left colic a.

T-12 (inter-
costal) nerve

1st lumbar
a. and v.

Iliohypo-
gastric n. (L-1)

Quadratus
lumborum m.

Ilioinguinal n.
(L-1)

Iliolumbar ligament;
4th lumbar a. and v.

Lat. femoral
cutan. n.

Psoas major m.;
Psoas minor m.

Iliacus m.

Middle sacral
a. and v.
sacral promontory

Sup. rectal
artery

Femoral nerve;
Iliac branches,
Iliolumbar
a. and v.

Genito-
femoral n.

Internal
iliac artery

Rectum

Urinary bladder

Fig. 218: The Abdominal Cavity (12): The Posterior Abdominal Wall

NOTE: 1) the kidneys, ureters, suprarenal glands, and the great vessels and their branches. The kidneys extend between vertebral levels T-12 and L-3. The ureters commence on the posterior aspect of the hilum of the kidneys, course inferiorly over the pelvic brim near the bifurcation of the common iliac arteries, eventually to terminate in the bladder.

2) the suprarenal glands as they cap the upper pole of each kidney. These are highly vascular and vital glands of internal secretion (endocrine).

3) the aorta which enters the abdomen through the aortic hiatus (T-12). The inferior vena cava lies to the right of the vertebral column. It is formed by the confluence of the two common iliac veins (at about L-5) and passes through the caval opening of the diaphragm.

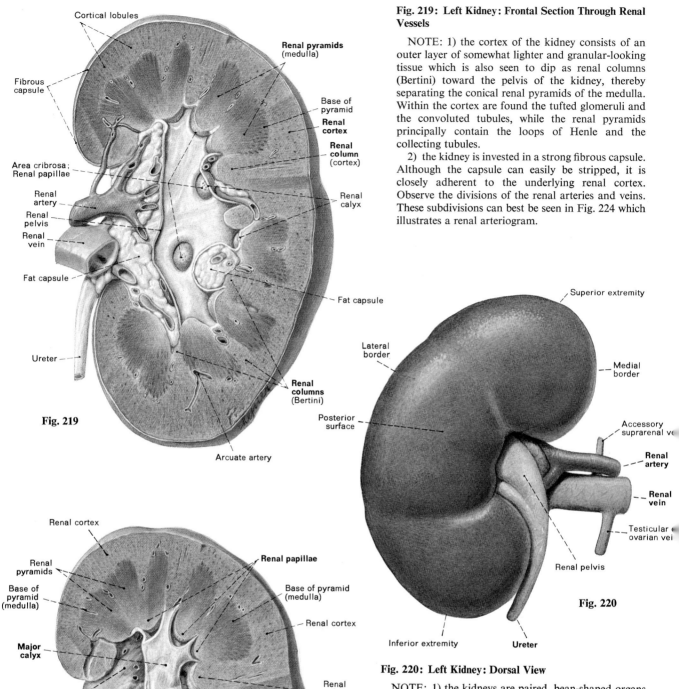

Cortical lobules

Renal pyramids
(medulla)

Fibrous
capsule

Base of
pyramid
**Renal
cortex**

**Renal
column**
(cortex)

Area cribrosa;
Renal papillae

Renal
calyx

Renal
artery

Renal
pelvis

Renal
vein

Fat capsule

Fat capsule

Ureter

**Renal
columns**
(Bertini)

Fig. 219

Arcuate artery

Fig. 219: Left Kidney: Frontal Section Through Renal Vessels

NOTE: 1) the cortex of the kidney consists of an outer layer of somewhat lighter and granular-looking tissue which is also seen to dip as renal columns (Bertini) toward the pelvis of the kidney, thereby separating the conical renal pyramids of the medulla. Within the cortex are found the tufted glomeruli and the convoluted tubules, while the renal pyramids principally contain the loops of Henle and the collecting tubules.

2) the kidney is invested in a strong fibrous capsule. Although the capsule can easily be stripped, it is closely adherent to the underlying renal cortex. Observe the divisions of the renal arteries and veins. These subdivisions can best be seen in Fig. 224 which illustrates a renal arteriogram.

Superior extremity

Lateral
border

Medial
border

Accessory
suprarenal ve

**Renal
artery**

**Renal
vein**

Posterior
surface

Testicular
ovarian vei

Renal pelvis

Fig. 220

Inferior extremity

Ureter

Fig. 220: Left Kidney: Dorsal View

NOTE: 1) the kidneys are paired, bean-shaped organs and normally weigh about 125 to 150 grams each. Their lateral borders are convex and their medial borders concave, the latter being interrupted by the renal vessels and the ureter.

2) that the ureter is the most posterior structure at the hilum. Generally the renal vein is the most anterior structure at the hilum. The renal artery frequently divides into anterior and posterior branches, however, this is variable.

Renal cortex

Renal papillae

Renal
pyramids

Base of pyramid
(medulla)

Base of
pyramid
(medulla)

Renal cortex

**Major
calyx**

Renal
columns
(Bertini)

**Renal
sinus**

**Renal
pelvis**

**Major
calyx**

**Minor
calyces**

Renal
pyramids

Ureter

Renal
pyramid
(medulla)

Fig. 221

Renal columns

Renal cortex

Fig. 221: Left Kidney: Frontal Section Through Renal Pelvis

NOTE: that this frontal section cuts through the renal pelvis and ureter. Observe that the renal papillae are cupped by small collecting tubes, the minor calyces. Several minor calyces unite to form a major calyx while the renal pelvis is formed by the union of two or three major calyces. Leading from the renal pelvis is the somewhat more narrowed ureter.

Fig. 222: Retrograde Pyelogram

NOTE: 1) a radioopaque substance has been introduced into each ureter and forced in a retrograde manner into the renal pelvis, major calyces and minor calyces of each side. Observe that into the minor calyces project the renal papillae (5), resulting in radiolucent invaginations into the radioopaque minor calyces.

2) the shadow of the superior extremity of the left kidney extending to the top of the body of the T-12 vertebra, while the right kidney is somewhat more inferior.

3) the lateral margins of the psoas major muscles. The ureters course toward the pelvis along the anterior surfaces of these muscles.

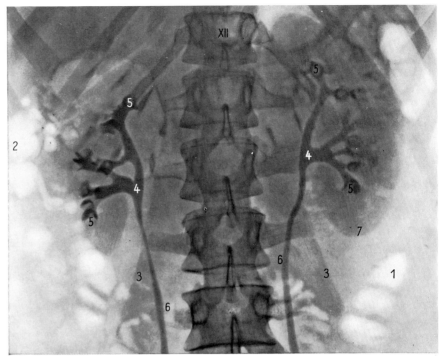

1 Descending colon	3 Psoas major muscle	5 Renal papilla	7 Inferior pole of
2 Ascending colon	(lateral border)	6 Ureter	left kidney
	4 Renal pelvis		XII 12th thoracic vertebra

Fig. 223: Left Kidney: Ventral View

NOTE: 1) although the stem of the renal artery initially lies dorsal to the stem of the renal vein at the hilum, the renal artery divides into anterior and posterior branches. The anterior branch generally enters the kidney ventral to the renal vein as is shown in this figure.

2) the anterior surfaces of the kidneys are covered by peritoneum and are in relationship to more ventrally located abdominal organs. In contrast, their posterior surfaces lie adjacent to the musculature of the posterior abdominal wall and the diaphragm.

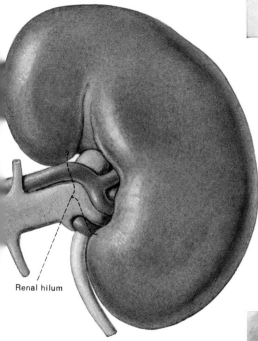

Renal hilum

1 Stomach	3 Right renal artery	5 Interlobular arteries	XII 12th thoracic
2 Superior (1st) part	4 Interlobar arteries	K Catheter	vertebra
of duodenum			

Fig. 224: Arteriogram of Right Renal Artery and its Branches

NOTE: 1) an arterial catheter (K) has been inserted into the femoral artery, passed through the abdominal aorta and into the right renal artery. Observe the division of the renal artery successively into interlobar arteries (4).

2) as the interlobar arteries reach the junction of the renal cortex and medulla, they arch over the bases of the pyramids forming the arcuate arteries (not numbered in this figure). From the arcuate arteries branch a series of interlobular arteries which extend through the afferent arterioles which enter the renal glomeruli.

3) the stomach (1) and superior (1st) part of the duodenum (2) which are filled with air.

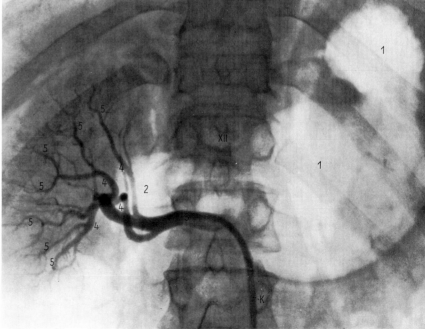

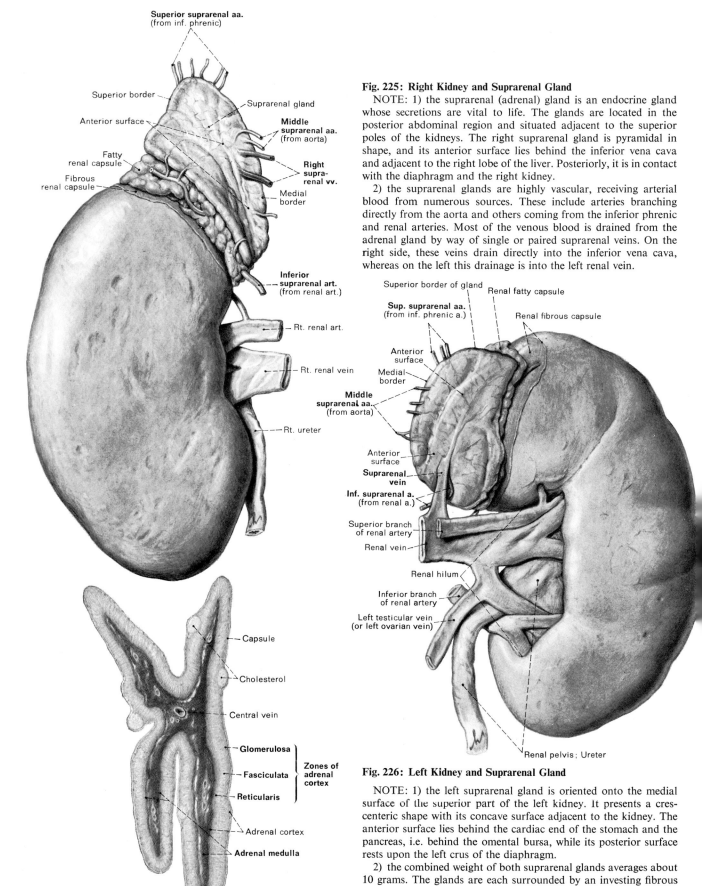

Fig. 225: Right Kidney and Suprarenal Gland

NOTE: 1) the suprarenal (adrenal) gland is an endocrine gland whose secretions are vital to life. The glands are located in the posterior abdominal region and situated adjacent to the superior poles of the kidneys. The right suprarenal gland is pyramidal in shape, and its anterior surface lies behind the inferior vena cava and adjacent to the right lobe of the liver. Posteriorly, it is in contact with the diaphragm and the right kidney.

2) the suprarenal glands are highly vascular, receiving arterial blood from numerous sources. These include arteries branching directly from the aorta and others coming from the inferior phrenic and renal arteries. Most of the venous blood is drained from the adrenal gland by way of single or paired suprarenal veins. On the right side, these veins drain directly into the inferior vena cava, whereas on the left this drainage is into the left renal vein.

Fig. 226: Left Kidney and Suprarenal Gland

NOTE: 1) the left suprarenal gland is oriented onto the medial surface of the superior part of the left kidney. It presents a crescenteric shape with its concave surface adjacent to the kidney. The anterior surface lies behind the cardiac end of the stomach and the pancreas, i.e. behind the omental bursa, while its posterior surface rests upon the left crus of the diaphragm.

2) the combined weight of both suprarenal glands averages about 10 grams. The glands are each surrounded by an investing fibrous capsule around which is a variable amount of areolar tissue.

Fig. 227: Section Through Suprarenal Gland

Note that the suprarenal gland is composed of an inner medulla and outer cortex. The cells of the medulla secrete epinephrine while the adrenal cortex secretes adrenal corticosteroids.

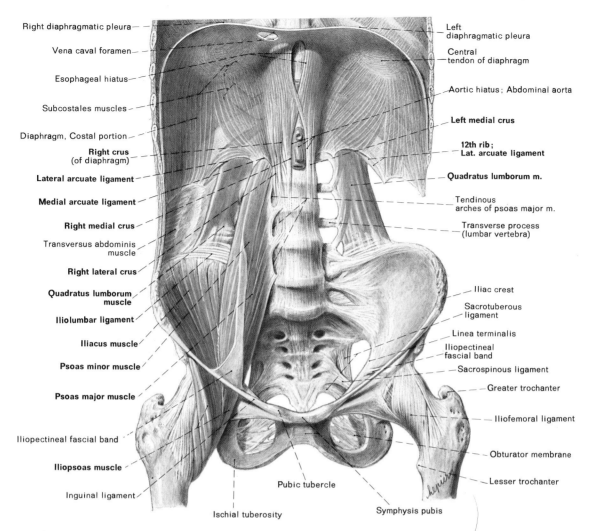

Right diaphragmatic pleura
Vena caval foramen
Esophageal hiatus
Subcostales muscles
Diaphragm, Costal portion
Right crus (of diaphragm)
Lateral arcuate ligament
Medial arcuate ligament
Right medial crus
Transversus abdominis muscle
Right lateral crus
Quadratus lumborum muscle
Iliolumbar ligament
Iliacus muscle
Psoas minor muscle
Psoas major muscle
Iliopectineal fascial band
Iliopsoas muscle
Inguinal ligament

Left diaphragmatic pleura
Central tendon of diaphragm
Aortic hiatus; Abdominal aorta
Left medial crus
12th rib; Lat. arcuate ligament
Quadratus lumborum m.
Tendinous arches of psoas major m.
Transverse process (lumbar vertebra)
Iliac crest
Sacrotuberous ligament
Linea terminalis
Iliopectineal fascial band
Sacrospinous ligament
Greater trochanter
Iliofemoral ligament
Obturator membrane
Lesser trochanter

Ischial tuberosity
Pubic tubercle
Symphysis pubis

Fig. 228: The Diaphragm and Posterior Abdominal Wall Muscles

NOTE: 1) the posterior attachments of the diaphragm include a) the right and left crura which arise from the anterior and lateral aspects of the bodies of the upper 3 or 4 lumbar vertebrae, b) the right and left medial arcuate ligaments which are thickenings in the psoas fascia, and c) the lateral arcuate ligaments along the 12th rib overlying the quadratus lumborum muscle.

2) the psoas major and minor muscles descending from the lumbar vertebrae to join the iliacus in the lateral wall of the pelvis to insert onto the lesser trochanter of the femur. The iliopsoas is the most powerful flexor of the thigh at the hip joint.

3) the rectangular quadratus lumborum intervening between the 12th rib, the transverse processes of the lumbar vertebrae and the posteromedial iliac crest.

Fig. 229: Posterior View of Diaphragm

NOTE: 1) the posterior half of the bony thorax (ribs and vertebral column) has been removed to reveal the diaphragm from behind. Observe that the caval opening is to the right of midline and more superior to those transmitting the esophagus and aorta.

2) that from their origin around the thoracic outlet, the muscular fibers of the diaphragm converge to insert into a central tendon. Observe the dome-shape of the diaphragm on each side and that the right dome extends more superiorly into the thoracic cavity because of the large right lobe of the liver.

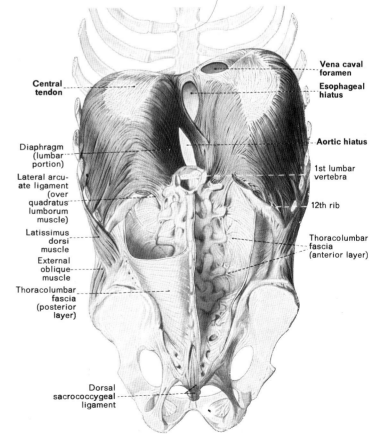

Central tendon
Vena caval foramen
Esophageal hiatus
Aortic hiatus
Diaphragm (lumbar portion)
1st lumbar vertebra
Lateral arcuate ligament (over quadratus lumborum muscle)
12th rib
Latissimus dorsi muscle
Thoracolumbar fascia (anterior layer)
External oblique muscle
Thoracolumbar fascia (posterior layer)
Dorsal sacrococcygeal ligament

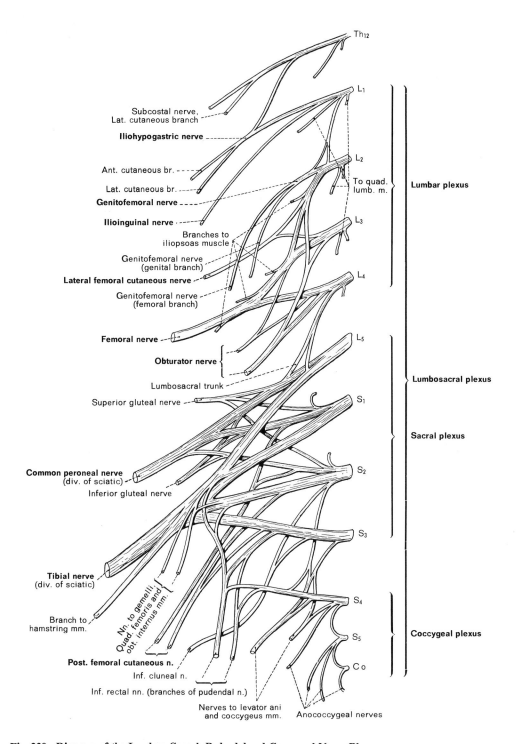

Fig. 230: Diagram of the Lumbar, Sacral, Pudendal and Coccygeal Nerve Plexuses

NOTE: 1) the 12th thoracic (subcostal) and 1st lumbar nerves are distributed principally to the lower abdominal wall. The anterior rami of the remaining segmental nerves of the lumbosacral plexus innervate the muscles and skin of the pelvis, perineum and lower extremity. L_1 divides into the iliohypogastric and ilioinguinal nerves.

2) L_2, L_3 and L_4 are the principal segments forming the lumbar plexus. L_1 contributes some fibers to the genitofemoral nerve. The main peripheral nerves derived from these segments include:

a) the genitofemoral nerve (L_1, L_2) c) the obturator nerve (L_2, L_3, L_4)
b) the lateral femoral cutaneous nerve (L_2, L_3) d) femoral nerve (L_2, L_3, L_4)

3) L_5, S_1, S_2 and S_3 with some contribution from L_4 form the sacral plexus. The principal peripheral nerves derived from these segments include:

a) the superior gluteal nerve (L_4, L_5, S_1) c) the sciatic nerve $\begin{cases} \text{common peroneal nerve } (L_4, L_5, S_1, S_2) \\ \text{tibial nerve} \hspace{2.5em} (L_4, L_5, S_1, S_2, S_3) \end{cases}$
b) the inferior gluteal nerve (L_5, S_1, S_2)

                                                  d) the posterior femoral cutaneous nerve (S_1, S_2, S_3)

4) S_2, S_3 and S_4 also contribute to the pudendal plexus while S_4, S_5 and the coccygeal nerve form fine nerve filaments which innervate the skin of the anococcygeal region. The pudendal nerve is the main sensory and motor nerve of the perineum. Other sensory (inferior cluneal) and motor (nerve to levator ani and coccygeus muscles) branches of the pudendal plexus also come from sacral segments.

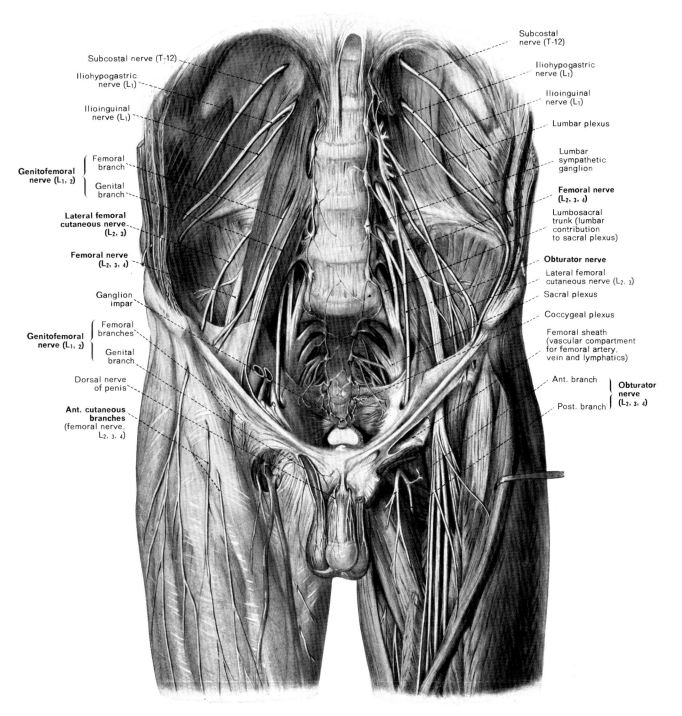

Subcostal nerve (T-12)

Iliohypogastric nerve (L₁)

Ilioinguinal nerve (L₁)

Genitofemoral nerve (L₁, ₂) { Femoral branch / Genital branch }

Lateral femoral cutaneous nerve (L₂, ₃)

Femoral nerve (L₂, ₃, ₄)

Ganglion impar

Genitofemoral nerve (L₁, ₂) { Femoral branches / Genital branch }

Dorsal nerve of penis

Ant. cutaneous branches (femoral nerve, L₂, ₃, ₄)

Subcostal nerve (T-12)

Iliohypogastric nerve (L₁)

Ilioinguinal nerve (L₁)

Lumbar plexus

Lumbar sympathetic ganglion

Femoral nerve (L₂, ₃, ₄)

Lumbosacral trunk (lumbar contribution to sacral plexus)

Obturator nerve

Lateral femoral cutaneous nerve (L₂, ₃)

Sacral plexus

Coccygeal plexus

Femoral sheath (vascular compartment for femoral artery, vein and lymphatics)

Ant. branch / Post. branch } **Obturator nerve (L₂, ₃, ₄)**

Fig. 231: The Lumbosacral Plexus: Posterior Abdominal Wall and Anterior Thigh

NOTE: 1) on the left side, the psoas major and minor muscles have been removed in order to reveal the plexus of lumbar nerves more completely. As can be seen on the right side, these nerves emerge from the spinal cord and descend along the posterior abdominal wall within the substance of the psoas muscles. Observe that the 12th thoracic nerve (subcostal nerve) courses around the abdominal wall below the 12th rib.

2) the 1st lumbar nerve divides into an iliohypogastric and an ilioinguinal branch. The ilioinguinal nerve descends obliquely toward the iliac crest, penetrates through the transversus and internal oblique muscles to join the spermatic cord, becoming cutaneous at the superficial inguinal ring.

3) the genitofemoral nerve can be found coursing superficially on the surface of the psoas major muscle. It divides into a genital branch (which innervates the cremaster muscle and the skin of the scrotum) and a femoral branch (which is sensory to the upper anterior thigh.)

4) the femoral and obturator nerves. These nerves are derived from L_2, L_3 and L_4 and descend to innervate the anterior and medial groups of femoral muscles, respectively. The femoral nerve enters the thigh beneath the inguinal ligament, dividing into both motor and sensory branches, whereas the obturator nerve courses more medially through the obturator foramen to become the principal nerve of the adductor muscle group.

5) L_4 and L_5 nerve roots (lumbosacral trunk) join with the upper three sacral nerves to form the sacral plexus. From most of this plexus is derived the large sciatic nerve which leaves the pelvis through the greater sciatic foramen to achieve the gluteal region and the posterior aspect of the lower limb.

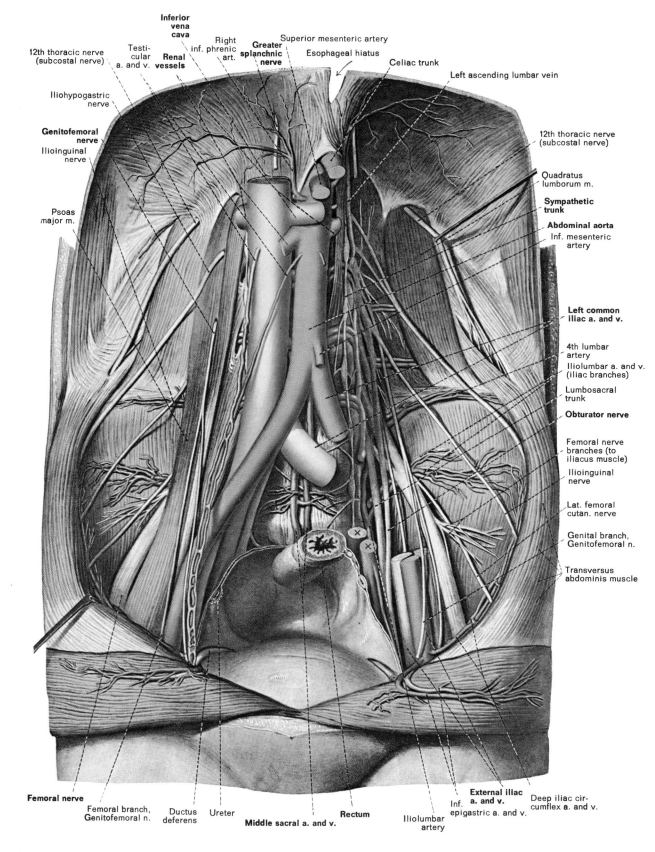

Fig. 232: The Posterior Abdominal Vessels and Nerves

NOTE: 1) the abdominal viscera have been removed as well as the psoas muscles on the left side. Observe the greater splanchnic nerves as they pierce the diaphragmatic crura to enter the abdomen. Also note the inferior phrenic arteries nearby. Identify the abdominal sympathetic chain of ganglia situated anterolaterally on the vertebral column.

2) the testicular arteries arising from the aorta just below the renal arteries. Inferiorly, the testicular artery and vein join the ductus deferens to enter the abdominal inguinal ring just lateral to the inferior epigastric vessels. Observe the middle sacral vessels descending into the pelvis in the midline. The middle sacral artery originates from the aorta at its bifurcation, whereas the vein usually drains into the left common iliac vein.

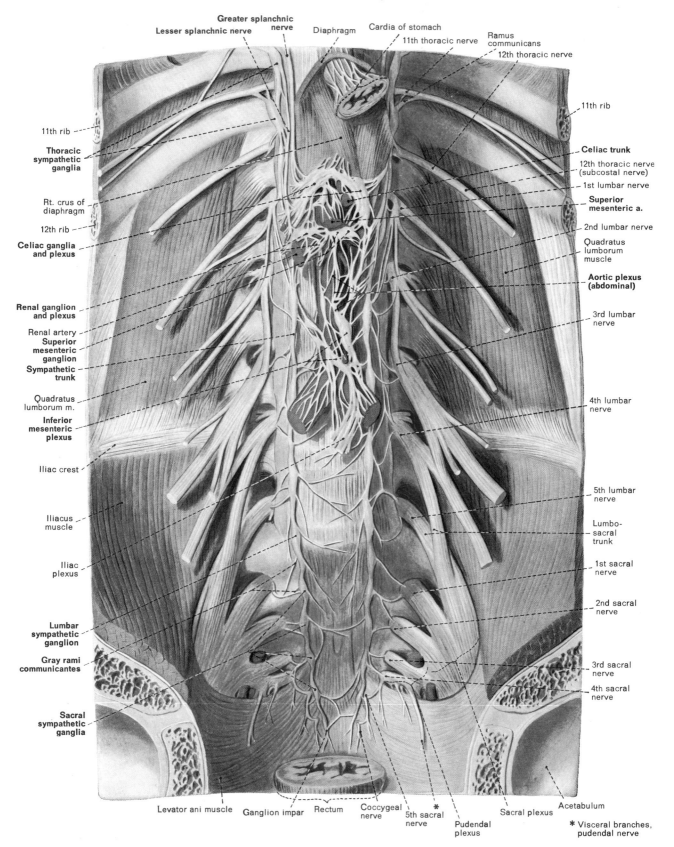

Greater splanchnic nerve
Lesser splanchnic nerve
Diaphragm
Cardia of stomach
11th thoracic nerve
Ramus communicans
12th thoracic nerve

11th rib
Thoracic sympathetic ganglia

Rt. crus of diaphragm
12th rib
Celiac ganglia and plexus

Renal ganglion and plexus
Renal artery
Superior mesenteric ganglion
Sympathetic trunk

Quadratus lumborum m.
Inferior mesenteric plexus

Iliac crest

Iliacus muscle

Iliac plexus

Lumbar sympathetic ganglion

Gray rami communicantes

Sacral sympathetic ganglia

11th rib
Celiac trunk
12th thoracic nerve (subcostal nerve)
1st lumbar nerve
Superior mesenteric a.
2nd lumbar nerve
Quadratus lumborum muscle
Aortic plexus (abdominal)
3rd lumbar nerve
4th lumbar nerve
5th lumbar nerve
Lumbo-sacral trunk
1st sacral nerve
2nd sacral nerve
3rd sacral nerve
4th sacral nerve
Acetabulum

Levator ani muscle
Ganglion impar
Rectum
Coccygeal nerve
5th sacral nerve
*
Pudendal plexus
Sacral plexus
* Visceral branches, pudendal nerve

Fig. 233: Lumbar Sympathetic Trunk and Abdominal Autonomic Ganglia

NOTE: 1) in addition to the two sympathetic chains of ganglia descending from the thorax through the abdomen and into the pelvis, the plexuses and their associated ganglia which overlie the major arteries branching from the aorta. Thus, the celiac plexuses along with the superior mesenteric, inferior mesenteric, renal, aortic and iliac plexuses form a dense network of autonomic fibers from which many of the abdominal and pelvic viscera receive sympathetic innervation.

2) the splanchnic nerves (containing preganglionic sympathetic fibers) as they join the upper abdominal ganglia where many of their fibers synapse with postganglionic sympathetic neurons.

3) that below L-2 only gray rami communicantes connect the ganglia of the sympathetic chain to the segmental nerves, since at these lower levels the rami consist only of postganglionic sympathetic fibers.

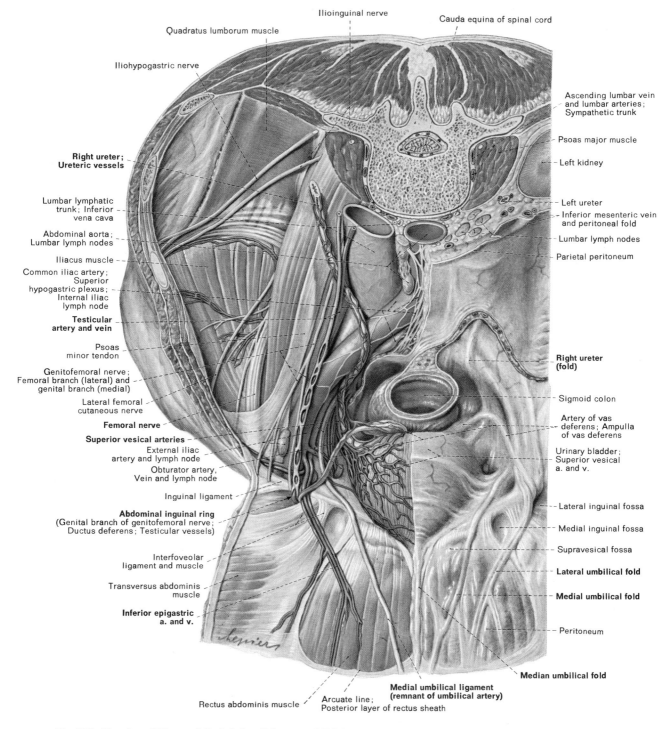

Quadratus lumborum muscle

Iliohypogastric nerve

Ilioinguinal nerve

Cauda equina of spinal cord

Ascending lumbar vein
and lumbar arteries;
Sympathetic trunk

Psoas major muscle

Left kidney

Left ureter

Inferior mesenteric vein
and peritoneal fold

Lumbar lymph nodes

Parietal peritoneum

**Right ureter;
Ureteric vessels**

Lumbar lymphatic
trunk; Inferior
vena cava

Abdominal aorta;
Lumbar lymph nodes

Iliacus muscle

Common iliac artery;
Superior
hypogastric plexus;
Internal iliac
lymph node

**Testicular
artery and vein**

Psoas
minor tendon

Genitofemoral nerve;
Femoral branch (lateral) and
genital branch (medial)

Lateral femoral
cutaneous nerve

Femoral nerve

Superior vesical arteries

External iliac
artery and lymph node

Obturator artery,
Vein and lymph node

Inguinal ligament

Abdominal inguinal ring
(Genital branch of genitofemoral nerve;
Ductus deferens; Testicular vessels)

Interfoveolar
ligament and muscle

Transversus abdominis
muscle

**Inferior epigastric
a. and v.**

**Right ureter
(fold)**

Sigmoid colon

Artery of vas
deferens; Ampulla
of vas deferens

Urinary bladder;
Superior vesical
a. and v.

Lateral inguinal fossa

Medial inguinal fossa

Supravesical fossa

Lateral umbilical fold

Medial umbilical fold

Peritoneum

Median umbilical fold

Rectus abdominis muscle

Arcuate line;
Posterior layer of rectus sheath

**Medial umbilical ligament
(remnant of umbilical artery)**

Fig. 234: Vessels and Nerves of the Inferior Abdomen and Pelvis

NOTE: 1) the anterior abdominal wall has been incised vertically on both sides and reflected inferiorly, thereby exposing its inner (posterior) surface. The body has been transected through the lumbar region at the caudal end of the 3rd lumbar vertebra. On the right side, the peritoneum investing the abdominal cavity has been stripped away whereas on the left it has been left intact.

2) this dissection reveals the intact male pelvic viscera viewed from above. Observe the course of the ureters as they cross the pelvic brim anterior to the common iliac arteries. Within the pelvis, the ureter curves medially toward the bladder. At the lateral angle of the bladder, the ductus deferens on its path to the seminal vesicle courses ventral to the ureter.

3) the convergence of the testicular vessels, ductus deferens and genital branch of the genitofemoral nerve (innervation of cremaster muscle) at the abdominal inguinal ring to form the spermatic cord of the inguinal canal.

4) the origins within the pelvis of the umbilical ligaments of the anterior abdominal wall: a) the median umbilical fold extending from the bladder to the umbilicus (urachus), b) the medial umbilical fold formed by a peritoneal reflection over the obliterated umbilical artery, and c) the lateral umbilical fold formed by peritoneum covering the inferior epigastric vessels.

5) the superior hypogastric plexus or presacral nerve lying anterior to the bifurcation of the aorta and descending behind the peritoneum into the pelvis.

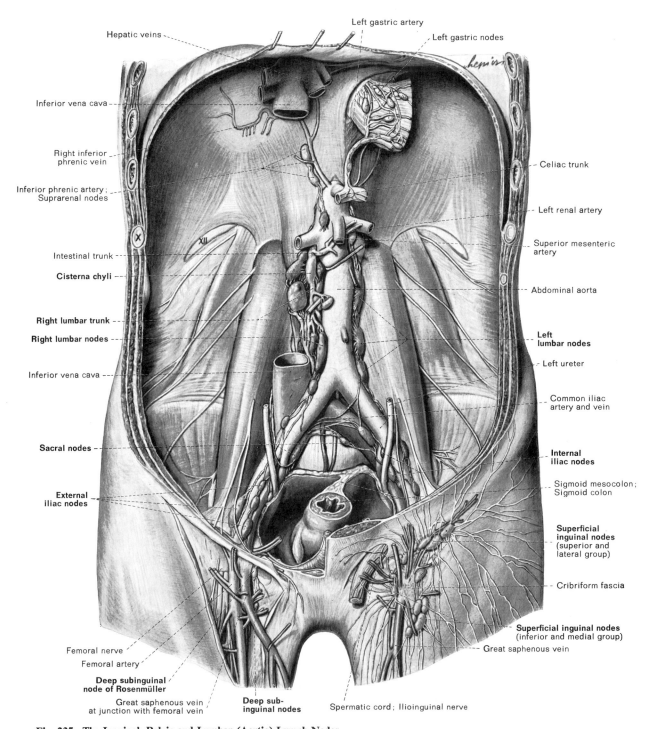

Left gastric artery

Hepatic veins

Left gastric nodes

Inferior vena cava

Celiac trunk

Right inferior phrenic vein

Left renal artery

Inferior phrenic artery; Suprarenal nodes

Superior mesenteric artery

Intestinal trunk

Abdominal aorta

Cisterna chyli

Right lumbar trunk

Left lumbar nodes

Right lumbar nodes

Left ureter

Inferior vena cava

Common iliac artery and vein

Sacral nodes

Internal iliac nodes

Sigmoid mesocolon; Sigmoid colon

External iliac nodes

Superficial inguinal nodes (superior and lateral group)

Cribriform fascia

Superficial inguinal nodes (inferior and medial group)

Great saphenous vein

Femoral nerve

Femoral artery

Deep subinguinal node of Rosenmüller

Great saphenous vein at junction with femoral vein

Deep sub-inguinal nodes

Spermatic cord; Ilioinguinal nerve

Fig. 235: The Inguinal, Pelvic and Lumbar (Aortic) Lymph Nodes

NOTE: 1) chains of lymph nodes from the inguinal region to the diaphragm lie along the paths of the major blood vessels. In the inguinal region, the superficial inguinal lymph nodes lie just distal to the inguinal ligament and in the subcutaneous superficial fascia. They range from 10 to 20 in number and receive drainage from the genitalia, perineum, gluteal region and the anterior abdominal wall. More deeply, the subinguinal nodes receive drainage from the lower extremity. One of the deep subinguinal nodes (node of Rosenmüller or Cloquet) lies in the femoral ring.

2) within the pelvis and abdomen, visceral lymph nodes lie close to the organs which they drain. These visceral nodes then channel lymph through chains of parietal nodes which generally are located along the paths of the major arteries and veins. Thus, external iliac, internal iliac (hypogastric) and common iliac nodes are located in proximity to these vessels in the pelvis.

3) along the posterior abdominal wall are found right and left lumbar chains which course along the sides of the abdominal aorta. Other groups of nodes, the preaortic, are arranged along the roots of the major unpaired branches of the aorta, forming the celiac and superior and inferior mesenteric node chains.

4) at about the level of the 2nd lumbar vertebra there is a confluence of lymph channels which forms a dilated sac, the cisterna chyli. This is located somewhat posterior and to the right of the aorta and marks the commencement of the thoracic duct.

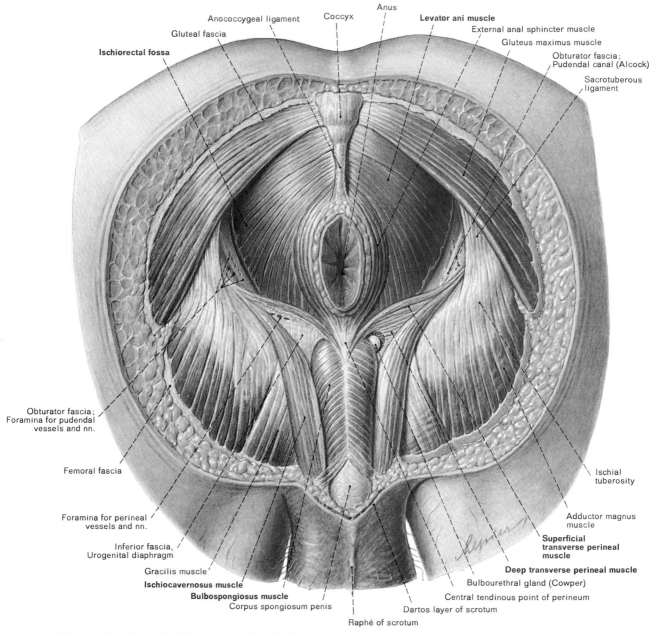

Anococcygeal ligament
Coccyx
Anus
Levator ani muscle
External anal sphincter muscle
Gluteus maximus muscle
Gluteal fascia
Ischiorectal fossa
Obturator fascia;
Pudendal canal (Alcock)
Sacrotuberous ligament

Obturator fascia;
Foramina for pudendal vessels and nn.
Femoral fascia
Foramina for perineal vessels and nn.
Inferior fascia, Urogenital diaphragm
Gracilis muscle
Ischiocavernosus muscle
Bulbospongiosus muscle
Corpus spongiosum penis
Raphé of scrotum
Dartos layer of scrotum
Central tendinous point of perineum
Bulbourethral gland (Cowper)
Deep transverse perineal muscle
Superficial transverse perineal muscle
Adductor magnus muscle
Ischial tuberosity

Fig. 236: The Superficial Muscles of the Male Perineum

Fig. 237: Diagram of Frontal Section Through Male Pelvis and Perineum

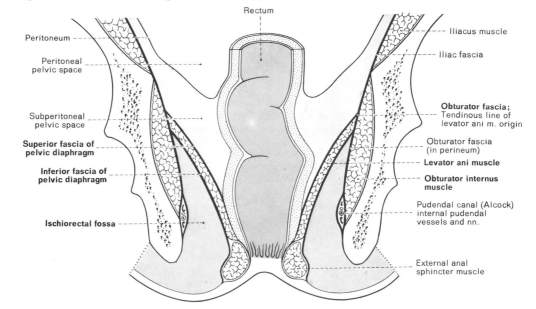

Rectum
Peritoneum
Iliacus muscle
Peritoneal pelvic space
Iliac fascia
Subperitoneal pelvic space
Obturator fascia;
Tendinous line of levator ani m. origin
Superior fascia of pelvic diaphragm
Obturator fascia (in perineum)
Inferior fascia of pelvic diaphragm
Levator ani muscle
Obturator internus muscle
Pudendal canal (Alcock) internal pudendal vessels and nn.
Ischiorectal fossa
External anal sphincter muscle

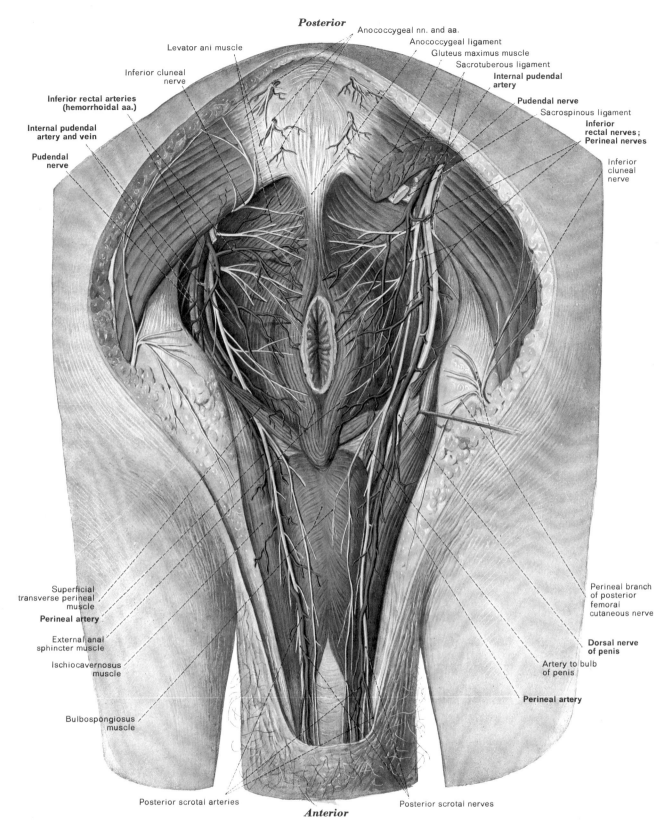

Fig. 238: Nerves and Blood Vessels of the Male Perineum

NOTE: 1) the skin of the male perineum as well as the fat of the ischiorectal fossae have been removed in order to expose the muscles, vessels and nerves of both the anal and urogenital regions of the perineum.

2) emerging from the pelvis through the lesser sciatic foramen by way of the pudendal canal (Alcock) are the internal pudendal vessels and the pudendal nerve. These structures enter the perineum at the lateral border of the ischiorectal fossa. There is an immediate branching of the inferior rectal (hemorrhoidal) vessels and nerves which course transversely across the ischiorectal fossa to supply the levator ani and external anal sphincter muscles.

3) the internal pudendal structures then continue anteriorly, pierce the urogenital diaphragm, and become the perineal vessels and nerve and the dorsal vessels and nerve of the penis. The muscles of the urogenital triangle are innervated by the perineal nerve while the dorsal nerve of the penis is the principal sensory nerve of that organ.

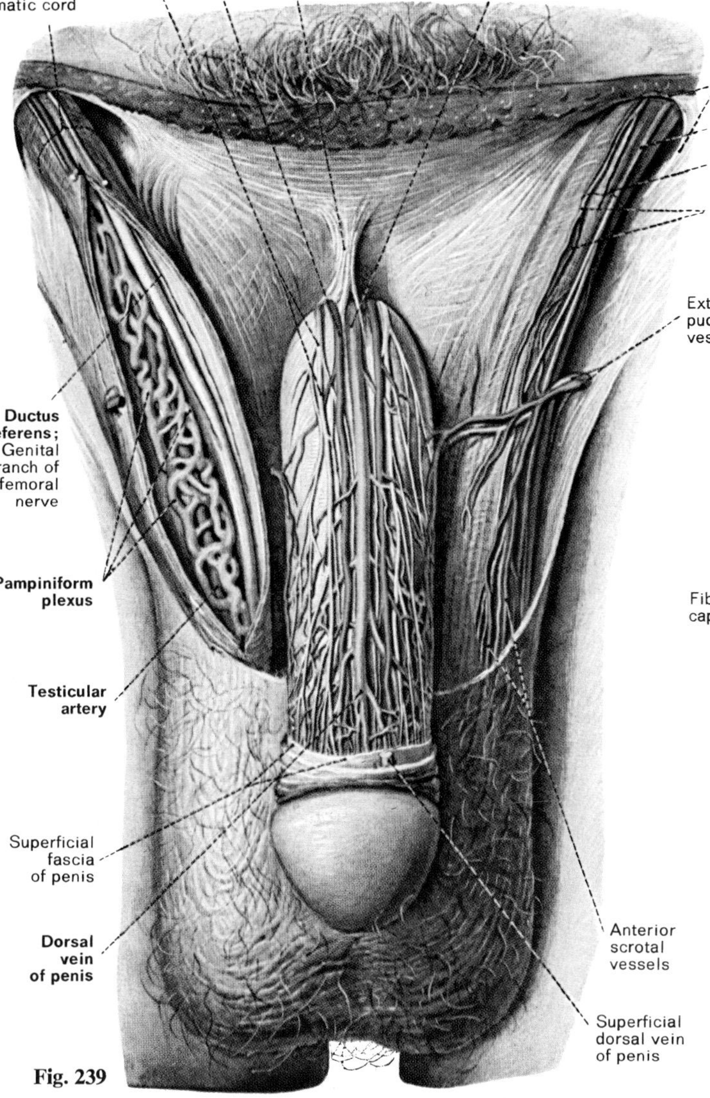

Dorsal artery of penis
Dorsal nerve of penis
Fundiform ligament of penis
Dorsal vein of penis
Spermatic cord

Superficial inguinal ring
Ilioinguinal nerve
Spermatic cord
Cremasteric art. and vein

External pudendal vessels

Ductus deferens; Genital branch of genitofemoral nerve

Pampiniform plexus

Testicular artery

Superficial fascia of penis

Dorsal vein of penis

Anterior scrotal vessels

Superficial dorsal vein of penis

Fig. 239

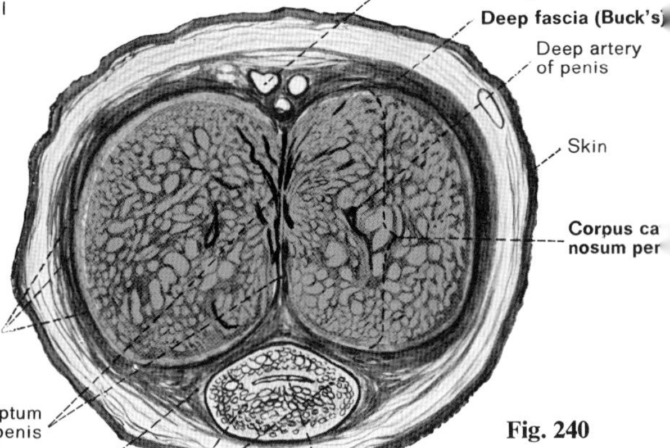

Dorsal vein of penis
Deep fascia (Buck's)
Deep artery of penis
Skin
Corpus ca nosum per

Fibrous capsule

Septum of penis

Deep fascia of penis

Corpus spongiosum penis   Penile urethra

Fig. 240

Fig. 239: Vessels and Nerves of the Penis and Spermatic cord

NOTE: 1) the skin has been removed from the anterior pubic region and the penis, revealing the superficial vessels and nerves of the penis and left spermatic cord. On the right side, the layers of the spermatic cord have been slit open in order to show the deeper structures of the cord.

2) along the surface of the spermatic cord course the ilioinguinal nerve and the cremasteric artery and vein. Within the cord is found the ductus deferens and the testicular artery surrounded by the pampiniform plexus of veins.

3) beneath the superficial fascia of the penis and in the midline courses the unpaired dorsal vein of the penis. Along the sides of the vein, note the paired dorsal arteries and nerves of the penis.

Cross Section of Penis

Fig. 240: Section Through Middle of Penis

NOTE that the penis is composed principally of two laterally situated corpora cavernosa penis containing erectile tissue and one corpus spongiosum penis placed ventrally and in the midline containing the penile portion of the urethra. These are surrounded by a closely investing layer of deep fascia. During erection, blood fills the erectile tissue (as is seen in this cross section), causing them to become rigid. This engorgement exerts pressure on the veins and maintains the erection by preventing the blood from draining back into the general circulation.

Fig. 241: Section at Neck of Glans Penis

This section is taken from the proximal part of the glans penis. Note that the corpora cavernosa penis becomes smaller distally while the corona of the glans penis is formed by the spongy tissue of the corpus spongiosum penis.

Fig. 242: Section Through Glans Penis

The expanded distal extremity of the corpus spongiosum penis is called the glans penis. At its distal end is the opening of the urethra. In the uncircumcised male, the glans penis is covered by a duplication of thin skin, the prepuce, which is attached to the glans penis ventrally by the frenulum.

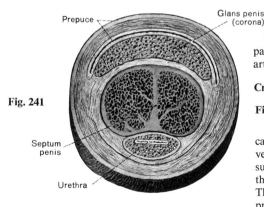

Prepuce
Glans penis (corona)

Fig. 241

Septum penis

Urethra

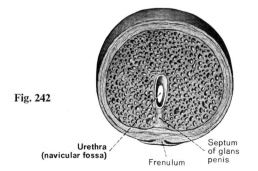

Fig. 242

Urethra (navicular fossa)
Septum of glans penis
Frenulum

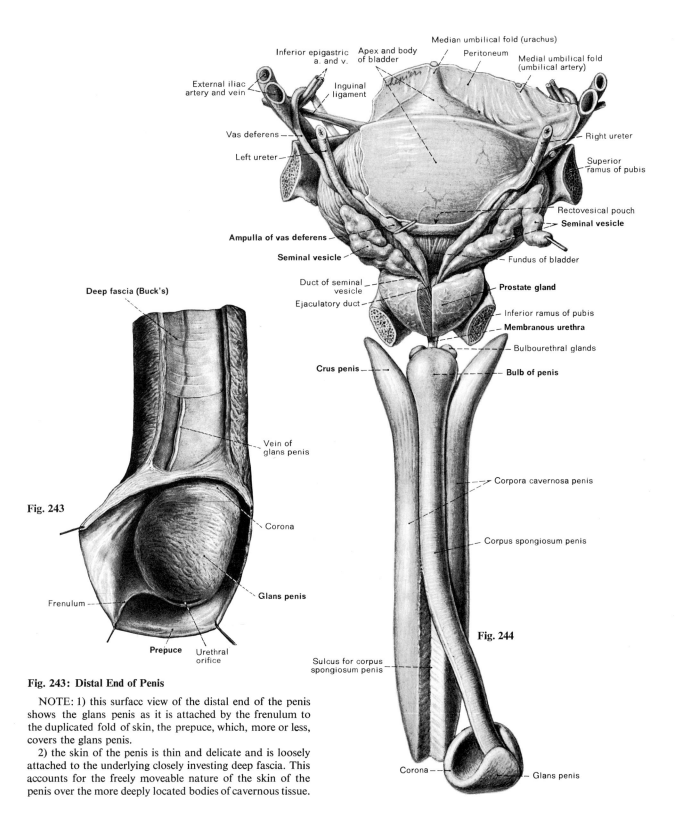

Fig. 243

Deep fascia (Buck's)

Vein of glans penis

Corona

Frenulum

Glans penis

Prepuce — Urethral orifice

Median umbilical fold (urachus)

Inferior epigastric a. and v.

Apex and body of bladder

Peritoneum

Medial umbilical fold (umbilical artery)

External iliac artery and vein

Inguinal ligament

Vas deferens

Right ureter

Left ureter

Superior ramus of pubis

Rectovesical pouch

Seminal vesicle

Ampulla of vas deferens

Seminal vesicle

Fundus of bladder

Duct of seminal vesicle

Prostate gland

Ejaculatory duct

Inferior ramus of pubis

Membranous urethra

Bulbourethral glands

Crus penis

Bulb of penis

Corpora cavernosa penis

Corpus spongiosum penis

Fig. 244

Sulcus for corpus spongiosum penis

Corona

Glans penis

Fig. 243: Distal End of Penis

NOTE: 1) this surface view of the distal end of the penis shows the glans penis as it is attached by the frenulum to the duplicated fold of skin, the prepuce, which, more or less, covers the glans penis.

2) the skin of the penis is thin and delicate and is loosely attached to the underlying closely investing deep fascia. This accounts for the freely moveable nature of the skin of the penis over the more deeply located bodies of cavernous tissue.

Fig. 244: The Erectile Bodies of the Penis Attached to the Bladder and Other Organs by the Membranous Urethra

NOTE: 1) the firmly investing deep fascia which surrounds the erectile bodies of the penis has been removed and the distal portion of the corpus spongiosum penis (which contains the penile urethra) has been displaced from its position between the two corpora cavernosa penis.

2) the posterior surface of the bladder and prostate and the associated seminal vesicles, vasa deferens, and bulbourethral glands are also demonstrated. These structures all communicate with the urethra, the membranous portion of which is in continuity with the penile urethra.

3) the tapered crura of the corpora cavernosa penis diverge laterally at their base to become adherent to the ischial and pubic rami. They are surrounded by the fibers of the ischiocavernosus muscles. The base of the corpus spongiosum penis is also expanded and is called the bulb. It is enclosed by the bulbocavernosus muscle.

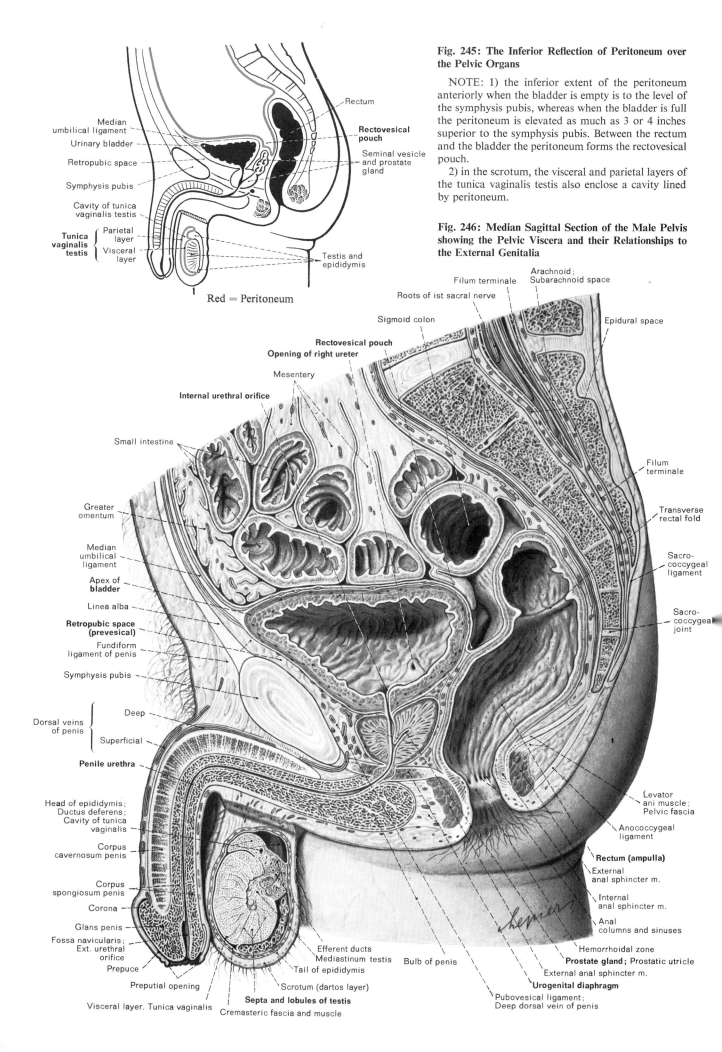

Median umbilical ligament
Urinary bladder
Retropubic space
Symphysis pubis
Cavity of tunica vaginalis testis
Tunica vaginalis testis { Parietal layer / Visceral layer

Rectum
Rectovesical pouch
Seminal vesicle and prostate gland
Testis and epididymis

Red = Peritoneum

Fig. 245: The Inferior Reflection of Peritoneum over the Pelvic Organs

NOTE: 1) the inferior extent of the peritoneum anteriorly when the bladder is empty is to the level of the symphysis pubis, whereas when the bladder is full the peritoneum is elevated as much as 3 or 4 inches superior to the symphysis pubis. Between the rectum and the bladder the peritoneum forms the rectovesical pouch.

2) in the scrotum, the visceral and parietal layers of the tunica vaginalis testis also enclose a cavity lined by peritoneum.

Fig. 246: Median Sagittal Section of the Male Pelvis showing the Pelvic Viscera and their Relationships to the External Genitalia

Filum terminale
Arachnoid; Subarachnoid space
Roots of ist sacral nerve
Epidural space
Sigmoid colon
Rectovesical pouch
Opening of right ureter
Mesentery
Internal urethral orifice
Small intestine
Filum terminale
Greater omentum
Transverse rectal fold
Median umbilical ligament
Sacro-coccygeal ligament
Apex of **bladder**
Linea alba
Sacro-coccygeal joint
Retropubic space (prevesical)
Fundiform ligament of penis
Symphysis pubis
Dorsal veins of penis { Deep / Superficial
Penile urethra
Head of epididymis; Ductus deferens; Cavity of tunica vaginalis
Levator ani muscle; Pelvic fascia
Anococcygeal ligament
Corpus cavernosum penis
Rectum (ampulla)
External anal sphincter m.
Corpus spongiosum penis
Internal anal sphincter m.
Corona
Anal columns and sinuses
Glans penis
Fossa navicularis; Ext. urethral orifice
Hemorrhoidal zone
Prepuce
Efferent ducts
Mediastinum testis
Tail of epididymis
Bulb of penis
Prostate gland; Prostatic utricle
External anal sphincter m.
Preputial opening
Scrotum (dartos layer)
Urogenital diaphragm
Visceral layer, Tunica vaginalis
Cremasteric fascia and muscle
Septa and lobules of testis
Pubovesical ligament; Deep dorsal vein of penis

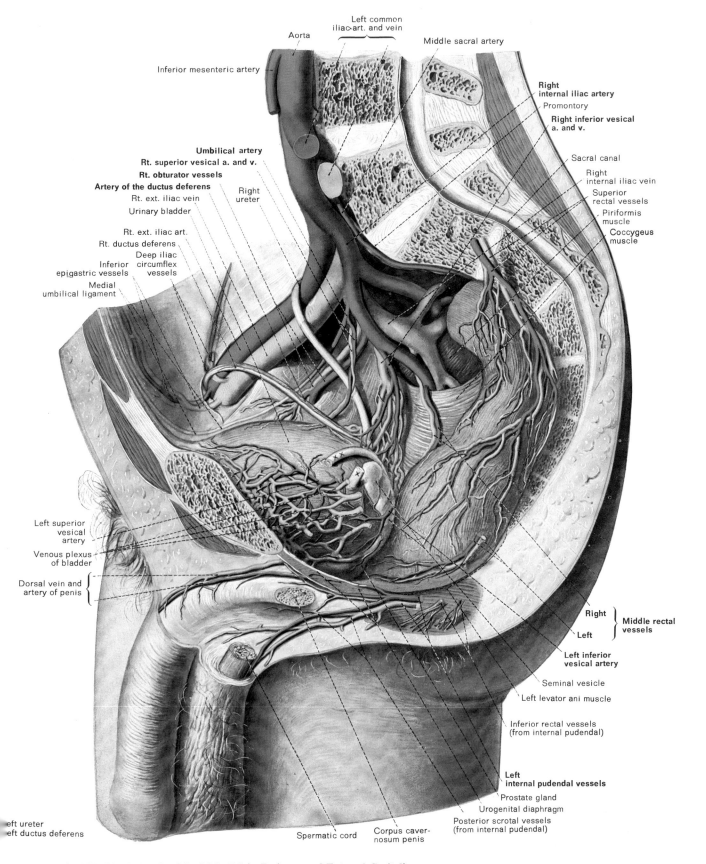

Fig. 247: Blood Vessels of the Male Pelvis, Perineum and External Genitalia

NOTE: 1) the aorta bifurcates into the common iliac arteries which then divide into the external and internal iliac arteries. The external iliac becomes the chief arterial trunk of the lower extremity, while the internal iliac artery supplies the organs of the pelvis and perineum.

2) the branches of the internal iliac artery include visceral and parietal vessels. The *visceral* branches are (a) the umbilical (from which is derived the superior vesical artery), (b) the inferior vesical, (c) the artery of the vas deferens (uterine in the female) and, (d) the middle rectal. The *parietal* branches include (a) the iliolumbar, (b) lateral sacral, (c) superior gluteal, (d) inferior gluteal, (e) obturator, and (f) internal pudendal.

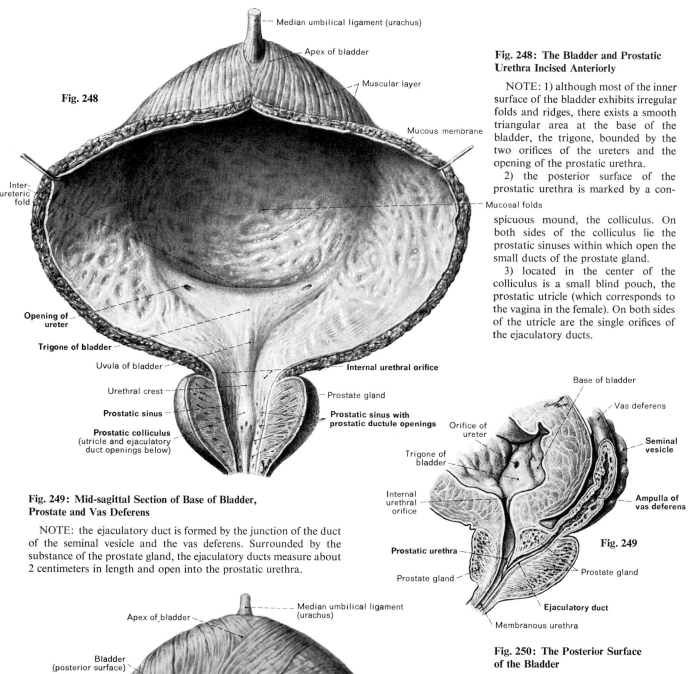

Fig. 248

Median umbilical ligament (urachus)

Apex of bladder

Muscular layer

Mucous membrane

Inter-ureteric fold

Mucosal folds

Opening of ureter

Trigone of bladder

Uvula of bladder

Internal urethral orifice

Urethral crest

Prostate gland

Prostatic sinus

Prostatic sinus with prostatic ductule openings

Prostatic colliculus (utricle and ejaculatory duct openings below)

Fig. 248: The Bladder and Prostatic Urethra Incised Anteriorly

NOTE: 1) although most of the inner surface of the bladder exhibits irregular folds and ridges, there exists a smooth triangular area at the base of the bladder, the trigone, bounded by the two orifices of the ureters and the opening of the prostatic urethra.

2) the posterior surface of the prostatic urethra is marked by a conspicuous mound, the colliculus. On both sides of the colliculus lie the prostatic sinuses within which open the small ducts of the prostate gland.

3) located in the center of the colliculus is a small blind pouch, the prostatic utricle (which corresponds to the vagina in the female). On both sides of the utricle are the single orifices of the ejaculatory ducts.

Fig. 249: Mid-sagittal Section of Base of Bladder, Prostate and Vas Deferens

NOTE: the ejaculatory duct is formed by the junction of the duct of the seminal vesicle and the vas deferens. Surrounded by the substance of the prostate gland, the ejaculatory ducts measure about 2 centimeters in length and open into the prostatic urethra.

Base of bladder

Vas deferens

Orifice of ureter

Seminal vesicle

Trigone of bladder

Internal urethral orifice

Ampulla of vas deferens

Prostatic urethra

Fig. 249

Prostate gland

Prostate gland

Ejaculatory duct

Membranous urethra

Fig. 250: The Posterior Surface of the Bladder

NOTE: 1) the ureters, vasa deferens, seminal vesicles and prostate gland are all in contact with the inferior aspect of the posterior surface of the bladder. The *ureters* penetrate the muscular wall of the bladder diagonally at points about two inches apart. At their sites of entrance into the *bladder,* the ureters are crossed anteriorly by the vasa deferens.

2) that the vasa deferens join the ducts of the lobulated seminal vesicles to form the two ejaculatory ducts. Observe that the prostate gland hugs the bladder at its outlet, thereby surrounding the prostatic urethra. The posterior surface of the bladder lies directly anterior to the rectum in the lower pelvis.

Median umbilical ligament (urachus)

Apex of bladder

Bladder (posterior surface)

Fig. 250

Right ureter

Vas deferens; Ampulla of vas deferens

Ampulla of vas deferens

Left seminal vesicle

Right seminal vesicle

Prostate gland

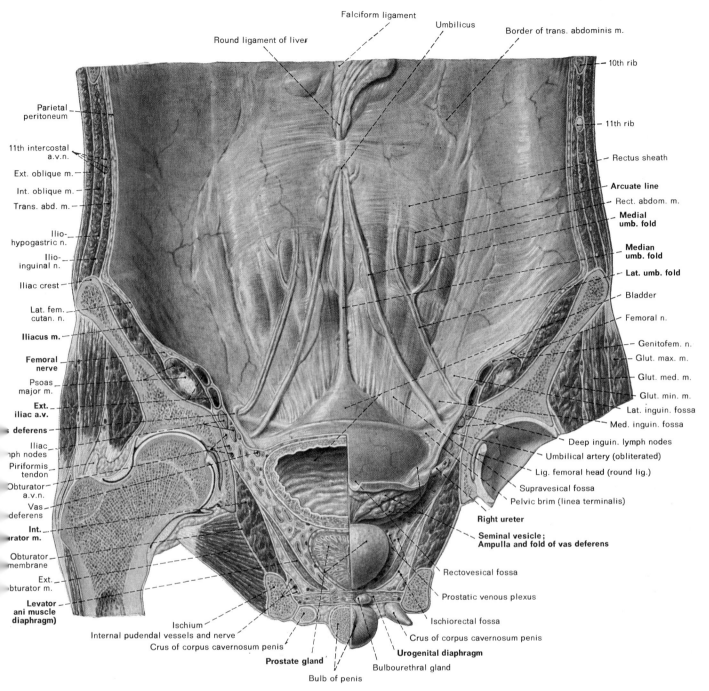

Labels on figure:

Round ligament of liver
Falciform ligament
Umbilicus
Border of trans. abdominis m.

Parietal peritoneum
11th intercostal a.v.n.
Ext. oblique m.
Int. oblique m.
Trans. abd. m.
Ilio-hypogastric n.
Ilio-inguinal n.
Iliac crest
Lat. fem. cutan. n.
Iliacus m.
Femoral nerve
Psoas major m.
Ext. iliac a.v.
Vas deferens
Iliac lymph nodes
Piriformis tendon
Obturator a.v.n.
Vas deferens
Int. obturator m.
Obturator membrane
Ext. obturator m.
Levator ani muscle (diaphragm)

10th rib
11th rib
Rectus sheath
Arcuate line
Rect. abdom. m.
Medial umb. fold
Median umb. fold
Lat. umb. fold
Bladder
Femoral n.
Genitofem. n.
Glut. max. m.
Glut. med. m.
Glut. min. m.
Lat. inguin. fossa
Med. inguin. fossa
Deep inguin. lymph nodes
Umbilical artery (obliterated)
Lig. femoral head (round lig.)
Supravesical fossa
Pelvic brim (linea terminalis)
Right ureter
Seminal vesicle; Ampulla and fold of vas deferens
Rectovesical fossa
Prostatic venous plexus
Ischiorectal fossa
Crus of corpus cavernosum penis

Ischium
Internal pudendal vessels and nerve
Crus of corpus cavernosum penis
Prostate gland
Bulb of penis
Urogenital diaphragm
Bulbourethral gland

Fig. 251: The Posterior Aspect of the Ventral Abdominal Wall and the Male Pelvic Organs

NOTE: 1) the inner aspect of the anterior abdominal wall shows the courses of the umbilical ligaments and the round ligament of the liver as well as the smooth contours of the rectus abdominis muscle and the arcuate line which marks the inferior limit of the posterior layer of the rectus sheath.

2) the frontal section through the bones of the pelvis and the femur. Observe the expanded wings (alae) of each ilium which extend laterally to reach the skin as the iliac crests. The wings of the ilia bound the greater (or false) pelvis. On their internal or pelvic surface lie the iliacus and psoas muscles along with the iliac vessels and the various nerves of the lumbar plexus. Their external surface is directed toward the gluteal region.

3) the lesser (or true) pelvis lies below the pelvic brim, is more restricted by bone and bounds more snugly the pelvic organs (bladder, prostate, seminal vesicle, etc.). Inferiorly the pelvic organs are separated from the perineum by the pelvic diaphragm (levator ani muscles) and, to a lesser extent, the urogenital diaphragm (deep transverse perineal muscles).

4) the reflection of peritoneum as it invests the inner surface of the anterior abdominal wall, curves over the superior surface of the bladder and dips somewhat posterior to the bladder (rectovesical pouch) to come into contact with the seminal vesicles and vasa deferens.

5) the obturator internus muscle which covers much of the inner surface of the lateral wall of the true pelvis. Extending into the perineum, this muscle also forms the lateral boundary of the ischiorectal fossa.

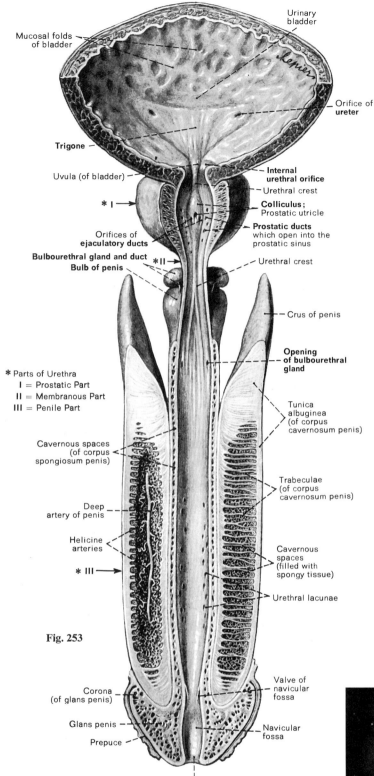

Mucosal folds
of bladder

Urinary
bladder

Orifice of
ureter

Trigone

Uvula (of bladder)

**Internal
urethral orifice**

Urethral crest

* I →

Colliculus;
Prostatic utricle

Prostatic ducts
which open into the
prostatic sinus

Orifices of
ejaculatory ducts

Bulbourethral gland and duct
Bulb of penis

* II →

Urethral crest

Crus of penis

* Parts of Urethra
 I = Prostatic Part
 II = Membranous Part
 III = Penile Part

**Opening
of bulbourethral
gland**

Tunica
albuginea
(of corpus
cavernosum penis)

Cavernous spaces
(of corpus
spongiosum penis)

Trabeculae
(of corpus
cavernosum penis)

Deep
artery of penis

Helicine
arteries

* III →

Cavernous
spaces
(filled with
spongy tissue)

Urethral lacunae

Fig. 253

Corona
(of glans penis)

Valve of
navicular
fossa

Glans penis

Prepuce

Navicular
fossa

External urethral orifice

Fig. 252: Radiograph of Bladder, Seminal Vesicles, Vasa Deferens and Ejaculatory Ducts

NOTE: 1) this figure is a positive print of an X-ray. The bladder has been filled with air and appears light, whereas the images of the seminal vesicles, vasa deferens and ejaculatory ducts stand out as dark.

2) that the convoluted seminal vesicles which secrete the seminal fluid consist of coiled tubes 4–5 mm in diameter and 2 to 3 inches in length.

3) the shadows of the vasa deferens. These cross the bladder surface toward the midline to join the seminal vesicles forming the ejaculatory ducts.

Fig. 253: The Male Urethra and its Associated Orifices

NOTE: 1) the male urethra is a canal that extends from its internal urethral orifice at the bladder to its external urethal orifice at the end of the glans penis. Since the male urethra transverses the prostate gland, the urogenital diaphragm (membrane) and the penis, it is divided into three parts: prostatic, membranous and penile.

2) urine passes through the urethra from the bladder. The urethra also transports the seminal fluid which is composed of a mixture of sperm from the testis and the secretions of the seminal vesicles and prostate. Just prior to ejaculation, the urethra is lubricated by a viscous fluid secreted by the bulbourethral glands (of Cowper). These glands are located in the urogenital diaphragm but their ducts open about one inch or more distally into the penile urethra.

3) the total urethra measures between 7 and 8 inches in length. The prostatic urethra is about 1½ inches long, the membranous urethra about ½ inch and the penile urethra 5 to 6 inches. On its posterior wall, the *prostatic urethra* is marked by a ridge, the urethral crest and a mound, the colliculus. It receives the secretions of the ejaculatory ducts along with those of the prostate. Enlargement of the prostate, often occurring in older men, tends to constrict the urethra at this site and frequently results in difficulty in urination.

4) the *membranous urethra* is short and narrow. In its course through the urogenital diaphragm, it is completely surrounded by the circular fibers of the urethral sphincter muscle (see Figure 258). Since this important sphincter is under voluntary control, its relaxation initiates urination while its tonic contraction constricts the urethra and maintains urinary continence.

5) the penile (or spongy) portion of the urethra at once is surrounded by the bulb of the penis and, thus, the bulbospongiosus muscle. It traverses the penile shaft embedded within the corpus spongiosum penis. In its course, it receives the ducts of the bulbourethral glands. The internal surface of its distal half is marked by a number of small recesses, the urethral lacunae. The distal portion of the penile urethra is somewhat narrowed and its external urethral orifice simply a vertical slit.

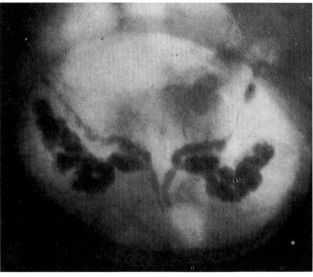

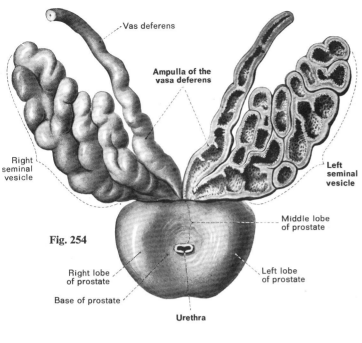

Vas deferens

Ampulla of the vasa deferens

Right seminal vesicle

Left seminal vesicle

Middle lobe of prostate

Fig. 254

Right lobe of prostate

Left lobe of prostate

Base of prostate

Urethra

Fig. 254: The Prostate Gland, Seminal Vesicles and Ampullae of the Vasa Deferens (Superior View)

NOTE: the left seminal vesicle and vas deferens were cut longitudinally while the urethra was cut transversely just distal to the bladder. The prostate gland is conical in shape and normally measures just over 1–½ inches across, 1 inch in thickness and slightly longer than 1 inch vertically. In the young adult male it weighs about 25 grams and is formed by two lateral lobes surrounding a middle lobe.

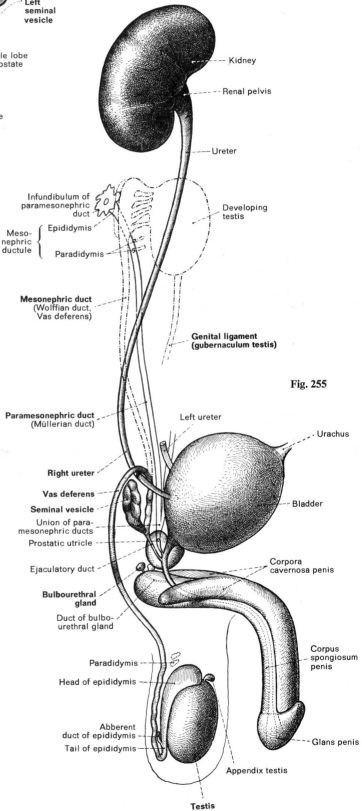

Kidney

Renal pelvis

Ureter

Infundibulum of paramesonephric duct

Developing testis

Meso-nephric ductule { Epididymis

Paradidymis

Mesonephric duct (Wolffian duct, Vas deferens)

Genital ligament (gubernaculum testis)

Fig. 255

Paramesonephric duct (Müllerian duct)

Left ureter

Urachus

Right ureter

Vas deferens

Bladder

Seminal vesicle

Union of para-mesonephric ducts

Prostatic utricle

Corpora cavernosa penis

Ejaculatory duct

Bulbourethral gland

Duct of bulbo-urethral gland

Corpus spongiosum penis

Paradidymis

Head of epididymis

Abberent duct of epididymis

Glans penis

Tail of epididymis

Appendix testis

Testis

Fig. 255: Diagram of the Male Genitourinary System

NOTE: 1) this figure shows:

a) the organs of the adult male genitourinary system;

b) the structures of the genital system prior to the descent of the testis (interrupted black lines);

c) those structures which partially or entirely became atrophic and disappeared during development (red lines).

2) the urinary system includes the *kidneys* which produce urine by filtration of the blood, the *ureters* which convey the urine to the *bladder* where it is stored and the *urethra* through which urine is discharged.

3) the adult male genital system includes the *testis* where sperm are generated, the *epididymis* and *vas deferens* which transport the sperm to the *ejaculatory duct* where the *seminal vesicle* joins the genital system. The *prostate* and *bulbourethral glands* along with ejaculatory ducts join the *urethra* which then courses through the male copulatory organ, the *penis*.

4) embryologically, structures capable of developing into both male and female genital systems exist in all individuals. In the male, the Wolffian or mesonephric duct (which becomes the epididymis, vas deferens ejaculatory duct and seminal vesicle) and the penis, develop while the paramesonephric or Müllerian duct becomes vestigial.

5) the testes are developed on the posterior abdominal wall and are attached by a fibrous genital ligament called the gubernaculum testis to the abdominal wall. As development continues, each testis gradually "migrates" from its site of formation so that by the 5th month it comes to lie adjacent to the abdominal inguinal ring. The gubernaculum testis is still attached to anterior abdominal wall tissue which by this time has evaginated as the developing scrotum. The testes then commence their descent through the inguinal canal so that by the 8th month they usually lie in the scrotum. During this "migration", the testes pass behind the peritoneum but are attached to it by its peritoneal reflection, the processus vaginalis testis. This becomes the *tunica vaginalis testis*.

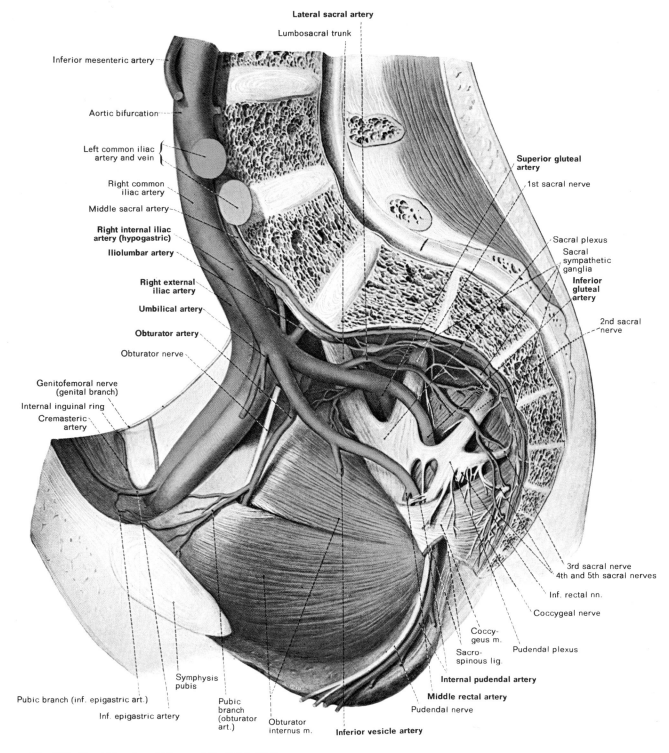

Fig. 256: Blood Vessels and Nerves of the Pelvic Wall

NOTE: 1) this is a mid-sagittal view of the right pelvic wall viewed from the left side. The pelvic viscera have been removed and the parietal blood vessels and nerves demonstrated.

2) the principal arteries of the pelvic wall are derived from the internal iliac artery. Although the branches of this vessel are quite variable, in at least 50% of cadavers it courses about 1-½ inches toward the greater sciatic foramen before branching into a posterior division of 4 vessels and an anterior division of 6 vessels.

3) the four posterior division vessels include a) the *iliolumbar* which courses superiorly toward the iliac fossa, b) the *lateral sacral* which courses inferiorly, anastomoses with the middle sacral artery and supplies branches to the upper sacral foramina, c) the *superior gluteal* which is the largest of the branches of the internal iliac and which leaves the pelvis above the border of the piriformis muscle, and d) the *inferior gluteal* which leaves the pelvis below the piriformis muscle.

4) the anterior division of the internal iliac artery gives rise to four visceral arteries (umbilical, inferior vesicle, middle rectal and uterine or deferential; see in Fig. 247). These are simply indicated by cut stumps in this figure. The two parietal vessels of this posterior division are the *obturator* artery which courses through the obturator canal to the medial thigh and the long *internal pudendal* artery which leaves the pelvis through the greater sciatic foramen, crosses the ischial spine to reenter the pelvis by way of the lesser sciatic foramen. It then courses toward the perineum by way of the pudendal canal to supply the anal and urogenital triangles.

Fig. 257: The Muscular Floor of the Pelvis: Pelvic Diaphragm

NOTE: 1) with the pelvic organs removed, this superior view of the floor of the pelvis emphasizes the muscular nature of the pelvic outlet. The *pelvic diaphragm* consists of the levator ani and coccygeus muscles along with two fascial layers which cover the pelvic (supra-anal fascia) and perineal (infraanal fascia) surfaces of these muscles.

2) the muscles and fascial layers composing the pelvic diaphragm stretch across the pelvic floor in a concave sling-like manner, thereby forming a separation between the structures of the pelvis and those of the perineum below.

3) the more caudal part of this "sling" is formed by the two coccygeus muscles. Since these muscles stretch from the ischial spines to the sacrum and coccyx, they are sometimes referred to as the ischiococcygeus muscles. The mid and anterior portions of the "sling" are formed by the iliococcygeus and pubococcygeus muscles These latter combine to form the levator ani muscle. The levator ani arises from the tendinous arc along the pelvic surface of the obturator internus and insert into the anococcygeal raphé, the central point of the perineum, the external spincter and the lower segments of the coccyx.

4) in the male, the pelvic diaphragm is perforated by the anal canal and urethra.

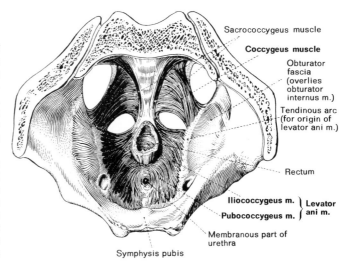

Sacrococcygeus muscle
Coccygeus muscle
Obturator fascia (overlies obturator internus m.)
Tendinous arc (for origin of levator ani m.)
Rectum
Iliococcygeus m. }
Pubococcygeus m. } Levator ani m.
Membranous part of urethra
Symphysis pubis

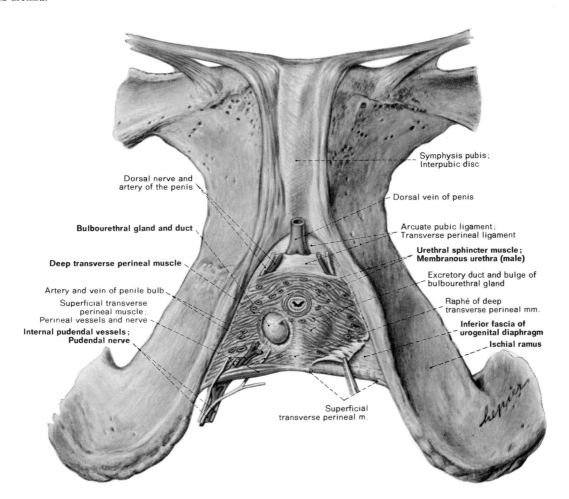

Symphysis pubis; Interpubic disc
Dorsal nerve and artery of the penis
Dorsal vein of penis
Bulbourethral gland and duct
Arcuate pubic ligament; Transverse perineal ligament
Deep transverse perineal muscle
Urethral sphincter muscle; Membranous urethra (male)
Artery and vein of penile bulb
Excretory duct and bulge of bulbourethral gland
Superficial transverse perineal muscle; Perineal vessels and nerve
Raphé of deep transverse perineal mm.
Internal pudendal vessels; Pudendal nerve
Inferior fascia of urogenital diaphragm
Ischial ramus
Superficial transverse perineal m.

Fig. 258: The Urogenital Diaphragm; Deep Transverse Perineal Muscle (Male)

NOTE: 1) the deep transverse perineal muscle, which stretches between the rami of the ischium, is covered by fascia on both its internal (pelvic or superior) surface and its external (perineal or inferior) surface. As such, this muscle and these two fascial sheaths constitute the urogenital diaphragm.

2) the region between the superior and inferior fascial planes is frequently referred to as the deep perineal compartment (pouch, cleft or space). In the male it contains a) the deep transverse perineal muscle, b) the membranous sphincter of the urethra, c) the bulbourethral glands and ducts, d) the membranous urethra and e) the various branches of the internal pudendal vessels and nerves.

3) the urogenital diaphragm assists somewhat in strengthening the anterior portion of the levator ani muscle where, in the midline at the so-called genital hiatus, it is penetrated by the urethra in the male and the urethra and vagina in the female.

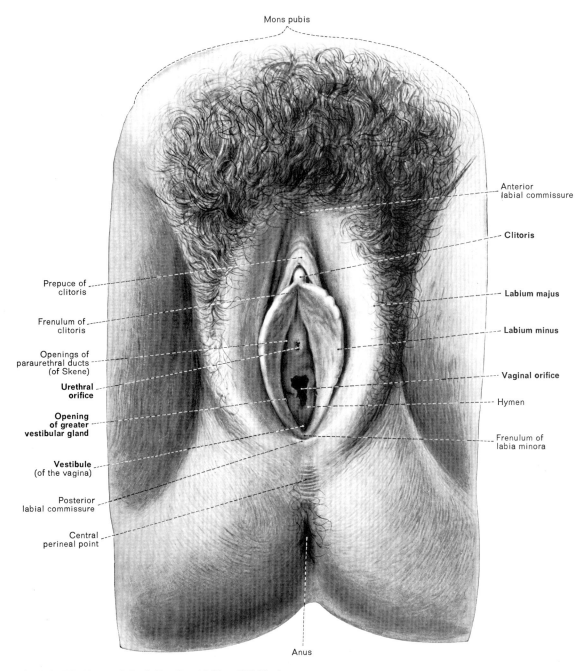

Mons pubis

Anterior
labial commissure

Clitoris

Prepuce of
clitoris

Labium majus

Frenulum of
clitoris

Labium minus

Openings of
paraurethral ducts
(of Skene)

Vaginal orifice

Urethral
orifice

Hymen

Opening
of greater
vestibular gland

Frenulum of
labia minora

Vestibule
(of the vagina)

Posterior
labial commissure

Central
perineal point

Anus

Fig. 259: The External Genitalia of an 18 Year Old Virgin

NOTE: 1) the female external genitalia include a) the labia majora, b) the labia minora, c) the clitoris and d) the vestibule of the vagina. The mons pubis, a rounded mound of adipose tissue anterior to the symphysis pubis and covered with hair in the adult, might also be considered an external genital organ. The orifices of the female perineum include the urethral orifice, the vaginal orifice, the two openings of the ducts of the greater vestibular glands, the orifices of the small paraurethral ducts (of Skene) and the anus.

2) the labia majora are two elongated folds of skin which form natural extensions from the mons pubis toward the anus. Although there is some variation in size and thickness dependent on age and obesity, the labia majora are in contact laterally with the thighs, unite both anteriorly and posteriorly to form integumentary commissures and represent the female homologous structures to the male scrotum. The anterior end of each labia majora receives the fibrous round ligament of the uterus as it leaves the superficial inguinal ring.

3) the labia minora are two thin folds of skin situated between the labia majora. Anteriorly the labia minora commence at the glans clitoris, although small extensions of the labia pass over the dorsum of the clitoris to unite and form the prepuce. Posteriorly the labia minora meet at the midline to form the frenulum of the labia.

4) the clitoris, homologous to the male penis, is an erectile organ and measures one inch or less in length. It is composed of two corpora cavernosa which are bound by dense connective tissue and which are attached by crura to the pubic rami; the crura are covered by small ischiocavernosus muscles. The clitoris is maintained by a suspensory ligament and capped by the glans.

5) the vestibule (of the vagina) is the region between the two labia minora. Into it open the urethra ventrally, the ducts of the greater vestibular glands bilaterally and the vagina. The vaginal orifice is partially closed in the virgin by a thin mucous membrane, the hymen, which separates the vestibule from the vagina proper. Generally, the hymen is ruptured at first copulation, however since its form and extent are quite variable, the establishment of virginity in this manner cannot be ascertained with certainty.

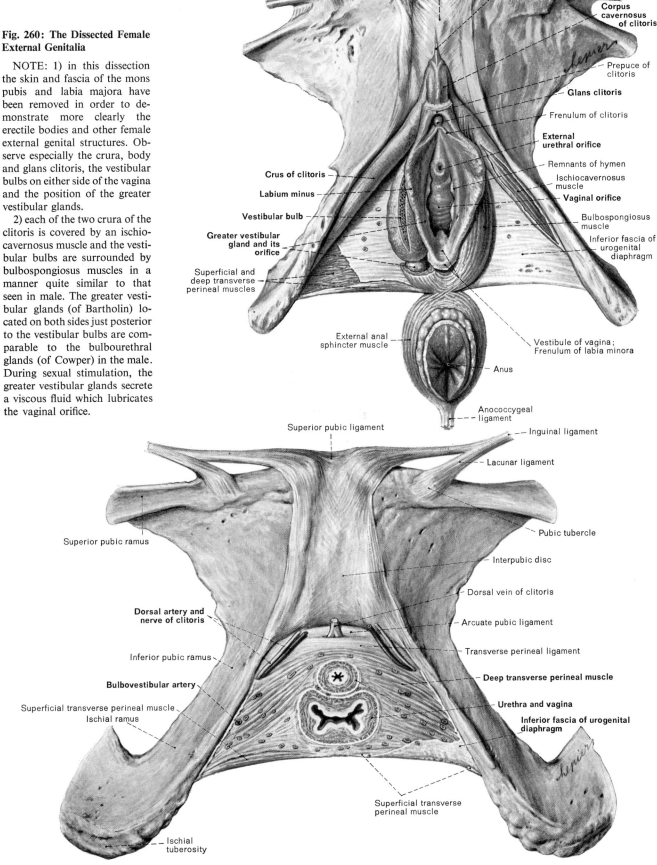

Fig. 260: The Dissected Female External Genitalia

NOTE: 1) in this dissection the skin and fascia of the mons pubis and labia majora have been removed in order to demonstrate more clearly the erectile bodies and other female external genital structures. Observe especially the crura, body and glans clitoris, the vestibular bulbs on either side of the vagina and the position of the greater vestibular glands.

2) each of the two crura of the clitoris is covered by an ischiocavernosus muscle and the vestibular bulbs are surrounded by bulbospongiosus muscles in a manner quite similar to that seen in male. The greater vestibular glands (of Bartholin) located on both sides just posterior to the vestibular bulbs are comparable to the bulbourethral glands (of Cowper) in the male. During sexual stimulation, the greater vestibular glands secrete a viscous fluid which lubricates the vaginal orifice.

Symphysis pubis

Suspensory ligament of clitoris

Corpus cavernosus of clitoris

Prepuce of clitoris

Glans clitoris

Frenulum of clitoris

External urethral orifice

Remnants of hymen

Ischiocavernosus muscle

Vaginal orifice

Bulbospongiosus muscle

Inferior fascia of urogenital diaphragm

Crus of clitoris

Labium minus

Vestibular bulb

Greater vestibular gland and its orifice

Superficial and deep transverse perineal muscles

External anal sphincter muscle

Vestibule of vagina; Frenulum of labia minora

Anus

Anococcygeal ligament

Superior pubic ligament

Inguinal ligament

Lacunar ligament

Pubic tubercle

Interpubic disc

Dorsal vein of clitoris

Arcuate pubic ligament

Transverse perineal ligament

Deep transverse perineal muscle

Urethra and vagina

Inferior fascia of urogenital diaphragm

Superior pubic ramus

Dorsal artery and nerve of clitoris

Inferior pubic ramus

Bulbovestibular artery

Superficial transverse perineal muscle

Ischial ramus

Ischial tuberosity

Superficial transverse perineal muscle

Fig. 261: The Urogenital Diaphragm in the Female

Note that in the female both the urethra and the vagina pass through the urogenital diaphragm. As in the male, the female urogenital diaphragm consists of the deep transverse perineal muscles and a layer of deep fascia on each of their superior and inferior surfaces. Observe the circular sphincter surrounding the membranous urethra.

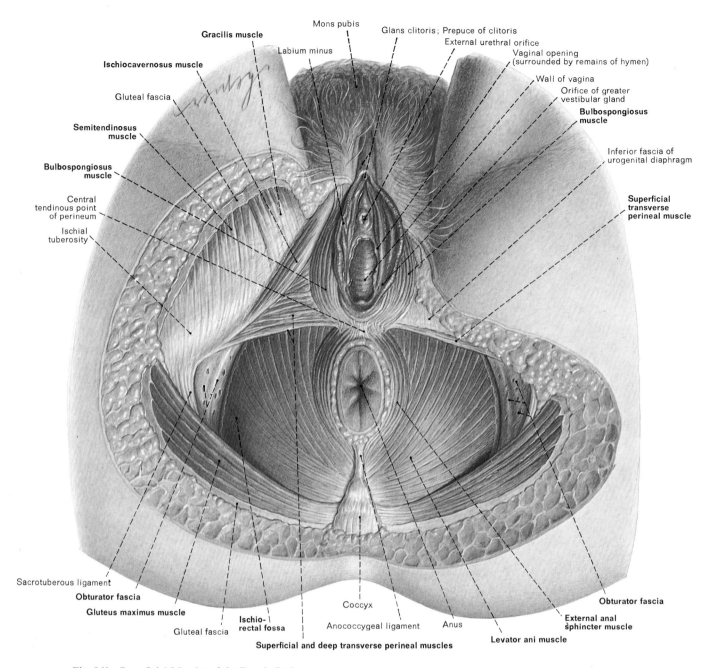

Gracilis muscle

Mons pubis

Glans clitoris; Prepuce of clitoris

External urethral orifice

Vaginal opening (surrounded by remains of hymen)

Ischiocavernosus muscle

Labium minus

Wall of vagina

Gluteal fascia

Orifice of greater vestibular gland

Semitendinosus muscle

Bulbospongiosus muscle

Bulbospongiosus muscle

Inferior fascia of urogenital diaphragm

Central tendinous point of perineum

Superficial transverse perineal muscle

Ischial tuberosity

Sacrotuberous ligament

Obturator fascia

Gluteus maximus muscle

Coccyx

Obturator fascia

Gluteal fascia

Ischio-rectal fossa

Anococcygeal ligament

Anus

External anal sphincter muscle

Superficial and deep transverse perineal muscles

Levator ani muscle

Fig. 262: Superficial Muscles of the Female Perineum

NOTE: 1) the perineum is a diamond-shaped region which is located inferior to the pelvis and separated from it by the muscular pelvic diaphragm. Four points limit the perineum: the symphysis pubis anteriorly; the tip of the coccyx posteriorly; the two ischial tuberosities laterally. A line drawn transversely across the perineum between the two ischial tuberosities, passing anterior to the anus through the central point of the perineum, divides the diamond-shaped region into an anterior urogenital region and a posterior anal region.

2) the urogenital region contains the external genital organs and the associated muscles and glands. A description of this region frequently refers to a superficial and deep perineal compartment (space, pouch). Simply stated the superficial perineal compartment lies superficial to the inferior layer of fascia of the urogenital diaphragm and contains the ischiocavernosus, bulbocavernosus and superficial transverse perineal muscles, plus a number of other structures related to the external genitalia. It is traversed by the perineal vessels and nerves and is limited superficially by a layer of deep fascia, the external perineal fascia which stretches just deep to Colles' fascia. The deep perineal compartment is that space enclosed between the superior and inferior layers of fascia of the urogenital diaphragm. Thus it contains the deep transverse perineal and urethral sphincter muscles (plus the bulbourethral glands in the male) and is traversed by the urethra and vagina in the female and the urethra in the male.

3) the anal region is situated posterior to the urogenital region. The anus, surrounded by the external anal sphincter muscle is located about 1½ inches anterior to the tip of the coccyx. A large portion of the anal region of the perineum is occupied on each side by the fat-filled ischiorectal fossae. Each fossa is wedge-shaped with the base of the wedge directed inferiorly toward the skin. The medial wall of the ischiorectal fossa is formed by the levator ani muscle, the lateral wall being the fascia over the obturator internus muscle. Recesses of each ischiorectal fossa extend anteriorly adjacent (superior) to the urogenital diaphragm.

Anterior

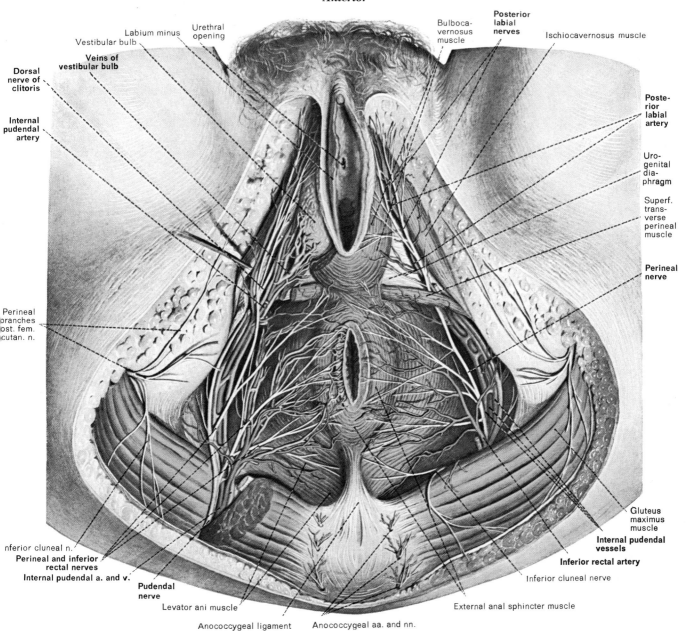

Vestibular bulb · Labium minus · Urethral opening · Bulbocavernosus muscle · Posterior labial nerves · Ischiocavernosus muscle

Veins of vestibular bulb

Dorsal nerve of clitoris

Internal pudendal artery

Posterior labial artery

Urogenital diaphragm

Superf. transverse perineal muscle

Perineal nerve

Perineal branches post. fem. cutan. n.

Gluteus maximus muscle

Internal pudendal vessels

Inferior rectal artery

nferior cluneal n.

Perineal and inferior rectal nerves

Internal pudendal a. and v.

Pudendal nerve

Levator ani muscle

Inferior cluneal nerve

External anal sphincter muscle

Anococcygeal ligament · Anococcygeal aa. and nn.

Posterior

Fig. 263: Nerves and Blood Vessels of the Female Perineum

NOTE: 1) in this dissection the skin and superficial fascia have been removed from both the urogenital and anal regions of the female perineum. The ischiorectal fossae have been cleared of fat as well.

2) the principal nerve from which most of the branches which innervate the perineum are derived is the *pudendal nerve*. It originates in the sacral cord and contains fibers of the S_2, S_3 and S_4 segments. In its course within the pelvis, it is joined by the *internal pudendal artery* and *vein* at the lower border of the piriformis muscle at the greater sciatic foramen. Together the vessels and nerve leave the pelvis through the greater sciatic foramen, cross the ischial spine (sacrospinous ligament) to enter the pelvis once again through the lesser sciatic foramen.

3) the pudendal structures course into the perineum from the pelvis by way of the pudendal canal (of Alcock) which courses beneath the fascia of the obturator internus muscle. Within the perineum, the pudendal structures are first seen at the lateral wall of the ischiorectal fossa. At this point the *inferior rectal vessels* and nerves branch and cross the ischiorectal fossa toward the midline thereby supplying the levator ani and external anal sphincter muscles along with the other structures in the anal region.

4) continuing anteriorly the pudendal nerve and internal pudendal vessels approach the urogenital diaphragm to become the perineal vessels and nerve. Upon entering the urogenital region, superficial and deep branches supply the structures of the superficial and deep perineal compartments.

5) the superficial perineal branches in the female supply the labia majora and the external genital structures while the deep branches supply the muscles of the urogenital region, the vestibular bulb and the clitoris.

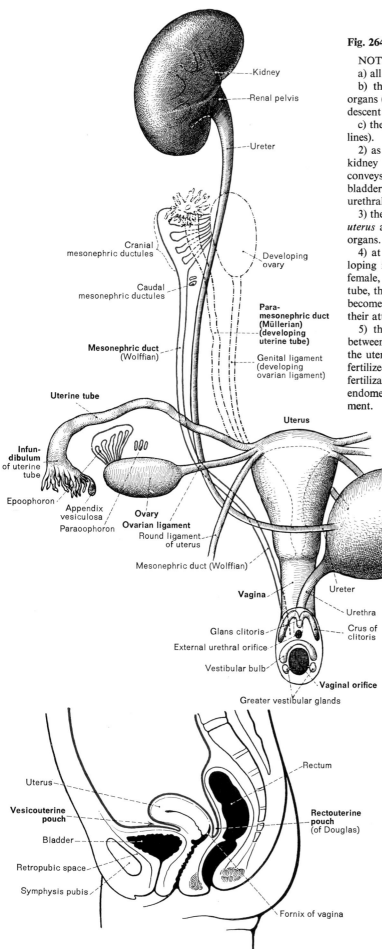

Fig. 264: Diagram of the Female Genitourinary System

NOTE: 1) this figure shows:

a) all the organs of the adult female genitourinary system;

b) the structures and relevant positions of the female genital organs (gonad and ovarian ligament and uterine tube) prior to their descent into the pelvis (interrupted black lines); and

c) the structures which became atrophic during development (red lines).

2) as in the male, the urinary system of the female includes the kidney which produces urine from the blood, the ureter which conveys the urine to the bladder where it is stored. Leading from the bladder is the urethra through which urine passes to the external urethral orifice during micturition.

3) the adult female genital system includes the *ovary, uterine tube, uterus* and *vagina*, plus the associated glands and external genital organs.

4) at one time during development, structures capable of developing into both male and female genital systems existed. In the female, the Müllerian or paramesonephric duct forms the uterine tube, the uterus and vagina while the Wolffian or mesonephric duct becomes vestigial. Also the developing gonads become ovaries while their attachments become the ovarian ligaments.

5) the ovaries produce ova which are discharged periodically between adolescence and the menopause. The ova are captured by the uterine tube where fertilization may occur. If this happens the fertilized ovum is transported to the uterus and about a week after fertilization, implantation occurs in the wall of the uterus. The endometrium nourishes the embryo in this early period of development.

Fig. 265: Diagram of Peritoneal Reflections Over Female Pelvic Organs (Mid-Sagittal Section)

Peritoneum in red

NOTE: 1) that the parietal peritoneum is reflected over the free abdominal surfaces of the pelvic organs. Observe that as the uterus and vagina are interposed between the bladder and rectum that peritoneal pouches are formed between the bladder and the uterus (vesicouterine) and between the rectum and the uterus (rectouterine pouch of Douglas).

2) the vesicouterine pouch is relatively shallow. The forward tilt or inclination of the uterus (anteversion) toward the superior surface of the bladder reduces the potential size of the vesicouterine pouch. This fossa does not extend as far inferiorly as the vagina whereas the deeper rectouterine pouch dips to the posterior surface of the fornix of the vagina. This important anatomical relationship stresses the fact that the fornix of the vagina is separated from the peritoneal cavity only by the thin vaginal wall and the peritoneum.

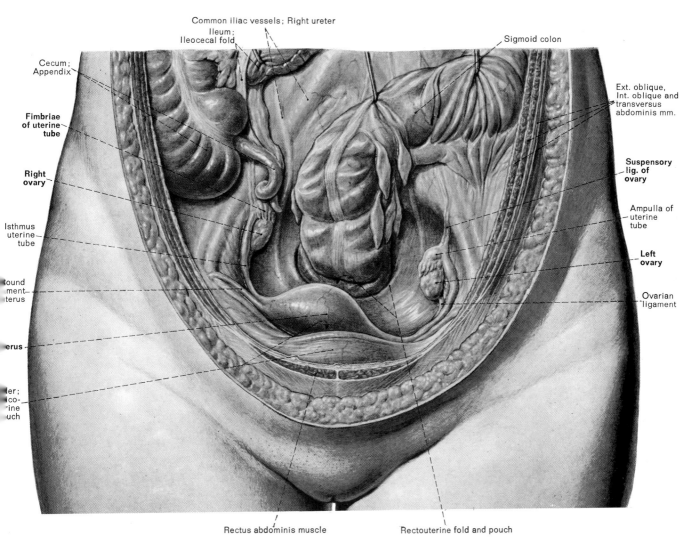

Common iliac vessels; Right ureter
Ileum;
Ileocecal fold

Sigmoid colon

Cecum;
Appendix

Fimbriae
of uterine
tube

Right
ovary

Isthmus
uterine
tube

Round
ment
terus

erus

ler;
co-
ine
uch

Ext. oblique,
Int. oblique and
transversus
abdominis mm.

Suspensory
lig. of
ovary

Ampulla of
uterine
tube

Left
ovary

Ovarian
ligament

Rectus abdominis muscle

Rectouterine fold and pouch

Fig. 266: Pelvic Viscera of an Adult Female: Anterior View

NOTE: 1) that the ovaries are situated on the posterolateral aspect of the true pelvis on each side. Having descended from the posterior abdominal wall to their location just below the pelvic brim, the ovaries are held in position by ligamentous attachments. The suspensory ligament transmits the ovarian vessels and nerves.

2) the position of the uterus interposed between the bladder and rectum. Observe that the uterus is frequently located somewhat to one or the other side of the midline.

3) the fimbriae of the uterine tubes as they extend from the ampullae of the tubes to encircle the upper medial surfaces of the ovaries. These tubes vary from 3 to 6 inches in length and, as extensions of the uterus, they convey the ova to the uterus. It is within the uterine tube that fertilization of the ovum usually occurs.

Fig. 267: Utero-Salpingogram

By means of a cannula (K) placed in the vagina, radiopaque material has been injected into the uterus and uterine tubes (salpinx). Observe the narrow lumen of the isthmus of the uterine tubes and note how the tubes enlarge at the ampullae. On the specimen's left side (reader's right side), even the fimbriated end of the tube is discernible, while on the specimen's right side (reader's left side) a small portion of the radiopaque material has been forced into the pelvis through the opening of the uterine tube.

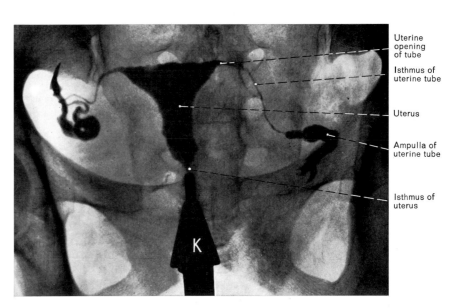

Uterine
opening
of tube

Isthmus of
uterine tube

Uterus

Ampulla of
uterine tube

Isthmus of
uterus

K

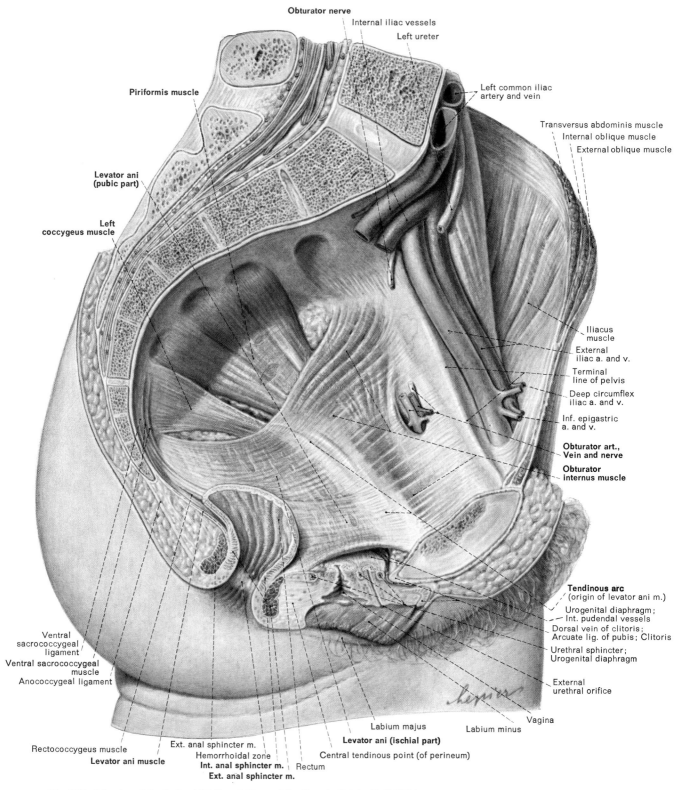

Obturator nerve
Internal iliac vessels
Left ureter
Piriformis muscle
Left common iliac artery and vein
Transversus abdominis muscle
Internal oblique muscle
External oblique muscle
Levator ani (pubic part)
Left coccygeus muscle
Iliacus muscle
External iliac a. and v.
Terminal line of pelvis
Deep circumflex iliac a. and v.
Inf. epigastric a. and v.
Obturator art., Vein and nerve
Obturator internus muscle
Tendinous arc (origin of levator ani m.)
Urogenital diaphragm;
Int. pudendal vessels
Dorsal vein of clitoris;
Arcuate lig. of pubis; Clitoris
Urethral sphincter;
Urogenital diaphragm
External urethral orifice
Ventral sacrococcygeal ligament
Ventral sacrococcygeal muscle
Anococcygeal ligament
Vagina
Rectococcygeus muscle
Levator ani muscle
Ext. anal sphincter m.
Hemorrhoidal zone
Int. anal sphincter m.
Ext. anal sphincter m.
Rectum
Labium majus
Labium minus
Levator ani (ischial part)
Central tendinous point (of perineum)

Fig. 268: Muscles of the Lateral Wall and Floor of the Female Pelvis (Left Side)

NOTE: 1) the lateral wall of the true pelvis is covered principally by the piriformis and obturator internus muscles while the floor of the pelvis is formed by both the pubic and ischial portions of the levator ani muscle and, more posteriorly, by the coccygeus muscle.

2) although the *piriformis muscle* arises from the ventral surface of the 2nd, 3rd and 4th sacral vertebrae, it is frequently studied with the gluteal muscles because its fibers converge and leave the pelvis through the greater sciatic foramen. The *obturator internus muscle,* covered by its fascia, has an extensive origin on the inner surface of the lateral and anterior wall of the true bony pelvis. It surrounds the obturator foramen (note the obturator vessels and nerve) and its fibers converge to form a tendon which passes out of the pelvis to enter the gluteal region through the lesser sciatic foramen.

3) both the pubic and ischial portions of the *levator ani* muscle arise principally from the tendinous arc of the obturator internus fascia. Observe the *internal* and *external* anal sphincters surrounding the anal orifice.

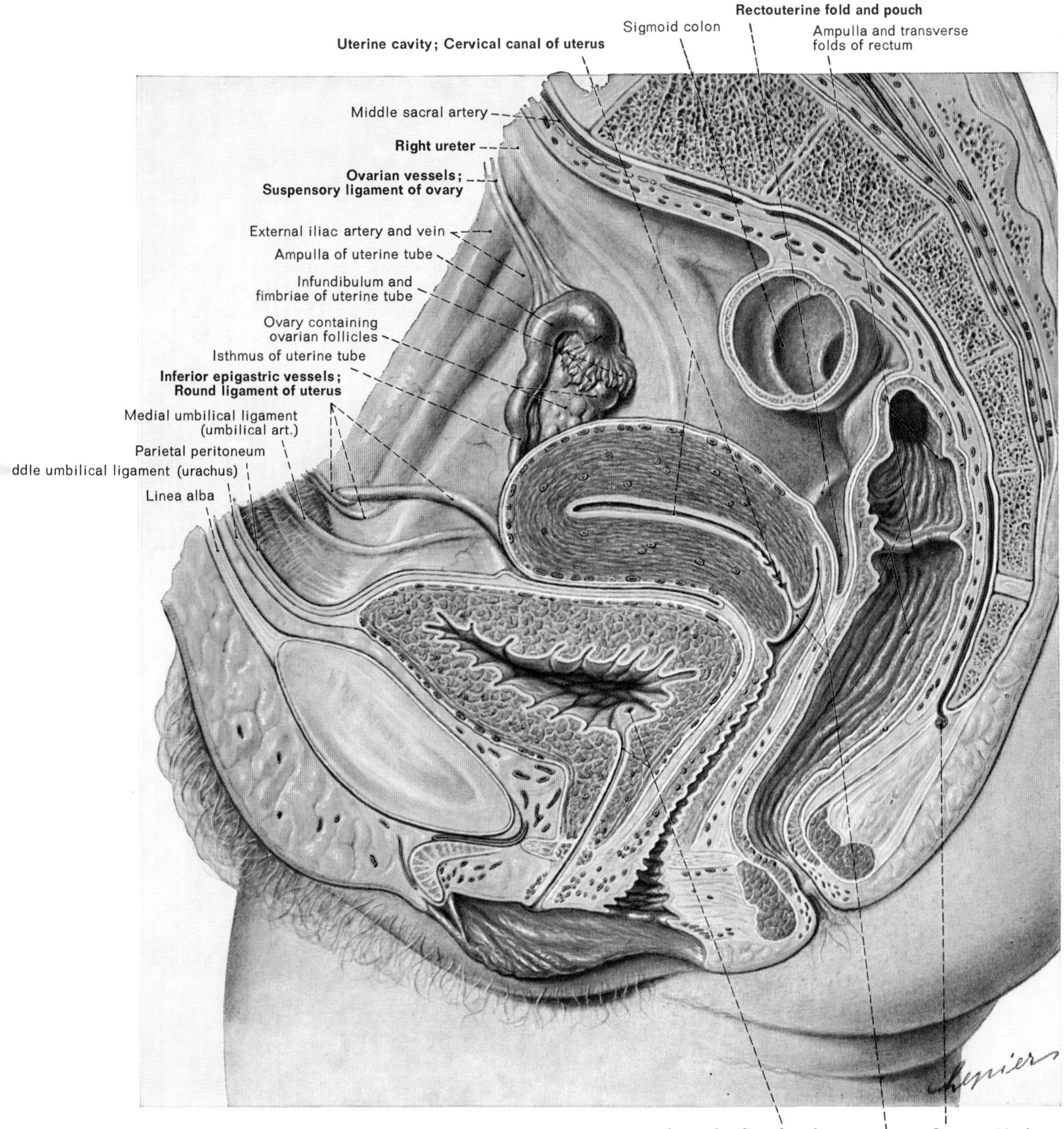

Fig. 269: The Adult Female Pelvis: Median Sagittal Section

NOTE: 1) this medial view of the right half of the female pelvis illustrates the relationships among the bladder, uterus and vagina, rectum, ovary and uterine tube. Observe the immediate retropubic position of the empty *bladder* and the relatively short course of the female *urethra,* which leads from the bladder through the urogenital diaphragm to open in the midline anterior to the vagina and between the labia minora.

2) the opening between the vagina and the uterus. An extension of the vagina, the posterior fornix reaches enough superiorly to lie just in front of the rectouterine pouch (of Douglas) and separated from it only by the vaginal wall. Note the interposition of the vagina and uterus between the bladder and rectum. The pear-shaped uterus is so positioned over the superior surface of the empty bladder that when the woman is standing erect, the uterus is horizontal.

3) that the round ligament is directed laterally and anteriorly to enter the abdominal inguinal ring and the course of the inferior epigastric vessels in relation to this ligament. Likewise observe the course of the ovarian vessels within the suspensory ligament of the ovary and their important relationship to the descending ureter on the posterolateral wall of the pelvis.

4) the sigmoid flexure of the large bowel and the relatively direct course of the rectum toward the anal canal. The peritoneum is reflected over the anterior surface of the rectum, thereby lining the rectouterine pouch.

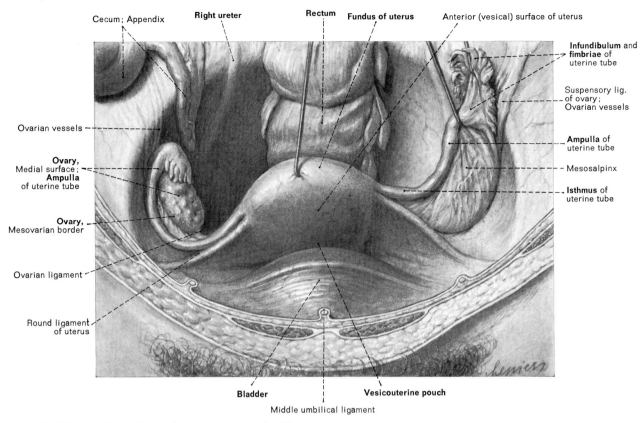

Cecum; Appendix — Right ureter — Rectum — Fundus of uterus — Anterior (vesical) surface of uterus

Infundibulum and fimbriae of uterine tube

Suspensory lig. of ovary; Ovarian vessels

Ovarian vessels —

Ampulla of uterine tube

Ovary, Medial surface; Ampulla of uterine tube

Mesosalpinx

Isthmus of uterine tube

Ovary, Mesovarian border

Ovarian ligament

Round ligament of uterus

Bladder — Vesicouterine pouch

Middle umbilical ligament

Fig. 270: The Female Pelvic Organs: Anterosuperior View

Observe that the body of the uterus has been elevated thereby exposing the vesicouterine pouch and demonstrating the broad ligaments.

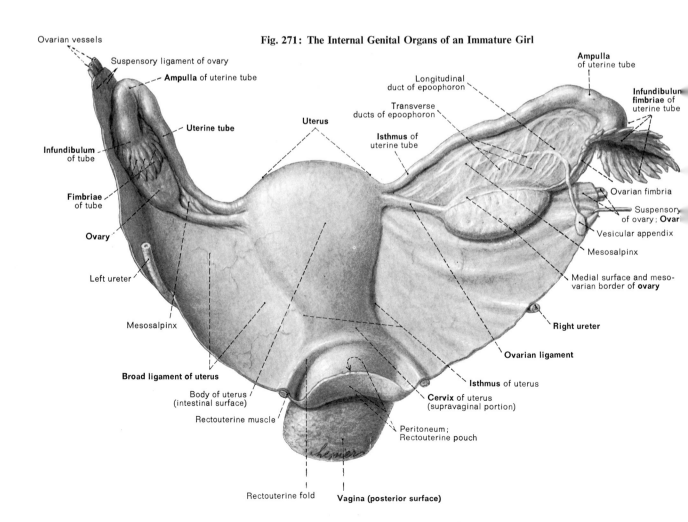

Fig. 271: The Internal Genital Organs of an Immature Girl

Ovarian vessels

Suspensory ligament of ovary

Ampulla of uterine tube

Uterus

Longitudinal duct of epoophoron

Ampulla of uterine tube

Infundibulum fimbriae of uterine tube

Transverse ducts of epoophoron

Isthmus of uterine tube

Uterine tube

Infundibulum of tube

Ovarian fimbria

Suspensory of ovary; Ovar

Fimbriae of tube

Vesicular appendix

Ovary

Mesosalpinx

Left ureter

Medial surface and mesovarian border of **ovary**

Right ureter

Mesosalpinx

Ovarian ligament

Broad ligament of uterus

Isthmus of uterus

Body of uterus (intestinal surface)

Cervix of uterus (supravaginal portion)

Rectouterine muscle

Peritoneum; Rectouterine pouch

Rectouterine fold

Vagina (posterior surface)

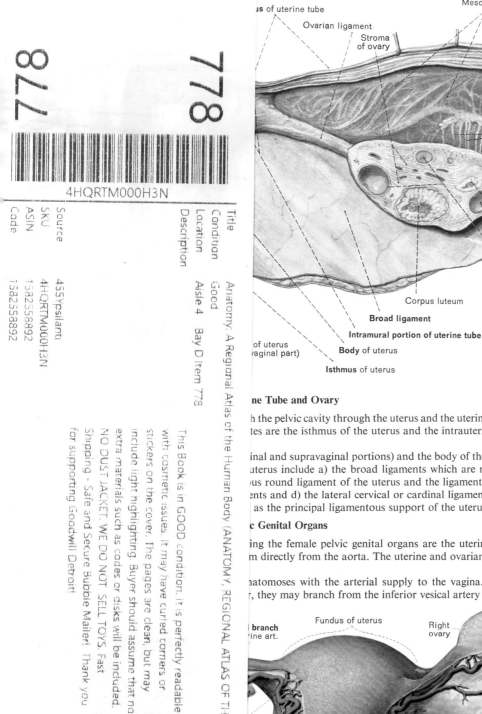

Fundus of uterine tube
Ovarian ligament
Stroma of ovary
Mesosalpinx
Longitudinal duct of epoophoron
Ampulla of uterine tube
Transverse ducts of epoophoron
Mucosal folds of tube
Fimbriae of uterine tube
Accessory hydatid
Ovarian vessels
Ovarian fimbria
Vesicular appendix
Corpus albicans
Ovarian follicles
Corpus luteum
Broad ligament
Intramural portion of uterine tube
Body of uterus
Isthmus of uterus
of uterus (vaginal part)

...ne Tube and Ovary

...h the pelvic cavity through the uterus and the uterine tube. The lumen of this pathway ...tes are the isthmus of the uterus and the intrauterine and most proximal portion of

...inal and supravaginal portions) and the body of the uterus. These are interconnected ...uterus include a) the broad ligaments which are mesentery-like attachments to the ...us round ligament of the uterus and the ligament of the ovary attached just below ...nts and d) the lateral cervical or cardinal ligaments (not shown in this figure). The ... as the principal ligamentous support of the uterus and upper vagina.

...c Genital Organs

...ing the female pelvic genital organs are the uterine arteries from the internal iliac ...m directly from the aorta. The uterine and ovarian arteries anastomose freely along

...natomoses with the arterial supply to the vagina. Frequently, the vaginal arteries ...r, they may branch from the inferior vesical artery or even directly from the internal iliac artery.

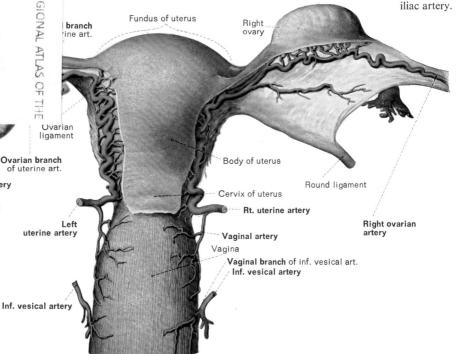

...l branch ...ine art.
Fundus of uterus
Right ovary
Ovarian ligament
Left ovary
Ovarian branch of uterine art.
Infundibulum
Left ovarian artery
Vesicular appendix
Body of uterus
Round ligament
Cervix of uterus
Rt. uterine artery
Right ovarian artery
Left uterine artery
Vaginal artery
Vagina
Vaginal branch of inf. vesical art.
Inf. vesical artery
Inf. vesical artery

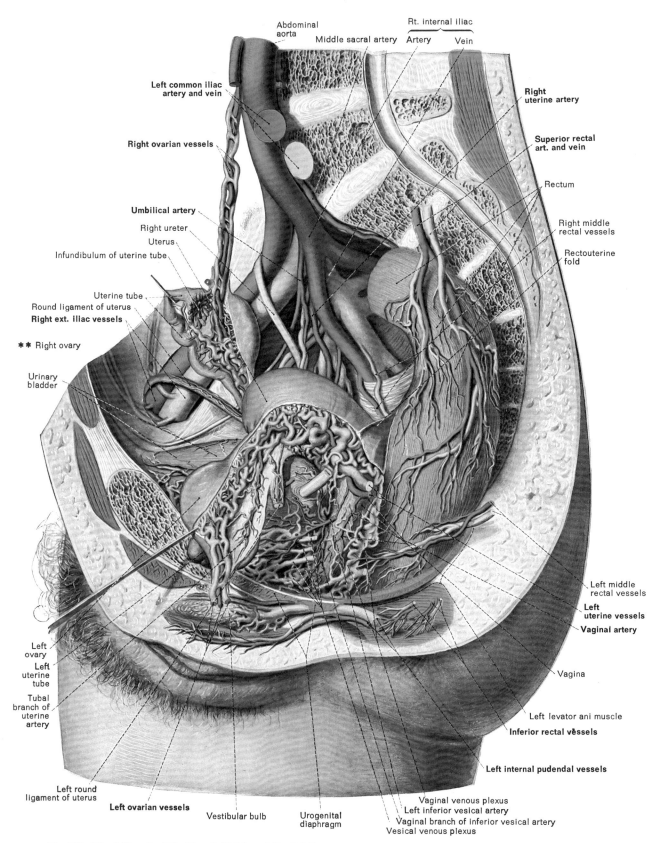

Abdominal aorta

Middle sacral artery

Rt. internal iliac Artery Vein

Left common iliac artery and vein

Right ovarian vessels

Umbilical artery

Right ureter

Uterus

Infundibulum of uterine tube

Uterine tube

Round ligament of uterus

Right ext. iliac vessels

∗∗ Right ovary

Urinary bladder

Left ovary

Left uterine tube

Tubal branch of uterine artery

Left round ligament of uterus

Left ovarian vessels

Vestibular bulb

Urogenital diaphragm

Right uterine artery

Superior rectal art. and vein

Rectum

Right middle rectal vessels

Rectouterine fold

Left middle rectal vessels

Left uterine vessels

Vaginal artery

Vagina

Left levator ani muscle

Inferior rectal vessels

Left internal pudendal vessels

Vaginal venous plexus

Left inferior vesical artery

Vaginal branch of inferior vesical artery

Vesical venous plexus

Fig. 274: Blood Vessels of the Female Pelvis and Genital System

NOTE: 1) the left half of the pelvis has been removed while most of the female pelvic organs are still in place. Observe the dense plexuses of veins. These include the ovarian, uterine, vaginal and vesical plexuses which accompany their respective arteries and which drain the pelvic organs.

2) with the exception of the *ovarian artery* which is derived from the aorta and the *superior rectal artery* (hemorrhoidal) which branches from the superior mesenteric, all the other arteries supplying blood to the pelvic organs, perineum and genital tract are derived from the *internal iliac artery* or its branches. Observe the anastomosis among the superior, middle and inferior rectal vessels.

3) the descending course of the ureter over the pelvic brim from the posterior abdominal wall. In its path it crosses the external iliac artery and vein as does the round ligament of the uterus more inferiorly.

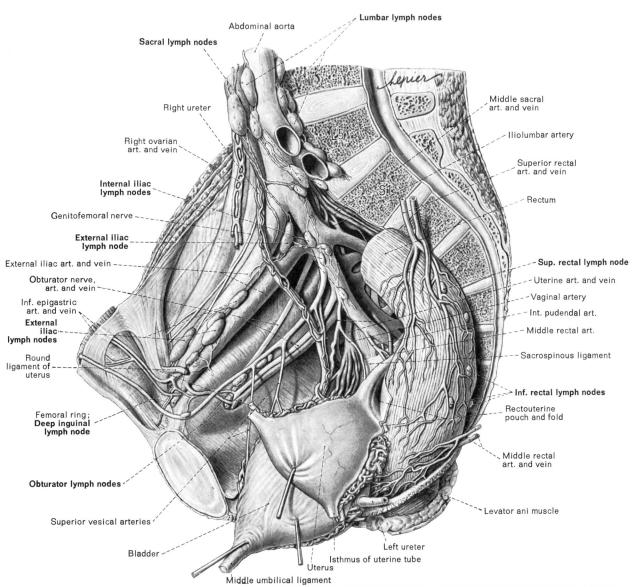

Abdominal aorta

Lumbar lymph nodes

Sacral lymph nodes

Middle sacral art. and vein

Right ureter

Iliolumbar artery

Right ovarian art. and vein

Superior rectal art. and vein

Internal iliac lymph nodes

Rectum

Genitofemoral nerve

External iliac lymph node

Sup. rectal lymph node

External iliac art. and vein

Uterine art. and vein

Obturator nerve, art. and vein

Vaginal artery

Inf. epigastric art. and vein

Int. pudendal art.

External iliac lymph nodes

Middle rectal art.

Round ligament of uterus

Sacrospinous ligament

Inf. rectal lymph nodes

Femoral ring; **Deep inguinal lymph node**

Rectouterine pouch and fold

Middle rectal art. and vein

Obturator lymph nodes

Levator ani muscle

Superior vesical arteries

Bladder

Left ureter

Isthmus of uterine tube

Uterus

Middle umbilical ligament

Fig. 275: Lymph Vessels and Nodes of the Female Pelvis

NOTE: 1) as a rule, the lymph nodes of the pelvis lie along the courses of the major vessels. Generally the lymphatics drain superiorly and posteriorly to achieve the right and left lumbar lymphatic chain of nodes which lie upon the psoas major muscles on both sides of the aorta.

2) the lymphatics of the bladder drain laterally to the external iliac nodes and posteriorly to the internal iliac nodes. These latter lymphatic channels and nodes also receive lymph from the fundus and body of the uterus in the female and the prostate and seminal vesicles in the male. Lymphatics of the cervix and vagina drain into both the external and internal iliac nodes.

Fig. 276: Lymphograph of Pelvis and Lumbar Region

This lymphograph displays the lymphatic channels from the deeper femoral vessels and nodes superiorly through to the lumbar and aortic nodes. Observe the profuse network along the iliac vessels and the concentration of nodes in the deep inguinal region.

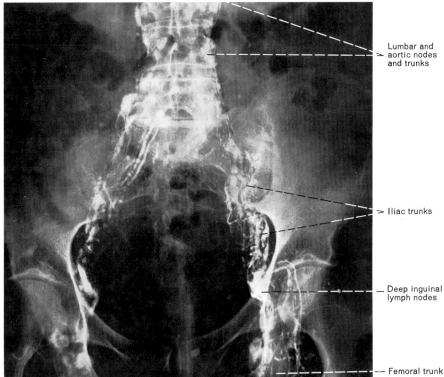

Lumbar and aortic nodes and trunks

Iliac trunks

Deep inguinal lymph nodes

Femoral trunk

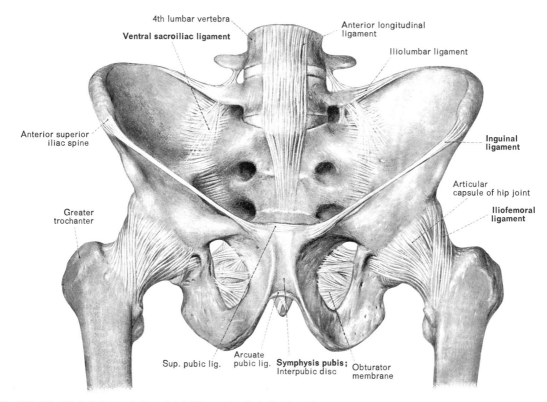

Fig. 277: The Male Pelvis and Associated Ligaments: Anterior Aspect

NOTE that the pelvis is formed by the articulation of the left and right hip bones anteriorly at the symphysis pubis and posteriorly with the sacrum and coccyx of the vertebral column. The articulations inferiorly of the pelvis with the two femurs allow the weight of the head, trunk and upper extremities to be transmitted to the lower limbs, thereby maintaining the upright posture characteristic of the human being.

Fig. 278: The Female Pelvis with Joints and Ligaments: Posterior Aspect

NOTE that the broad ligamentous bands articulating the two hip bones posteriorly with the sacrum and coccyx. This sacroiliac joint is bound by the extremely strong dorsal sacroiliac ligament. Attaching the sacrum to the ischial tuberosity is the broad sacrotuberous ligament. Additionally, the sacrospinous ligament stretches between the sacrum and the ischium (ischial spine).

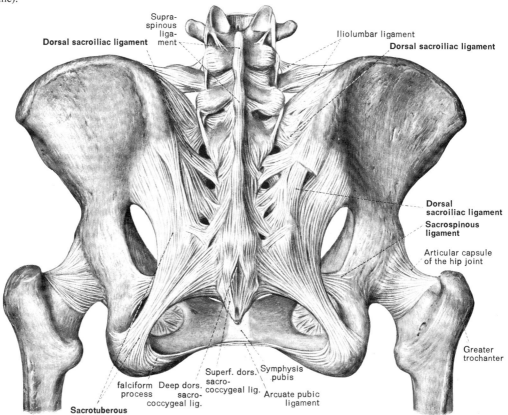

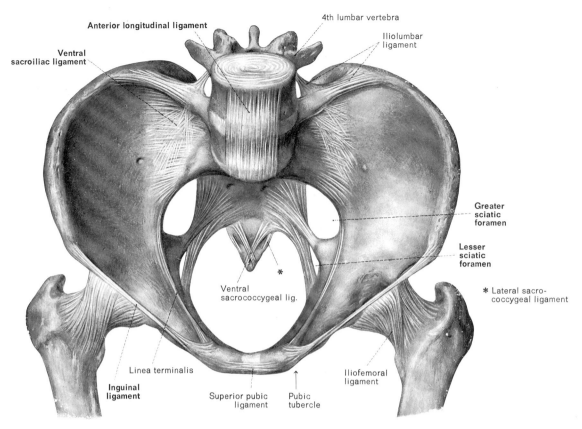

Fig. 279: The Male Pelvis and Ligaments Viewed from Above

NOTE that the size of both the pelvic inlet (superior aperture of the minor pelvis) and inferior outlet of the male pelvis is smaller than that in the female (see Figure 280, below). Thus, the minor pelvis is deeper and narrower in the male and its cavity has a smaller capacity than the female. In the male, however, pelvic bones are thicker and heavier and generally the major pelvis (above the pelvic brim) is larger than in the female.

Fig. 280: The Female Pelvis and Ligaments Viewed from Above

NOTE that in addition to having wider diameters, both the pelvic inlet and outlet of the female pelvis minor are more circular in shape than in the male. The female pelvic bones are more delicate and the sacrum less curved. The larger capacity of the true pelvis in the female and the fact that the female hormones of pregnancy tend to relax the pelvic ligaments serve to facilitate the function of child bearing.

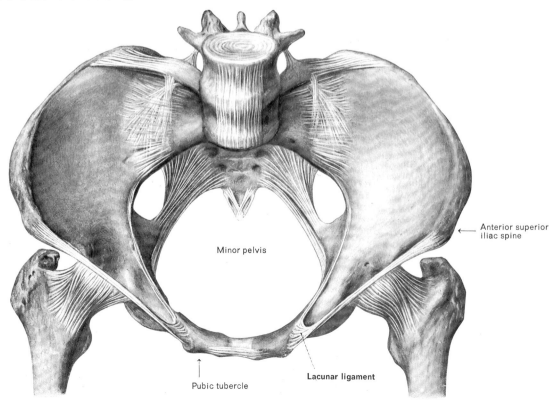

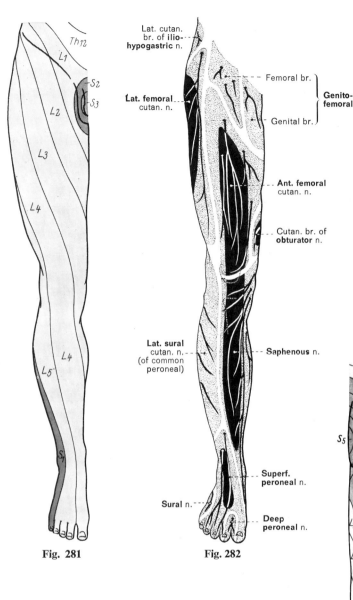

Fig. 281 **Fig. 282**

Fig. 281: Dermatomes of the Anterior Aspect of the Lower Extremity

Note that as a rule the lumbar segments of the spinal cord supply the cutaneous innervation ot the anterior aspect of the lower extremity and that the dermatomes are segmentally arranged in order from L-1 to S-1. Observe that the genital region is supplied by the sacral segments.

Fig. 282: The Distribution of Cutaneous Nerves: Anterior Aspect of the Lower Extremity

The segmental distribution of the cutaneous nerves supplying the anterior aspect of the lower extremity is as follows:

iliohypogastric nerve: (T_{12}), L_1
genitofemoral nerve: L_1, L_2
lateral femoral cutaneous nerve: L_2, L_3
femoral nerve: L_2, L_3, L_4
obturator nerve: L_2, L_3, L_4
saphenous nerve (femoral): L_2, L_3, L_4
deep peroneal (cutaneous br.): L_4, L_5
superficial peroneal: L_4, L_5, S_1
lateral sural cutaneous n.: L_5, S_1, S_2
(common peroneal n.)
sural nerve (tibial): S_1, S_2

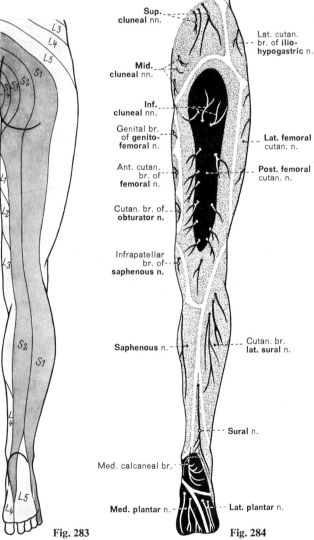

Fig. 283 **Fig. 284**

Fig. 283: Dermatomes of the Posterior Aspect of the Lower Extremity

Note that the skin on the posterior aspect of the lower extremity receives its sensory innervation principally from L5, S1 and S2. Observe, however, how the posterior medial border of the limb consecutively has the L1, L2, L3 and L4 segments represented. Segments S3, S4 and S5 are more limited to the perineal and anal regions.

Fig. 284: The Distribution of Cutaneous Nerves: Posterior Aspect of the Lower Extremity

NOTE: 1) the principal nerve supplying cutaneous innervation to the posterior aspect of the thigh is the posterior femoral cutaneous nerve (S1, S2, S3). The skin of the medial calf is supplied by the saphenous (femoral) nerve (L2, L3, L4) while the lateral calf receives the sural nerve (S1, S2).

2) the heel of the foot is innervated by the tibial nerve through S1 and S2 segments and the plantar surface of the foot receives L4 and L5 fibers medially (medial plantar nerve) and S1 and S2 laterally (lateral plantar nerve).

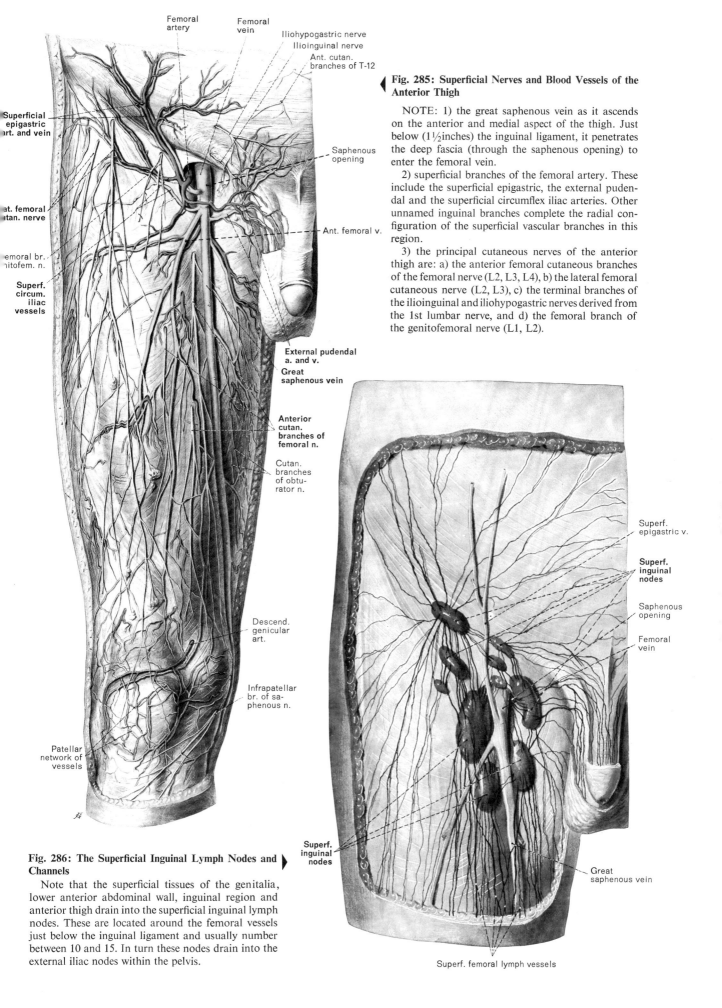

Femoral artery
Femoral vein
Iliohypogastric nerve
Ilioinguinal nerve
Ant. cutan. branches of T-12
Superficial epigastric art. and vein
Saphenous opening
at. femoral utan. nerve
Ant. femoral v.
emoral br. nitofem. n.
Superf. circum. iliac vessels
External pudendal a. and v.
Great saphenous vein
Anterior cutan. branches of femoral n.
Cutan. branches of obturator n.
Descend. genicular art.
Infrapatellar br. of saphenous n.
Patellar network of vessels
Superf. epigastric v.
Superf. inguinal nodes
Saphenous opening
Femoral vein
Superf. inguinal nodes
Great saphenous vein
Superf. femoral lymph vessels

Fig. 285: Superficial Nerves and Blood Vessels of the Anterior Thigh

NOTE: 1) the great saphenous vein as it ascends on the anterior and medial aspect of the thigh. Just below (1½ inches) the inguinal ligament, it penetrates the deep fascia (through the saphenous opening) to enter the femoral vein.

2) superficial branches of the femoral artery. These include the superficial epigastric, the external pudendal and the superficial circumflex iliac arteries. Other unnamed inguinal branches complete the radial configuration of the superficial vascular branches in this region.

3) the principal cutaneous nerves of the anterior thigh are: a) the anterior femoral cutaneous branches of the femoral nerve (L2, L3, L4), b) the lateral femoral cutaneous nerve (L2, L3), c) the terminal branches of the ilioinguinal and iliohypogastric nerves derived from the 1st lumbar nerve, and d) the femoral branch of the genitofemoral nerve (L1, L2).

Fig. 286: The Superficial Inguinal Lymph Nodes and Channels

Note that the superficial tissues of the genitalia, lower anterior abdominal wall, inguinal region and anterior thigh drain into the superficial inguinal lymph nodes. These are located around the femoral vessels just below the inguinal ligament and usually number between 10 and 15. In turn these nodes drain into the external iliac nodes within the pelvis.

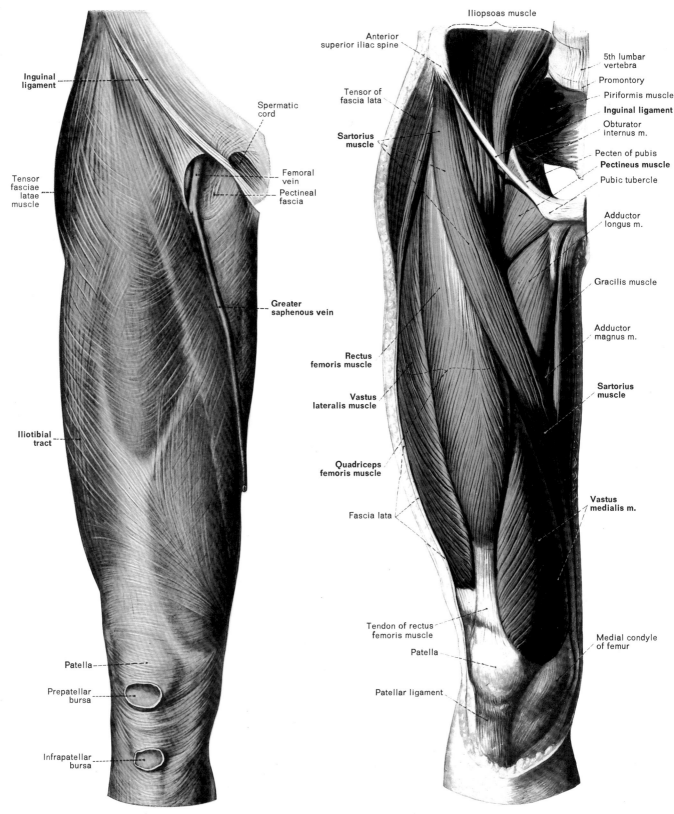

Fig. 287: The Fascia of the Anterior Thigh, the Fascia Lata (right)

NOTE: 1) the dense fascia which invests the muscles of the hip and thigh is called the fascia lata. It is attached above to the ischial and pubic rami and inguinal ligament anteriorly, the crest of the ilium laterally and the ischial tuberosity, sacrotuberous ligament, sacrum and coccyx posteriorly.

2) in the inguinal region the fascia lata is pierced by the greater saphenous vein and inferiorly it extends to the investing fascia below the knee.

Fig. 288: The Anterior Muscles of the Thigh: Superficial View (right)

NOTE: 1) the long narrow sartorius muscle which arises on the anterior superior iliac spine and passes obliquely across the anterior femoral muscles to insert on the medial aspect of the body of the tibia. The sartorius flexes the thigh and rotates it laterally. It also flexes the knee and rotates it medially.

2) the quadriceps muscle forms the bulk of the anterior femoral muscles and both the sartorius and quadriceps are innervated by the femoral nerve.

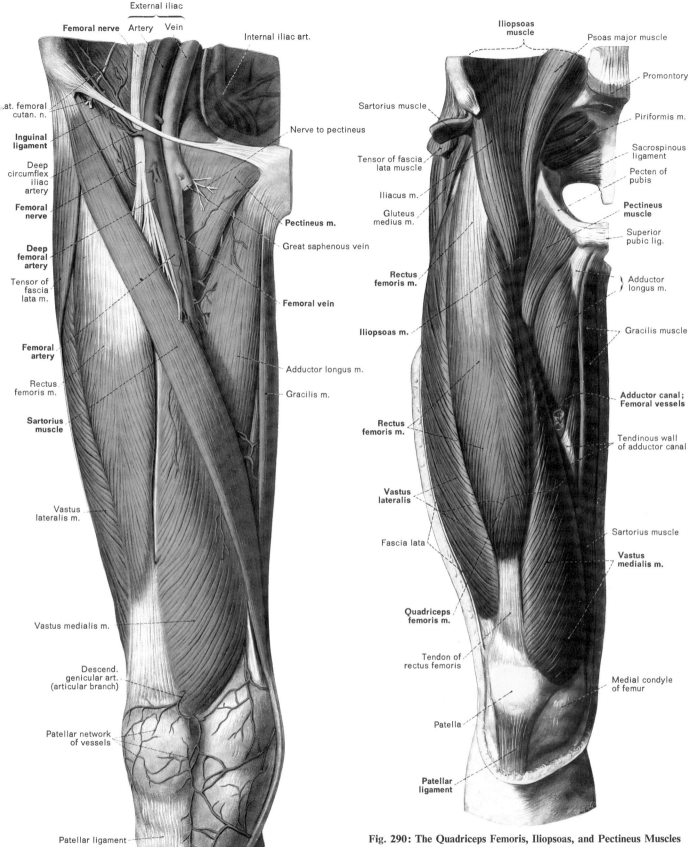

Femoral nerve External iliac Artery Vein

Internal iliac art.

at. femoral cutan. n.

Inguinal ligament

Deep circumflex iliac artery

Femoral nerve

Deep femoral artery

Tensor of fascia lata m.

Femoral artery

Rectus femoris m.

Sartorius muscle

Vastus lateralis m.

Vastus medialis m.

Descend. genicular art. (articular branch)

Patellar network of vessels

Patellar ligament

Nerve to pectineus

Pectineus m.

Great saphenous vein

Femoral vein

Adductor longus m.

Gracilis m.

Iliopsoas muscle Psoas major muscle

Promontory

Sartorius muscle

Piriformis m.

Tensor of fascia lata muscle

Sacrospinous ligament

Pecten of pubis

Iliacus m.

Pectineus muscle

Gluteus medius m.

Superior pubic lig.

Rectus femoris m.

Adductor longus m.

Iliopsoas m.

Gracilis muscle

Adductor canal; Femoral vessels

Rectus femoris m.

Tendinous wall of adductor canal

Vastus lateralis

Fascia lata

Sartorius muscle

Vastus medialis m.

Quadriceps femoris m.

Tendon of rectus femoris

Medial condyle of femur

Patella

Patellar ligament

Fig. 289: The Femoral Triangle

NOTE: the boundaries of the femoral triangle are the inguinal ligament, the sartorius muscle and the medial border of the adductor longus. The floor is formed by the iliopsoas and pectineus muscles. The femoral nerve, artery and vein descend beneath the inguinal ligament and traverse the femoral triangle.

Fig. 290: The Quadriceps Femoris, Iliopsoas, and Pectineus Muscles

NOTE: 1) the quadriceps femoris (rectus femoris and vastus lateralis, intermedius and medialis) as it converges inferiorly to form a powerful tendon which encases the patella and which is inserted onto the tuberosity of the tibia. The entire quadriceps extends the leg while the rectus femoris also flexes the thigh.

2) the iliopsoas muscle is a powerful flexor of the thigh and inserts on the lesser trochanter.

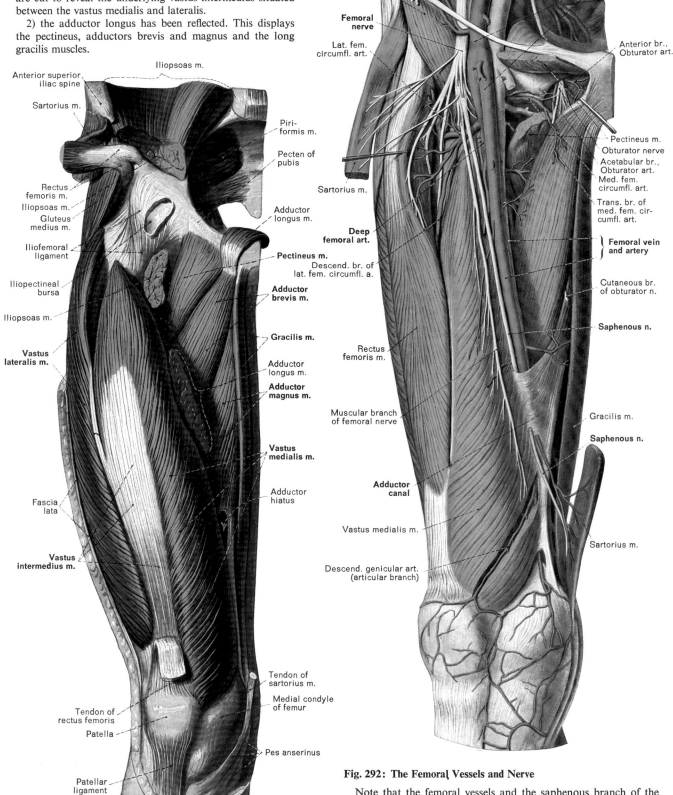

Fig. 291: The Intermediate Layer of Anterior and Medial Thigh Muscles

NOTE: 1) that the rectus femoris and iliopsoas muscles are cut to reveal the underlying vastus intermedius situated between the vastus medialis and lateralis.

2) the adductor longus has been reflected. This displays the pectineus, adductors brevis and magnus and the long gracilis muscles.

Anterior superior iliac spine
Iliopsoas m.
Sartorius m.
Piriformis m.
Pecten of pubis
Rectus femoris m.
Iliopsoas m.
Gluteus medius m.
Adductor longus m.
Iliofemoral ligament
Pectineus m.
Iliopectineal bursa
Adductor brevis m.
Iliopsoas m.
Gracilis m.
Vastus lateralis m.
Adductor longus m.
Adductor magnus m.
Vastus medialis m.
Adductor hiatus
Fascia lata
Vastus intermedius m.
Tendon of sartorius m.
Medial condyle of femur
Tendon of rectus femoris
Patella
Pes anserinus
Patellar ligament

Obturator nerve
Iliopsoas m.
Femoral artery
Femoral nerve
Lat. fem. circumfl. art.
Anterior br., Obturator art.
Sartorius m.
Pectineus m.
Obturator nerve
Acetabular br., Obturator art.
Med. fem. circumfl. art.
Trans. br. of med. fem. circumfl. art.
Deep femoral art.
Descend. br. of lat. fem. circumfl. a.
Femoral vein and artery
Rectus femoris m.
Cutaneous br. of obturator n.
Saphenous n.
Muscular branch of femoral nerve
Gracilis m.
Saphenous n.
Adductor canal
Vastus medialis m.
Sartorius m.
Descend. genicular art. (articular branch)

Fig. 292: The Femoral Vessels and Nerve

Note that the femoral vessels and the saphenous branch of the femoral nerve descend in the thigh and enter the adductor canal (of Hunter). Whereas the saphenous nerve then penetrates the overlying fascia to reach the superficial leg region, the vessels continue through the adductor magnus to reach the popliteal fossa on the posterior aspect.

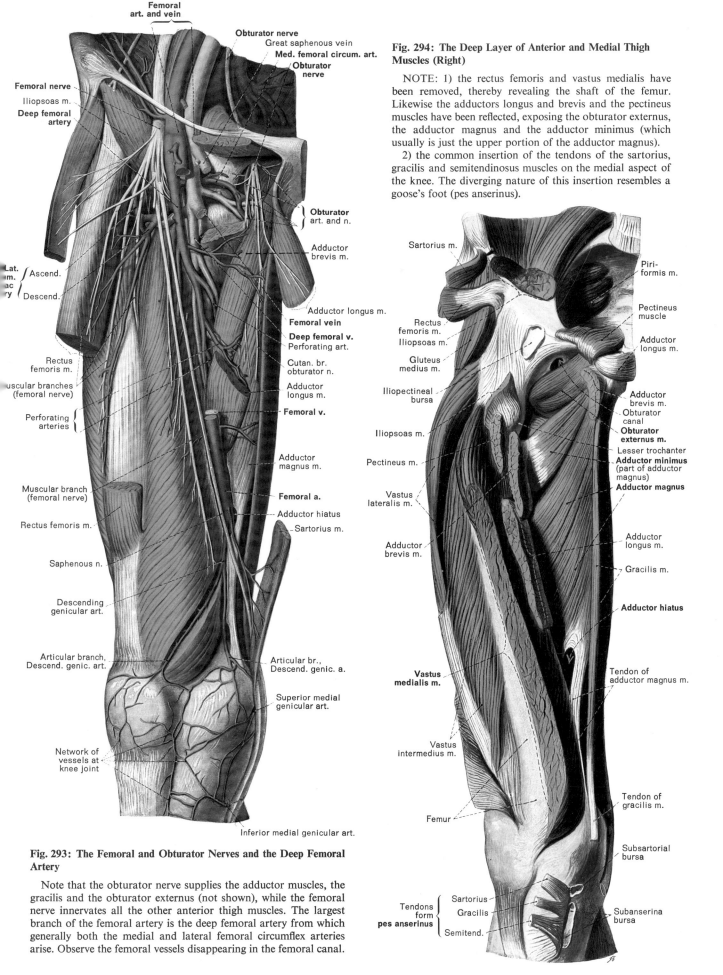

Femoral art. and vein

Obturator nerve

Great saphenous vein

Med. femoral circum. art.

Obturator nerve

Femoral nerve

Iliopsoas m.

Deep femoral artery

Obturator art. and n.

Adductor brevis m.

Lat. fm. iac ry { Ascend. / Descend.

Adductor longus m.

Femoral vein

Deep femoral v.

Perforating art.

Cutan. br. obturator n.

Adductor longus m.

Femoral v.

Rectus femoris m.

uscular branches (femoral nerve)

Perforating arteries

Adductor magnus m.

Femoral a.

Muscular branch (femoral nerve)

Adductor hiatus

Sartorius m.

Rectus femoris m.

Saphenous n.

Descending genicular art.

Articular branch, Descend. genic. art.

Articular br., Descend. genic. a.

Superior medial genicular art.

Network of vessels at knee joint

Inferior medial genicular art.

Fig. 293: The Femoral and Obturator Nerves and the Deep Femoral Artery

Note that the obturator nerve supplies the adductor muscles, the gracilis and the obturator externus (not shown), while the femoral nerve innervates all the other anterior thigh muscles. The largest branch of the femoral artery is the deep femoral artery from which generally both the medial and lateral femoral circumflex arteries arise. Observe the femoral vessels disappearing in the femoral canal.

Fig. 294: The Deep Layer of Anterior and Medial Thigh Muscles (Right)

NOTE: 1) the rectus femoris and vastus medialis have been removed, thereby revealing the shaft of the femur. Likewise the adductors longus and brevis and the pectineus muscles have been reflected, exposing the obturator externus, the adductor magnus and the adductor minimus (which usually is just the upper portion of the adductor magnus).

2) the common insertion of the tendons of the sartorius, gracilis and semitendinosus muscles on the medial aspect of the knee. The diverging nature of this insertion resembles a goose's foot (pes anserinus).

Sartorius m.

Piri-formis m.

Rectus femoris m.

Iliopsoas m.

Gluteus medius m.

Iliopectineal bursa

Iliopsoas m.

Pectineus m.

Vastus lateralis m.

Adductor brevis m.

Pectineus muscle

Adductor longus m.

Adductor brevis m.

Obturator canal

Obturator externus m.

Lesser trochanter

Adductor minimus (part of adductor magnus)

Adductor magnus

Adductor longus m.

Gracilis m.

Adductor hiatus

Vastus medialis m.

Tendon of adductor magnus m.

Vastus intermedius m.

Femur

Tendon of gracilis m.

Subsartorial bursa

Tendons form **pes anserinus** { Sartorius / Gracilis / Semitend.

Subanserina bursa

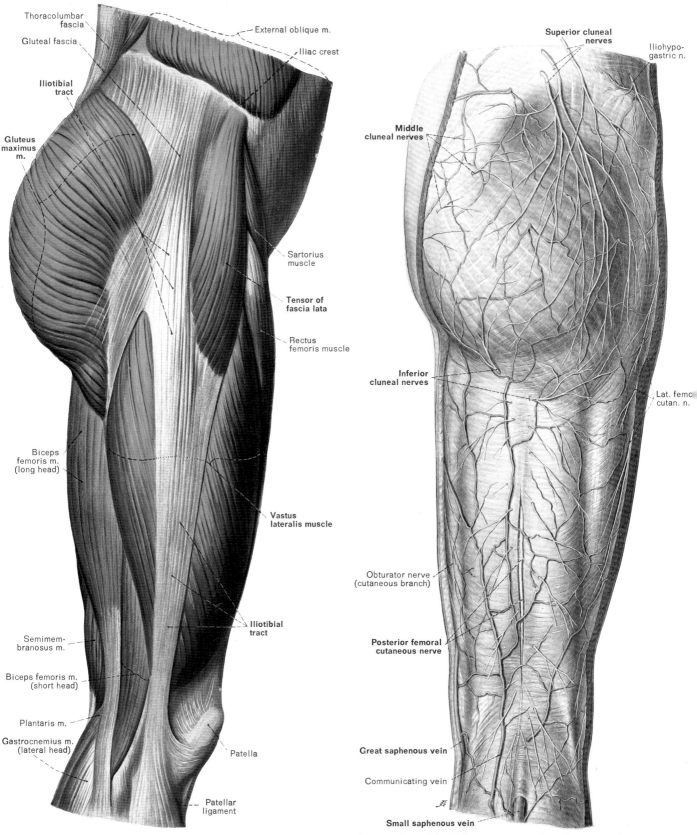

Fig. 295: Superficial Thigh and Gluteal Muscles (Lateral View)

Note the massive nature of the vastus lateralis and gluteus maximus muscles. Superficially, the iliotibial tract (band) stretches the length of the thigh, and its muscle, the tensor of the fascia lata, helps to keep the dense fascial sheet taut, thereby assisting in the maintenance of an erect posture.

Fig. 296: Superficial Veins and Nerves of the Gluteal Region and Posterior Thigh

Note that the principal cutaneous nerves of the gluteal region are the a) superior cluneal (L1, L2, L3, posterior rami), b) middle cluneal (S1, S2, S3, posterior rami), and c) inferior cluneal (S1, S2, S3 from posterior femoral cutaneous nerve). The skin of the posterior aspect of the thigh is innervated primarily by the posterior femoral cutaneous nerve (S1, S2, S3).

Fig. 313: Arteriogram of Lower Femoral and Popliteal Arteries

NOTE: 1) this arteriogram shows the arterial tree of the lower third of the thigh and the upper third of the calf. Note the course of the femoral artery as it becomes the popliteal artery just above the intercondylar fossa in the popliteal space. The genicular arteries supplying the knee joint, and the sural arteries descending to supply both superficial and muscular tissues in the calf can be seen arising from the popliteal artery.

2) below the popliteal fossa the popliteal artery becomes the posterior tibial artery. Soon, the anterior tibial artery branches from the posterior tibial to course toward the anterior compartment in the leg, while the posterior tibial continues to descend in the posterior compartment. About 3 inches below the knee the peroneal artery arises from the posterior tibial artery and descends in the lateral portion of the deep calf.

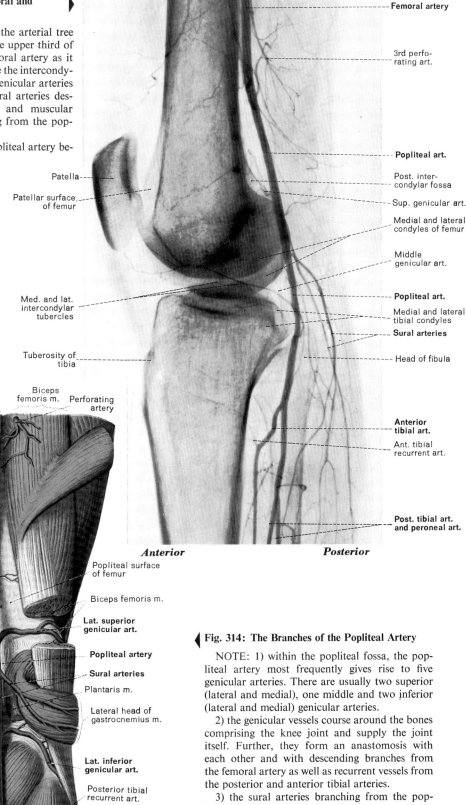

Anterior   Posterior

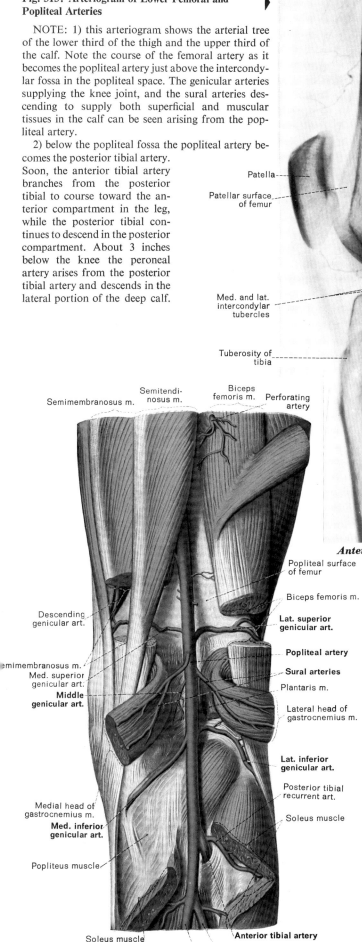

Fig. 314: The Branches of the Popliteal Artery

NOTE: 1) within the popliteal fossa, the popliteal artery most frequently gives rise to five genicular arteries. There are usually two superior (lateral and medial), one middle and two inferior (lateral and medial) genicular arteries.

2) the genicular vessels course around the bones comprising the knee joint and supply the joint itself. Further, they form an anastomosis with each other and with descending branches from the femoral artery as well as recurrent vessels from the posterior and anterior tibial arteries.

3) the sural arteries branching from the popliteal to supply the two heads of the gastrocnemius muscle.

4) the anterior tibial artery branching from the posterior tibial and penetrating an aperture above the interosseous membrane achieves the anterior compartment. Somewhat lower the peroneal artery also branches from the posterior tibial.

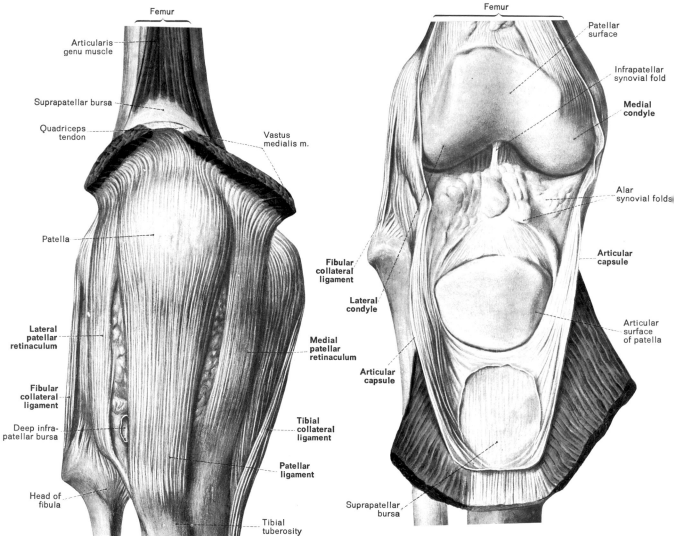

Fig. 315: Right Knee Joint (Anterior View)

Femur

Articularis genu muscle

Suprapatellar bursa

Quadriceps tendon

Vastus medialis m.

Patella

Lateral patellar retinaculum

Medial patellar retinaculum

Fibular collateral ligament

Deep infrapatellar bursa

Tibial collateral ligament

Patellar ligament

Head of fibula

Tibial tuberosity

Femur

Patellar surface

Infrapatellar synovial fold

Medial condyle

Alar synovial folds

Articular capsule

Fibular collateral ligament

Lateral condyle

Articular capsule

Articular surface of patella

Suprapatellar bursa

Fig. 316: Extended Right Knee Joint, opened from Anterior Side

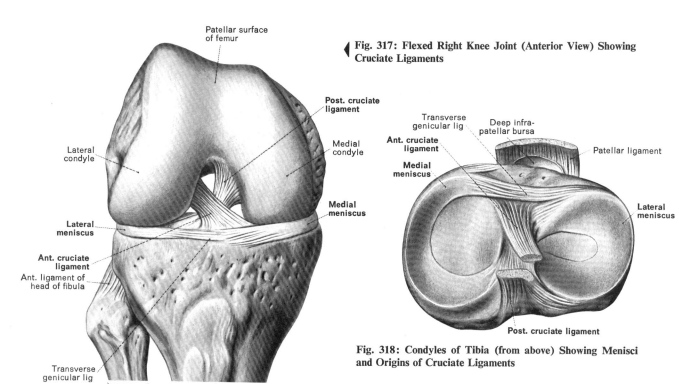

Patellar surface of femur

◀ **Fig. 317: Flexed Right Knee Joint (Anterior View) Showing Cruciate Ligaments**

Post. cruciate ligament

Lateral condyle

Medial condyle

Medial meniscus

Lateral meniscus

Ant. cruciate ligament

Ant. ligament of head of fibula

Transverse genicular lig

Fibula

Tibia

Transverse genicular lig

Deep infrapatellar bursa

Ant. cruciate ligament

Patellar ligament

Medial meniscus

Lateral meniscus

Post. cruciate ligament

Fig. 318: Condyles of Tibia (from above) Showing Menisci and Origins of Cruciate Ligaments

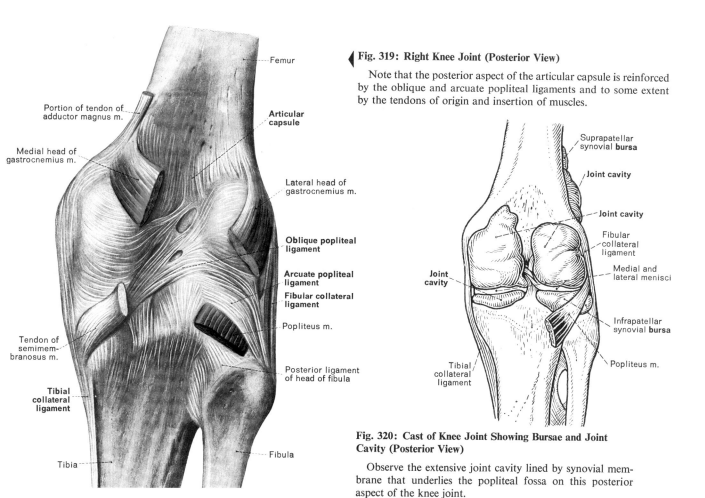

Femur

Portion of tendon of
adductor magnus m.

Medial head of
gastrocnemius m.

**Articular
capsule**

Lateral head of
gastrocnemius m.

**Oblique popliteal
ligament**

**Arcuate popliteal
ligament**

**Fibular collateral
ligament**

Popliteus m.

Tendon of
semimem-
branosus m.

Posterior ligament
of head of fibula

**Tibial
collateral
ligament**

Tibia

Fibula

◀ **Fig. 319: Right Knee Joint (Posterior View)**

Note that the posterior aspect of the articular capsule is reinforced
by the oblique and arcuate popliteal ligaments and to some extent
by the tendons of origin and insertion of muscles.

Suprapatellar
synovial **bursa**

Joint cavity

Joint cavity

Fibular
collateral
ligament

Medial and
lateral menisci

Joint
cavity

Infrapatellar
synovial **bursa**

Tibial
collateral
ligament

Popliteus m.

**Fig. 320: Cast of Knee Joint Showing Bursae and Joint
Cavity (Posterior View)**

Observe the extensive joint cavity lined by synovial membrane that underlies the popliteal fossa on this posterior
aspect of the knee joint.

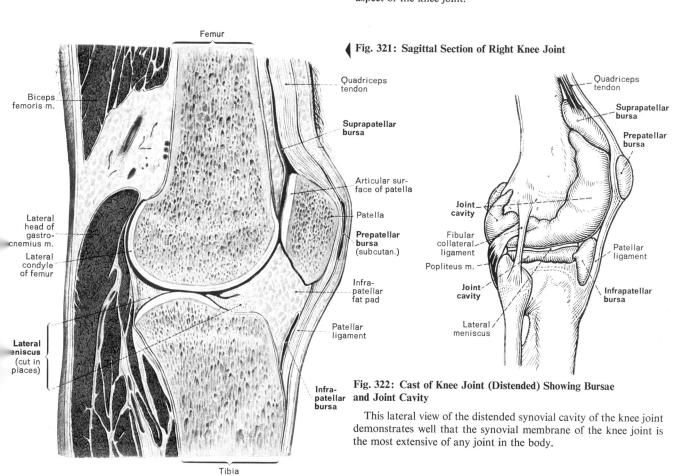

Femur

Biceps
femoris m.

Lateral
head of
gastro-
cnemius m.

Lateral
condyle
of femur

**Lateral
meniscus**
(cut in
places)

Tibia

Quadriceps
tendon

**Suprapatellar
bursa**

Articular sur-
face of patella

Patella

**Prepatellar
bursa**
(subcutan.)

Infra-
patellar
fat pad

Patellar
ligament

Infra-
patellar
bursa

◀ **Fig. 321: Sagittal Section of Right Knee Joint**

Quadriceps
tendon

**Suprapatellar
bursa**

**Prepatellar
bursa**

Joint
cavity

Fibular
collateral
ligament

Popliteus m.

Joint
cavity

Lateral
meniscus

Patellar
ligament

**Infrapatellar
bursa**

**Fig. 322: Cast of Knee Joint (Distended) Showing Bursae
and Joint Cavity**

This lateral view of the distended synovial cavity of the knee joint
demonstrates well that the synovial membrane of the knee joint is
the most extensive of any joint in the body.

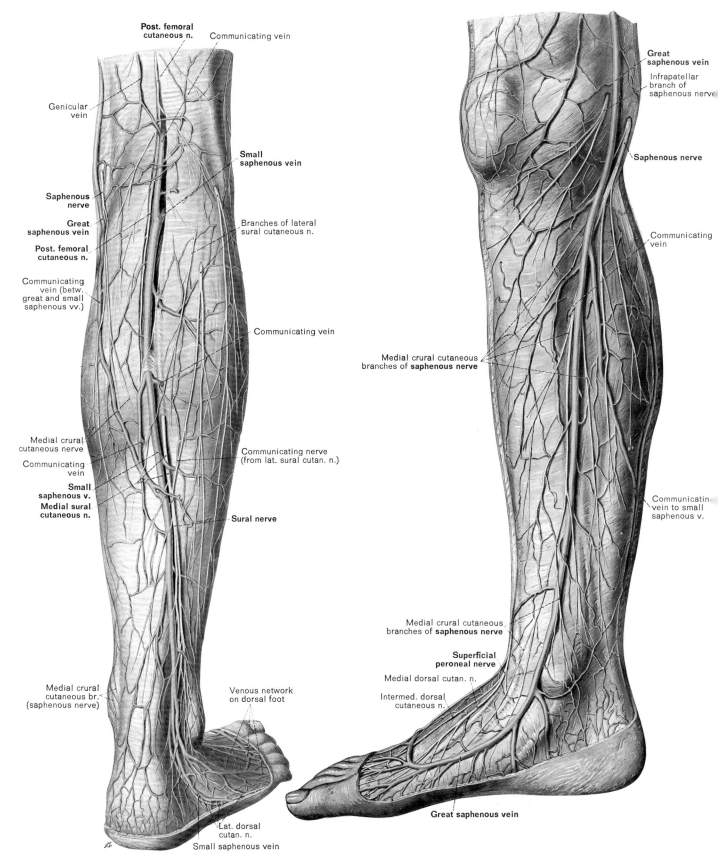

Post. femoral cutaneous n.

Communicating vein

Genicular vein

Small saphenous vein

Saphenous nerve

Branches of lateral sural cutaneous n.

Great saphenous vein

Post. femoral cutaneous n.

Communicating vein (betw. great and small saphenous vv.)

Communicating vein

Medial crural cutaneous nerve

Communicating vein

Communicating nerve (from lat. sural cutan. n.)

Small saphenous v.
Medial sural cutaneous n.

Sural nerve

Medial crural cutaneous br. (saphenous nerve)

Venous network on dorsal foot

Lat. dorsal cutan. n.

Small saphenous vein

Great saphenous vein

Infrapatellar branch of saphenous nerve

Saphenous nerve

Communicating vein

Medial crural cutaneous branches of **saphenous nerve**

Communicating vein to small saphenous v.

Medial crural cutaneous branches of **saphenous nerve**

Superficial peroneal nerve

Medial dorsal cutan. n.

Intermed. dorsal cutaneous n.

Great saphenous vein

Fig. 323: Superficial Veins and Nerves of the Posterior Leg and Foot

Note: the small saphenous vein which forms on the dorsolateral aspect of the foot and ascends to the popliteal fossa and the sural nerve which is formed by the junction of the medial sural cutaneous nerve and a communicating branch from the lateral sural cutaneous nerve.

Fig. 324: Superficial Veins and Nerves on the Medial Aspect of the Leg and Foot

Note the formation of the great saphenous vein on the medial aspect of the foot and its course anterior to the medial malleolus and up the medial aspect of the leg. Branches of the saphenous nerve accompany the great saphenous vein below the knee. The saphenous nerve is the largest branch of the femoral nerve.

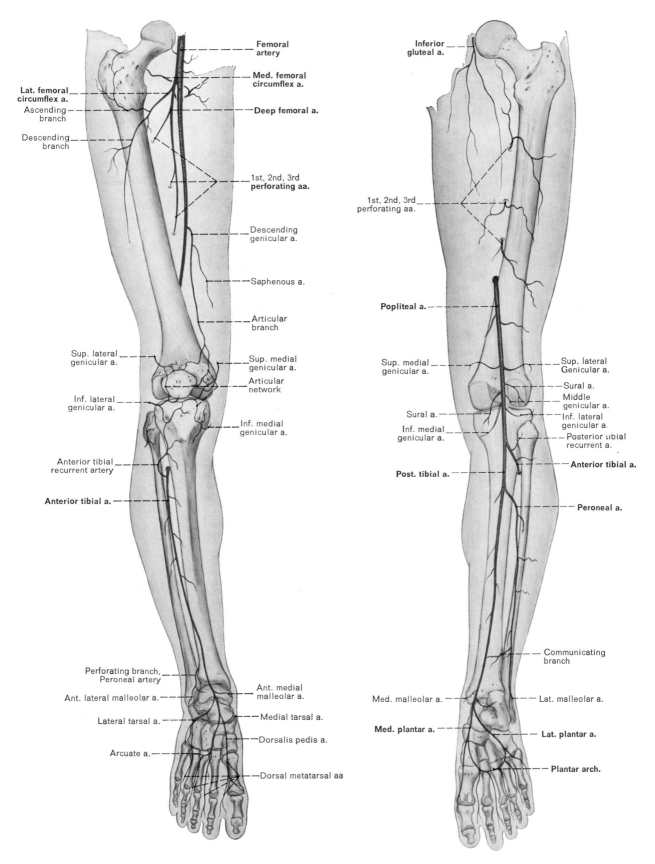

Fig. 325: Arteries and Bones of the Lower Limb (Anterior View)

Note the anastomosis of vessels in the hip and knee joint regions. Observe the perforating branches of the deep femoral artery which supply the musculature of the thigh. In the anterior leg region, the anterior tibial artery descends between the tibia and fibula to achieve the malleolar region and the dorsum of the foot.

Fig. 326: Arteries and Bones of the Lower Limb (Posterior View)

Note the participation of the inferior gluteal artery in the anastomosis of the hip region. Observe the branches of the popliteal artery in the knee region and its continuation as the posterior tibial. In the foot, the posterior tibial artery becomes the medial and lateral plantar arteries which are joined by the plantar arch.

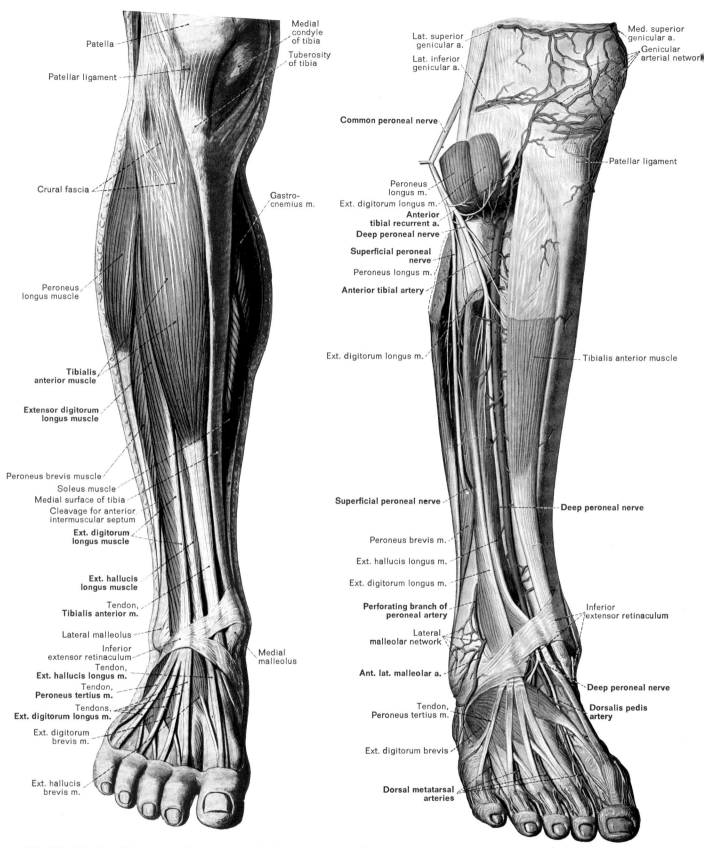

Fig. 327: Muscles of the Anterior Compartment of the Leg

NOTE: 1) the four anterior compartment muscles are the tibialis anterior, extensor hallucis longus, extensor digitorum longus and peroneus tertius.

2) the tibialis anterior dorsally flexes and supinates the foot. The other muscles extend the toes as well as dorsiflex the foot. Additionally, the extensor hallucis longus assists in supination while the extensor digitorum longus and peroneus tertius are pronators.

Fig. 328: Nerves and Arteries of the Anterior and Lateral Compartments of the Leg

NOTE: 1) as the common peroneal nerve courses laterally around the head of the fibula it divides into the superficial and deep peroneal nerves which innervate the muscles of the lateral and anterior compartments.

2) the deep peroneal nerve is joined by the anterior tibial artery which descends toward the foot.

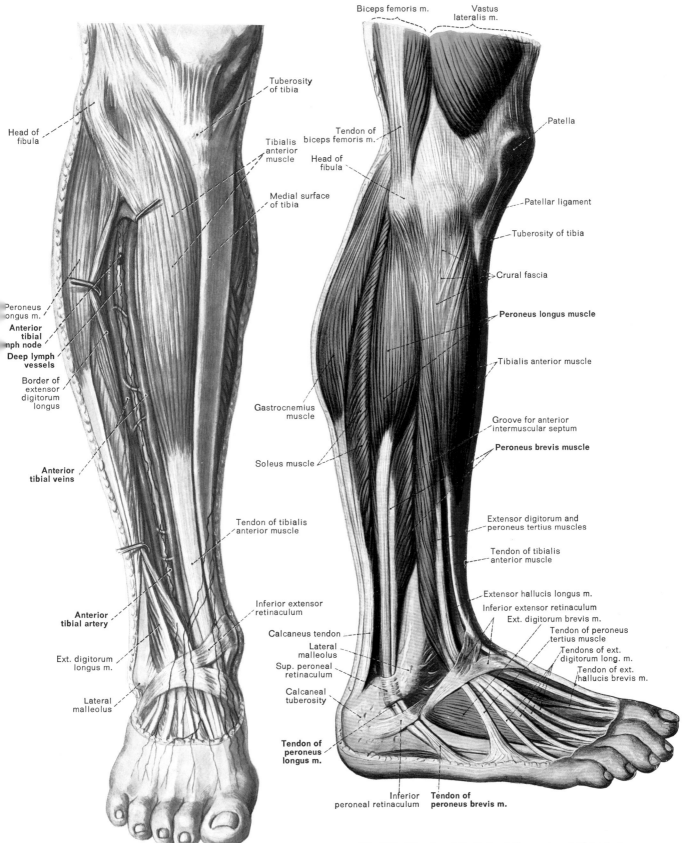

Fig. 329: Deep Lymphatic Channels and Nodes of the Anterior Leg

Note that lymphatic channels from the dorsum of the foot course superiorly and collect along the path of the more deeply situated anterior tibial vessels and nerve. At times a lymph node can be found just ventral to the anterior tibial artery below the knee.

Fig. 330: Muscles of the Lateral Compartment of the Leg

Note that the peroneus longus and brevis occupy the lateral compartment of the leg. Their tendons descend into the foot behind the lateral malleolus. The peroneus longus tendon crosses the sole of the foot to insert on the base of the 1st metatarsal bone while the peroneus brevis inserts directly onto the 5th metatarsal bone.

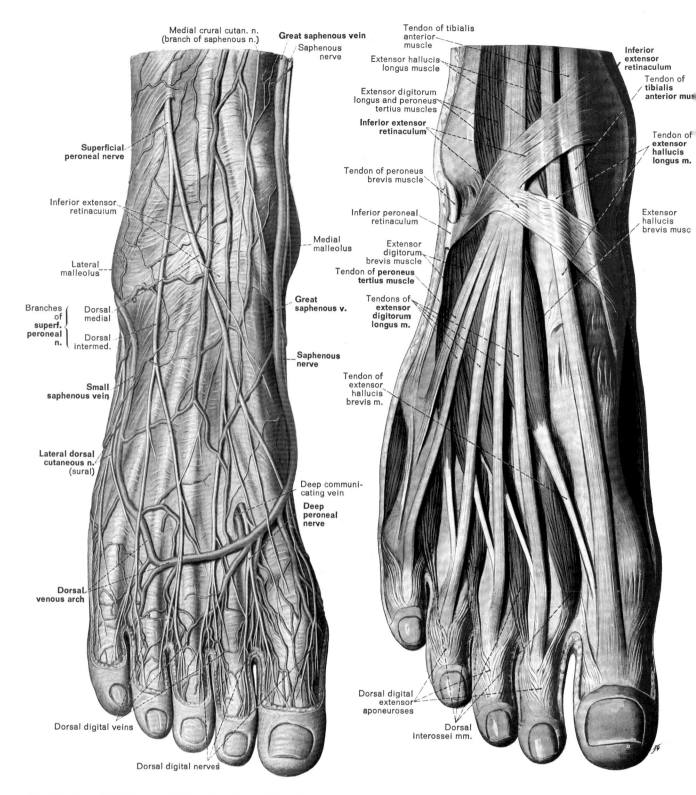

Fig. 331: Superficial Nerves and Veins of the Dorsal Right Foot

NOTE: 1) cutaneous innervation of the dorsal foot is supplied principally by the superficial peroneal nerve (L 4, L 5, S 1). Additionally, the deep peroneal nerve (L 4, L 5) supplies the adjacent sides of the 1st and 2nd toes while the lateral dorsal cutaneous nerve (S 1, S 2; terminal branch of the sural nerve in the foot) supplies the lateral and dorsal aspect of the 5th digit.

2) the digital and metatarsal veins drain back from the toes to form the dorsal venous arch of the foot. From this arch, the great saphenous vein ascends medially and the small saphenous vein laterally on the foot dorsum.

Fig. 332: Muscles and Tendons of the Dorsal Right Foot (Superficial View)

NOTE: 1) the tendons of the tibialis anterior, extensor hallucis longus and extensor digitorum longus are bound by the Y-shaped inferior extensor retinaculum as they enter the dorsum of the foot at the level of the ankle joint.

2) the long extensor tendons insert onto the dorsal aspect of the distal phalanx of each toe. In addition, the tendons of the extensor digitorum longus also insert onto the dorsum of the middle phalanx of the lateral four toes.

3) the tendon of the peroneus tertius inserts on the base of the 5th metatarsal bone (and at times the 4th also).

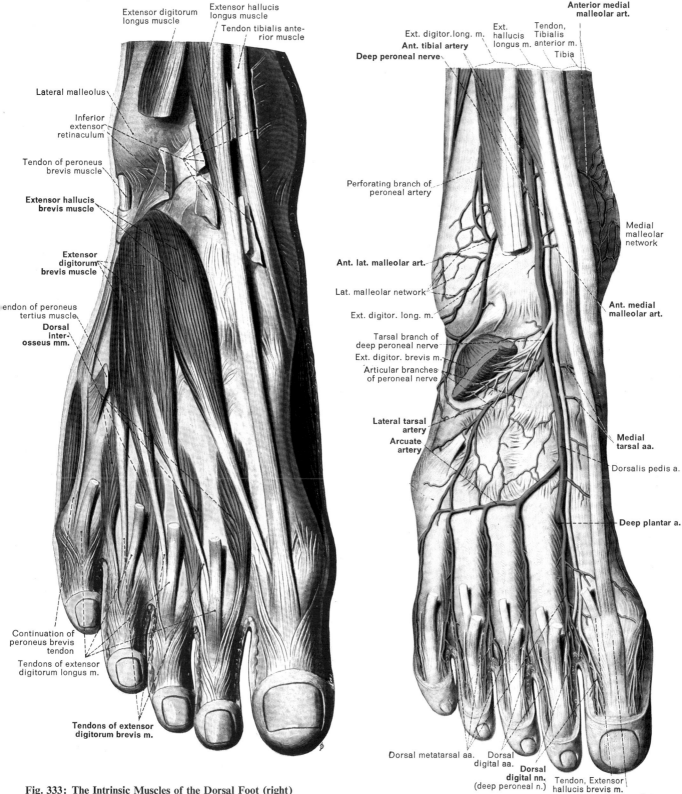

Fig. 333: The Intrinsic Muscles of the Dorsal Foot (right)

NOTE: 1) the inferior extensor retinaculum has been opened and the tendons of the extensor digitorum longus and peroneus tertius have been severed.

2) the extensor hallucis brevis and the three small bellies of the extensor digitorum brevis. The delicate tendons of these muscles insert on the proximal phalanx of the medial four toes.

3) the four dorsal interossei muscles. These muscles abduct the toes from the longitudinal axis of the foot (down the middle of the 2nd toe).

Fig. 334: Deep Nerves and Arteries of the Dorsal Foot

NOTE: 1) the deep coursing anterior tibial artery and deep peroneal nerve and their branches have been exposed. They enter the foot between the tendons of the extensor hallucis longus and extensor digitorum.

2) the anterior tibial artery becomes the dorsalis pedis artery below the ankle joint. Observe the malleolar, tarsal, arcuate, dorsal metatarsal and digital arteries.

3) the deep peroneal nerve supplies the extensor brevis muscle in the foot and continues distally to terminate as two dorsal digital nerves supplying the adjacent sides of the 1st and 2nd toes.

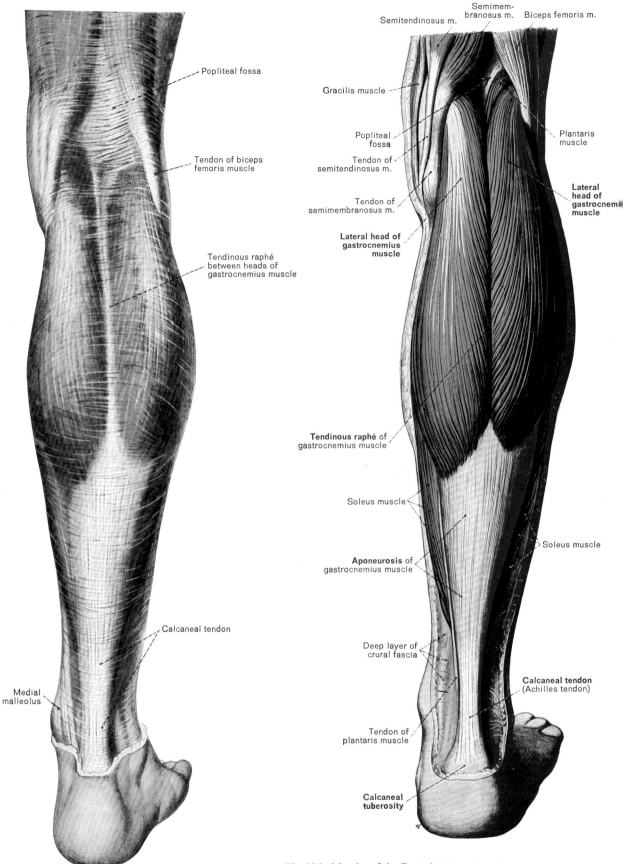

Semitendinosus m.
Semimembranosus m.
Biceps femoris m.

Gracilis muscle

Popliteal fossa

Popliteal fossa

Tendon of biceps femoris muscle

Tendon of semitendinosus m.

Plantaris muscle

Tendon of semimembranosus m.

Lateral head of gastrocnemius muscle

Lateral head of gastrocnemius muscle

Tendinous raphé between heads of gastrocnemius muscle

Tendinous raphé of gastrocnemius muscle

Soleus muscle

Soleus muscle

Aponeurosis of gastrocnemius muscle

Calcaneal tendon

Deep layer of crural fascia

Calcaneal tendon (Achilles tendon)

Medial malleolus

Tendon of plantaris muscle

Calcaneal tuberosity

Fig. 335: The Deep Fascia of the Leg (the Crural Fascia), Posterior View

Note that the deep fascia of the leg closely invests all of the muscles between the knee and ankle and forms the fascial covering over the popliteal fossa. It is continuous above with the fascia lata of the thigh and inferiorly with the retinacula which bind the tendons close to the bones.

Fig. 336: Muscles of the Posterior Leg: Superficial Calf Muscles

NOTE: 1) the gastrocnemius muscle arises by two heads from the condyles and posterior popliteal surface of the femur and its fibers are oriented inferomedially toward a central tendinous raphe. It inserts by means of the strong calcaneal tendon onto the calcaneal tuberosity.

2) the gastrocnemius is a powerful plantar flexor of the foot and its continued action also tends to flex the leg at the knee joint.

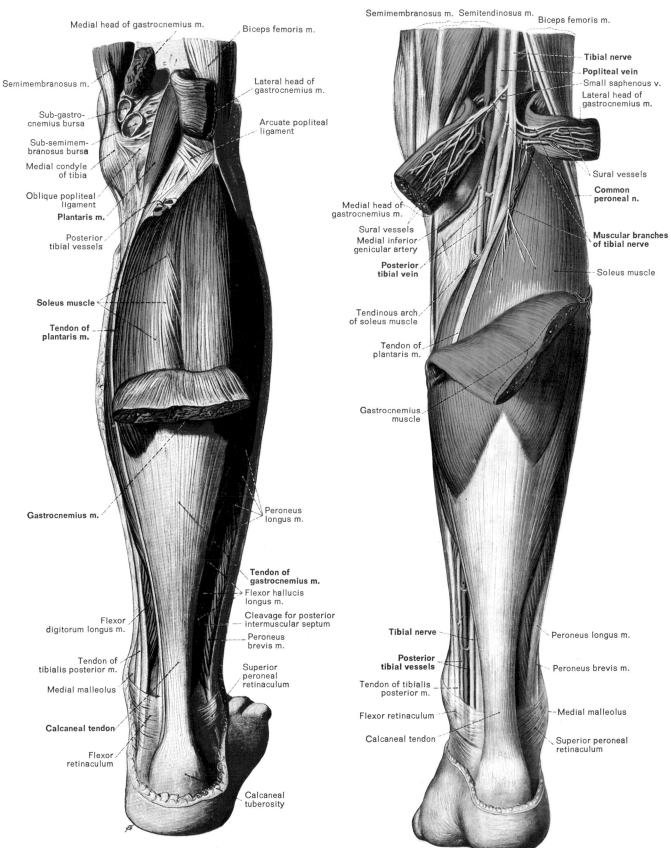

Fig. 337: Muscles of the Posterior Leg, Second Layer of Calf Muscles

NOTE: 1) both heads of the gastrocnemius have been severed to uncover the underlying soleus and plantaris muscles. The soleus is broad and thick, arising from the posterior surface of the fibula, the intermuscular septum and the dorsal aspect of the tibia. Its fibers join the calcaneal tendon.

2) the plantaris courses between the gastrocnemius and soleus. Both muscles are plantar flexors of the foot.

Fig. 338: Nerves and Vessels of the Posterior Leg: Superficial Layer

Note that the popliteal vessels and tibial nerve, descending from the popliteal fossa into the posterior compartment of the leg, commence in the middle of the leg and course medially in a gradual fashion so that at the ankle they lie behind the medial malleolus.

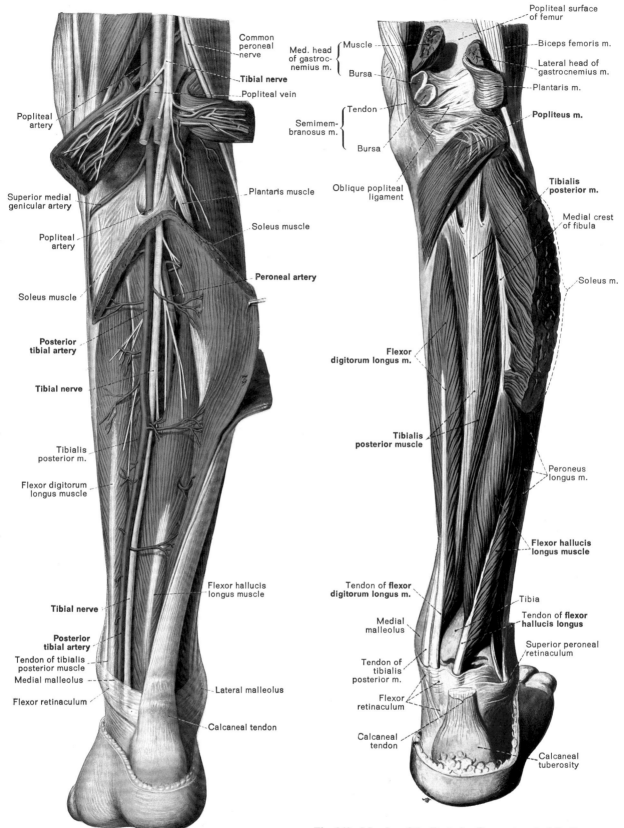

Fig. 339 labels:

Common peroneal nerve

Tibial nerve

Popliteal vein

Popliteal artery

Superior medial genicular artery

Popliteal artery

Soleus muscle

Posterior tibial artery

Tibial nerve

Tibialis posterior m.

Flexor digitorum longus muscle

Tibial nerve

Posterior tibial artery

Tendon of tibialis posterior muscle

Medial malleolus

Flexor retinaculum

Plantaris muscle

Soleus muscle

Peroneal artery

Flexor hallucis longus muscle

Lateral malleolus

Calcaneal tendon

Fig. 340 labels:

Popliteal surface of femur

Biceps femoris m.

Lateral head of gastrocnemius m.

Plantaris m.

Med. head of gastroc-nemius m. { Muscle / Bursa

Popliteus m.

Tendon

Semimem-branosus m. { Tendon / Bursa

Tibialis posterior m.

Oblique popliteal ligament

Medial crest of fibula

Soleus m.

Flexor digitorum longus m.

Tibialis posterior muscle

Peroneus longus m.

Flexor hallucis longus muscle

Tendon of **flexor digitorum longus m.**

Tibia

Tendon of **flexor hallucis longus**

Medial malleolus

Superior peroneal retinaculum

Tendon of tibialis posterior m.

Flexor retinaculum

Calcaneal tendon

Calcaneal tuberosity

Fig. 339: Nerves and Vessels of the Right Posterior Leg, Intermediate Layer

NOTE: 1) the soleus muscle has been severed and reflected laterally, exposing the course of the tibial artery and posterior tibial nerve as far as the medial malleolus.

2) that this vessel and nerve descend in the leg between the flexor hallucis longus and the flexor digitorum longus and dorsal to the tibialis posterior muscle.

Fig. 340: Muscles of the Posterior Compartment of the Leg: Deep Group: Four Muscles

NOTE: 1) the four deep posterior compartment muscles are: a) the popliteus, b) the flexor digitorum longus, c) the tibialis posterior and d) the flexor hallucis longus.

2) the popliteus is a femorotibial muscle and tends to rotate the leg medially and flex the leg at the knee joint. The other three muscles are cruropedal muscles and, as a group, they invert the foot, flex the toes and assist in plantarflexion at the ankle joint.

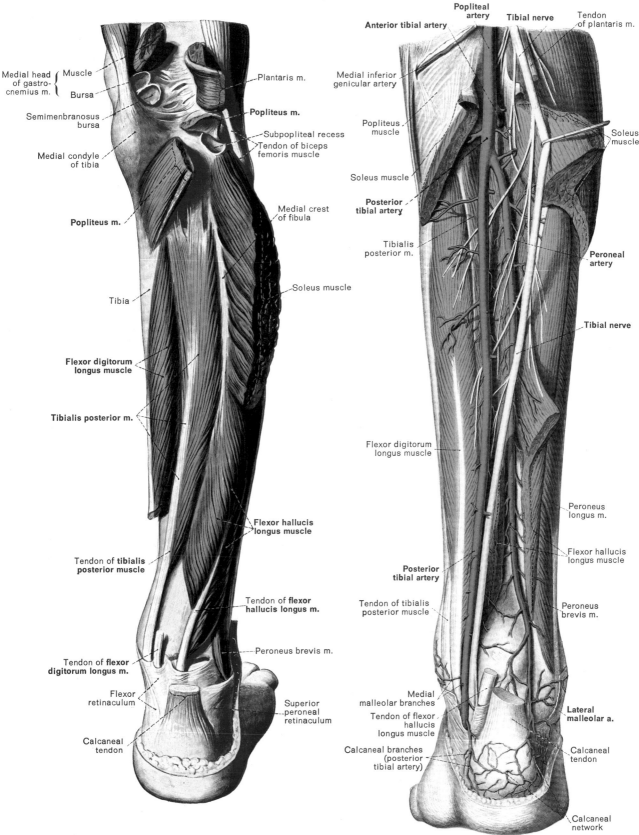

Fig. 341: The Tibialis Posterior and Flexor Hallucis Longus Muscles

NOTE: 1) the tendon of the flexor digitorum longus and the popliteus muscle have been severed. The tendon of the tibialis posterior crosses beneath that of the flexor digitorum longus just before entering the foot.

2) the flexor hallucis longus muscle arises from the distal 2/3rds of the fibula and the intermuscular septa. Its tendon lies in a groove on the posterior surface of the talus.

Fig. 342: Nerves and Muscles of the Deep Posterior Leg

NOTE: 1) the soleus muscle was resected and the tibial nerve pulled aside. Observe the branching of the peroneal artery from the posterior tibial and its descending course toward the lateral malleolus.

2) in the popliteal fossa, the tibial nerve courses superficial to the popliteal artery, whereas at the ankle, the posterior tibial artery is superficial to the tibial nerve.

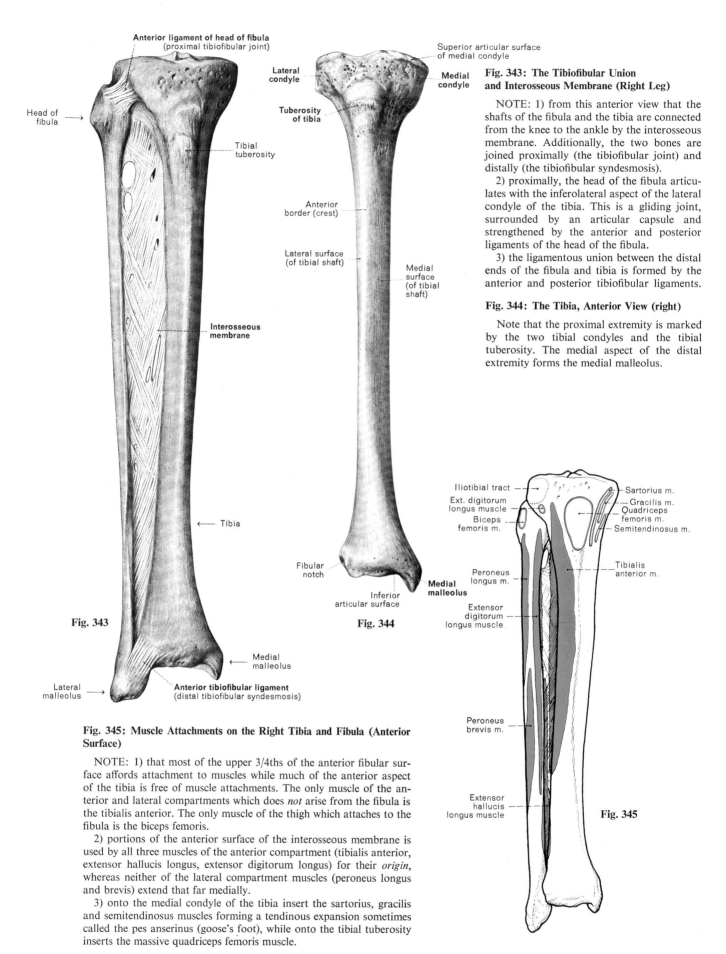

Anterior ligament of head of fibula
(proximal tibiofibular joint)

Head of fibula

Tibial tuberosity

Interosseous membrane

Tibia

Lateral malleolus

Medial malleolus

Anterior tibiofibular ligament
(distal tibiofibular syndesmosis)

Fig. 343

Superior articular surface of medial condyle

Lateral condyle

Medial condyle

Tuberosity of tibia

Anterior border (crest)

Lateral surface (of tibial shaft)

Medial surface (of tibial shaft)

Fibular notch

Medial malleolus

Inferior articular surface

Fig. 344

Iliotibial tract

Ext. digitorum longus muscle

Biceps femoris m.

Sartorius m.

Gracilis m.

Quadriceps femoris m.

Semitendinosus m.

Tibialis anterior m.

Peroneus longus m.

Medial malleolus

Extensor digitorum longus muscle

Peroneus brevis m.

Extensor hallucis longus muscle

Fig. 345

Fig. 343: The Tibiofibular Union and Interosseous Membrane (Right Leg)

NOTE: 1) from this anterior view that the shafts of the fibula and the tibia are connected from the knee to the ankle by the interosseous membrane. Additionally, the two bones are joined proximally (the tibiofibular joint) and distally (the tibiofibular syndesmosis).

2) proximally, the head of the fibula articulates with the inferolateral aspect of the lateral condyle of the tibia. This is a gliding joint, surrounded by an articular capsule and strengthened by the anterior and posterior ligaments of the head of the fibula.

3) the ligamentous union between the distal ends of the fibula and tibia is formed by the anterior and posterior tibiofibular ligaments.

Fig. 344: The Tibia, Anterior View (right)

Note that the proximal extremity is marked by the two tibial condyles and the tibial tuberosity. The medial aspect of the distal extremity forms the medial malleolus.

Fig. 345: Muscle Attachments on the Right Tibia and Fibula (Anterior Surface)

NOTE: 1) that most of the upper 3/4ths of the anterior fibular surface affords attachment to muscles while much of the anterior aspect of the tibia is free of muscle attachments. The only muscle of the anterior and lateral compartments which does *not* arise from the fibula is the tibialis anterior. The only muscle of the thigh which attaches to the fibula is the biceps femoris.

2) portions of the anterior surface of the interosseous membrane is used by all three muscles of the anterior compartment (tibialis anterior, extensor hallucis longus, extensor digitorum longus) for their *origin*, whereas neither of the lateral compartment muscles (peroneus longus and brevis) extend that far medially.

3) onto the medial condyle of the tibia insert the sartorius, gracilis and semitendinosus muscles forming a tendinous expansion sometimes called the pes anserinus (goose's foot), while onto the tibial tuberosity inserts the massive quadriceps femoris muscle.

Fig. 346: Muscle Attachments on the Right Tibia and Fibula (Posterior Surface)

NOTE: 1) that of the posterior compartment muscles, only the gastrocnemius and plantaris muscles do not attach to the posterior surface of the tibia, fibula or interosseous membrane.

2) that virtually the entire posterior surface of the fibula serves for the origin of muscles. The soleus arises from the upper one-third of the posterior fibular surface and along the soleal line of the tibia. Inferior to the origin of the soleus which spans across both bones, the flexor hallucis longus arises principally from the fibula, while the flexor digitorum longus arises primarily from the tibia.

3) the tibialis posterior is interposed between the flexors hallucis longus and digitorum longus, thereby arising from the posterior surface of the interosseous membrane.

4) the arrows indicating the course of the tendons into the foot from the posterior surface. Observe that the tendon of the tibialis posterior crosses from lateral to medial beneath the tendon of the flexor digitorum longus and enters the foot immediately behind the medial malleolus.

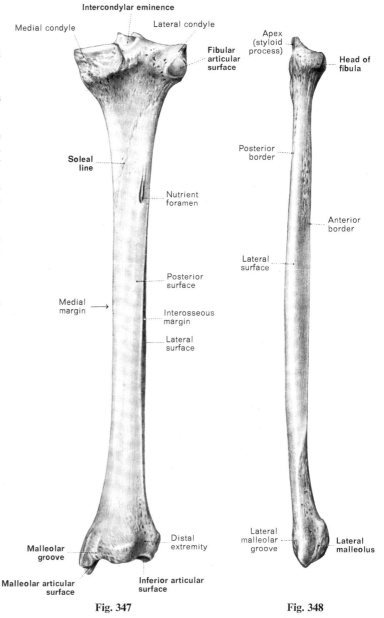

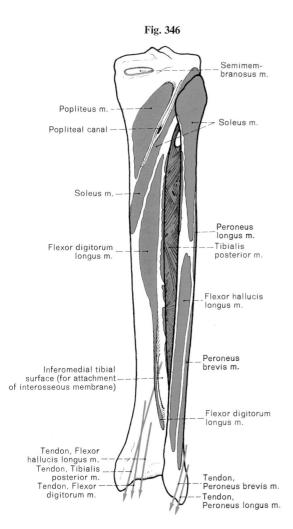

Fig. 346

Fig. 347: The Tibia, Posterior View (right)

NOTE: 1) the smooth posterior surface of the shaft of the tibia is marked by a prominent ridge (the soleal line) and a large oblong foramen (the nutrient foramen). The tibial shaft tapers toward a larger proximal extremity and somewhat less pronounced distal extremity.

2) at the proximal extremity the rounded medial and lateral condyles are separated by the intercondylar eminence, anterior and posterior to which attach the cruciate ligaments. At its distal extremity, the tibia articulates with the talus and, on this posterior surface, presents grooves for the passage of the tendons of the tibialis posterior, flexor digitorum longus and flexor hallucis longus.

Fig. 348: The Right Fibula (Lateral View)

NOTE: 1) the fibula is a long slender bone situated lateral to the tibia to which it articulates proximally (see Figure 345). Distally, the fibula expands to form the lateral malleolus. The medial aspect of its inferior articular surface participates with the tibia in forming the talocrural or ankle joint.

2) although the fibula does not bear any weight of the trunk (since it does not participate in the knee joint articulation), it is important because of the numerous muscles which attach to its surfaces (see Figures 345 and 346) and because it assists in the formation of the ankle joint.

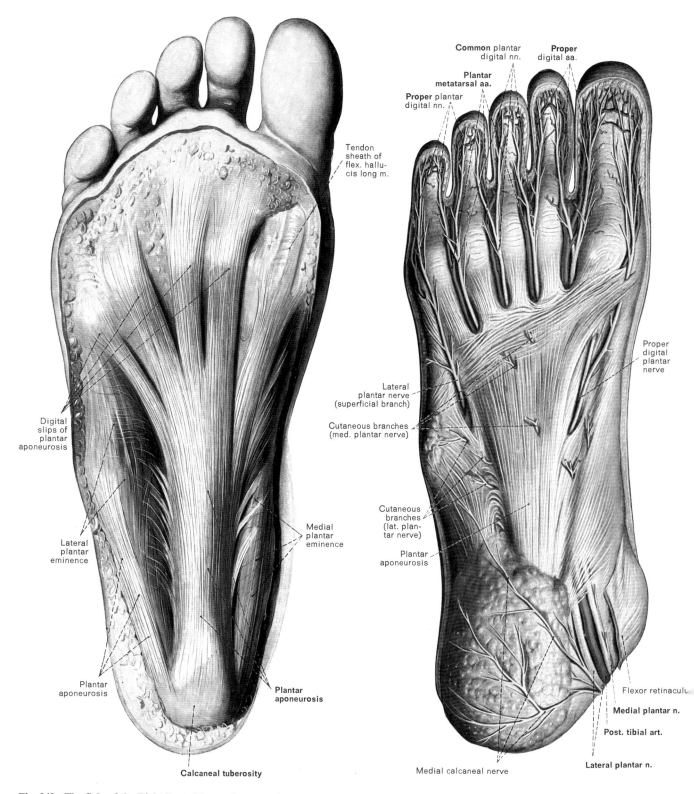

Fig. 349: The Sole of the Right Foot: Plantar Aponeurosis

NOTE: 1) the plantar aponeurosis which stretches across the sole of the foot. Similar to the palmar aponeurosis in the hand, the plantar aponeurosis is a thickened layer of deep fascia which serves both a protective and supportive function to the underlying muscles, vessels and nerves.

2) the longitudinal orientation of the fibers of the plantar aponeurosis and their attachment to the calcaneal tuberosity. Distally, the aponeurosis divides into five digital slips, one of which courses to each toe. Fibers extend from the margins of the aponeurosis to cover partially both the medial and lateral plantar eminences.

Fig. 350: The Sole of the Right Foot: Superficial Nerves and Arteries

NOTE: 1) the medial and lateral plantar nerves and posterior tibial artery as they enter the foot behind the medial malleolus and immediately course beneath the plantar aponeurosis toward the digits. Sensory branches of the nerves penetrate the aponeurosis to innervate the overlying skin and superficial fascia.

2) between the digital slips of the plantar aponeurosis the vessels and the nerves course superficially toward the toes. Metatarsal arteries and common plantar digital nerves divide to supply adjacent portions of the toes as proper plantar digital arteries and nerves.

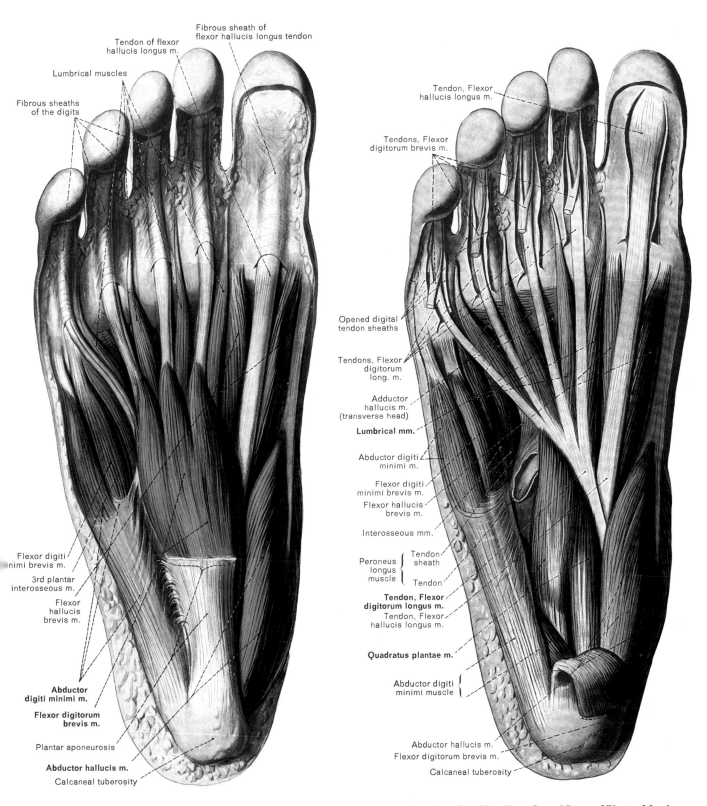

Fibrous sheath of
flexor hallucis longus tendon

Tendon of flexor
hallucis longus m.

Lumbrical muscles

Fibrous sheaths
of the digits

Flexor digiti
inimi brevis m.

3rd plantar
interosseous m.

Flexor
hallucis
brevis m.

**Abductor
digiti minimi m.**

**Flexor digitorum
brevis m.**

Plantar aponeurosis

Abductor hallucis m.
Calcaneal tuberosity

Tendon, Flexor
hallucis longus m.

Tendons, Flexor
digitorum brevis m.

Opened digital
tendon sheaths

Tendons, Flexor
digitorum
long. m.

Adductor
hallucis m.
(transverse head)

Lumbrical mm.

Abductor digiti
minimi m.

Flexor digiti
minimi brevis m.

Flexor hallucis
brevis m.

Interosseous mm.

Peroneus
longus
muscle

Tendon
sheath

Tendon

**Tendon, Flexor
digitorum longus m.**
Tendon, Flexor
hallucis longus m.

Quadratus plantae m.

Abductor digiti
minimi muscle

Abductor hallucis m.
Flexor digitorum brevis m.

Calcaneal tuberosity

Fig. 351: The Sole of the Right Foot: First Layer of Plantar Muscles

NOTE: 1) with most of the plantar aponeurosis removed, three muscles comprising the first layer of the sole are exposed. These are the abductor hallucis, the flexor digitorum brevis, and the abductor digiti minimi.

2) all three muscles arise from the tuberosity of the calcaneus. The abductor hallucis inserts on the first phalanx of the large toe. The flexor digiti brevis separates into four tendons which insert onto the middle phalanges of the lateral four toes. The abductor digiti minimi inserts onto the proximal phalanx of the little toe.

Fig. 352: The Sole of the Right Foot: Second Layer of Plantar Muscles

NOTE: 1) the tendons of the flexor hallucis brevis muscle were severed and removed, thereby exposing the underlying tendons of the flexor digitorum longus muscle.

2) the muscles of the second layer in the plantar foot include the quadratus plantae muscle and the four lumbrical muscles. The quadratus plantae arises by two heads from the calcaneus and inserts into the tendon of the flexor digitorum longus.

3) the four lumbrical muscles arising from the tendons of the flexor digitorum longus muscle. They insert on the medial aspect of the first phalanx of the lateral four toes as well as on the dorsal extensor hoods.

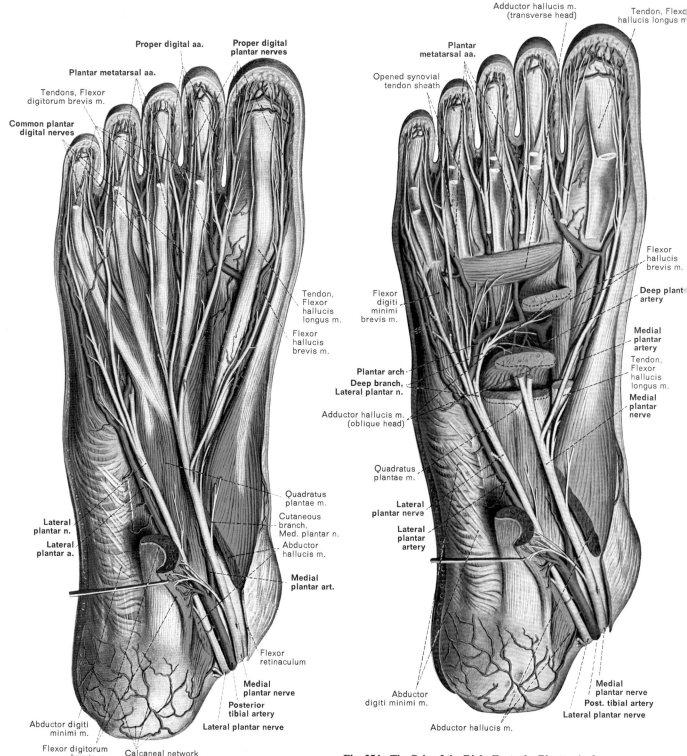

Fig. 353: The Sole of the Right Foot: the Plantar Nerves and Arteries

NOTE: 1) whereas the tibial nerve divides into medial and lateral plantar nerves just inferior to the medial malleolus, the posterior tibial artery enters the plantar surface of the foot as a single vessel and divides into medial and lateral plantar arteries beneath or at the medial border of the abductor hallucis muscle.

2) the lateral plantar nerve supplies the lateral 1–1/2 digits while the medial plantar nerve supplies the medial 3–1/2 digits. Observe the formation of the common digital plantar nerves which then divide into the proper digital plantar nerves.

Fig. 354: The Sole of the Right Foot: the Plantar Arch and Deep Vessels and Nerves

NOTE: 1) the formation of the deep plantar arch principally from the lateral plantar artery, and the junction of the deep plantar arch with the deep plantar artery from the foot dorsum (see Fig. 334). From the plantar arch branch plantar metatarsal arteries which then divide into proper digital arteries.

2) the muscles of the foot are innervated in the following manner:

	medial plantar nerve	*lateral plantar nerve*
1st layer	abductor hallucis flexor digitorum brevis	abductor digiti minimi
2nd layer	1st lumbrical	quadratus plantae 2nd, 3rd and 4th lumbrical
3rd layer	flexor hallucis brevis	adductor hallucis flexor digiti minimi brevis
4th layer	– – – – – –	plantar interossei dorsal interossei

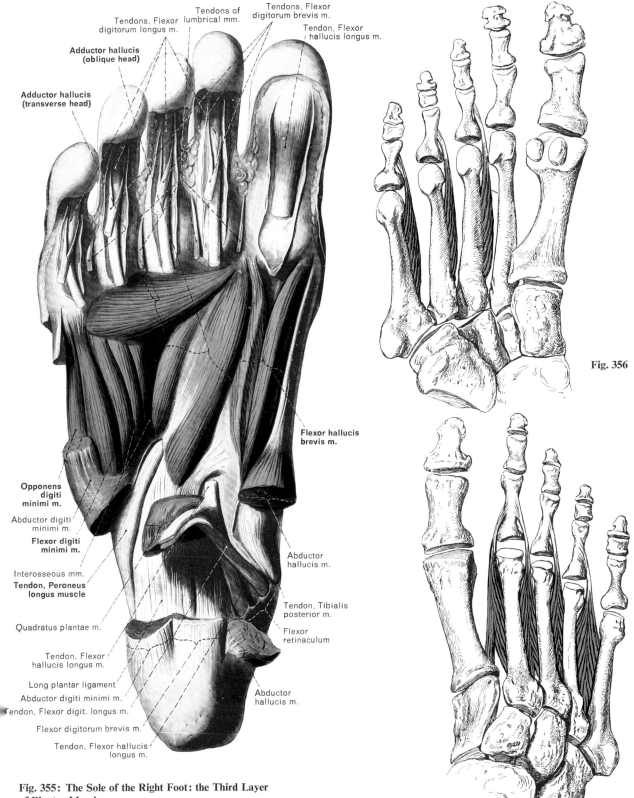

Tendons, Flexor digitorum longus m.

Tendons of lumbrical mm.

Tendons, Flexor digitorum brevis m.

Tendon, Flexor hallucis longus m.

Adductor hallucis (oblique head)

Adductor hallucis (transverse head)

Flexor hallucis brevis m.

Opponens digiti minimi m.

Abductor digiti minimi m.

Flexor digiti minimi m.

Interosseous mm.
Tendon, Peroneus longus muscle

Quadratus plantae m.

Abductor hallucis m.

Tendon, Tibialis posterior m.

Flexor retinaculum

Tendon, Flexor hallucis longus m.

Long plantar ligament

Abductor digiti minimi m.

Abductor hallucis m.

Tendon, Flexor digit. longus m.

Flexor digitorum brevis m.

Tendon, Flexor hallucis longus m.

Fig. 356

Fig. 357

Fig. 355: The Sole of the Right Foot: the Third Layer of Plantar Muscles

NOTE: 1) the third layer of plantar muscles consists of two flexors and an adductor in contrast to the first layer which contains one flexor and two abductors. Thus, the flexor hallucis brevis, flexor digiti minimi brevis and the two heads (oblique and transverse) of the adductor hallucis form the third layer of plantar muscles.

2) at times those fibers of the flexor digiti minimi brevis muscle which insert on the lateral side of the first phalanx of the 5th toe are referred to as a separate muscle, the opponens digiti minimi.

3) the tendon of the peroneus longus muscle which crosses the plantar aspect of the foot obliquely to insert on the lateral side of the base of the first metatarsal and the first (medial) cuneiform bone.

Fig. 356: The Plantar Interossei

Note that there are three plantar interossei. These muscles adduct the 3rd, 4th and 5th toes toward the 2nd toe which acts as the longitudinal axis of the foot.

Fig. 357: The Dorsal Interossei

Note that there are four dorsal interossei. These muscles abduct the toes from the reference axis. Both plantar and dorsal interossei flex the metatarsophalangeal joints and extend the interphalangeal joints.

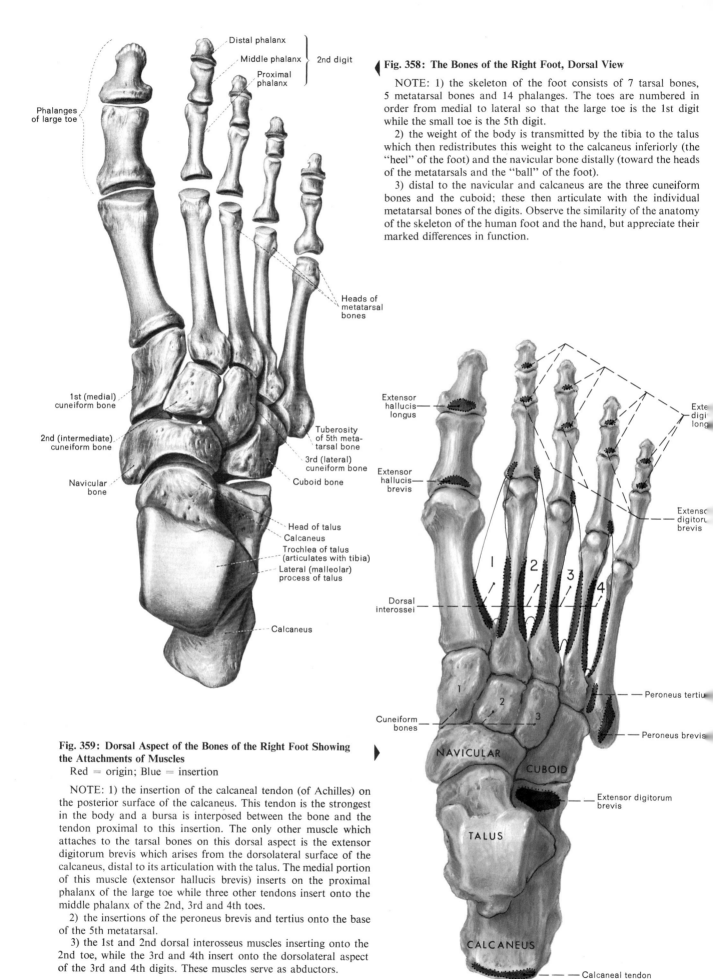

Distal phalanx
Middle phalanx } 2nd digit
Proximal phalanx

Phalanges of large toe

1st (medial) cuneiform bone

2nd (intermediate) cuneiform bone

Navicular bone

Heads of metatarsal bones

Tuberosity of 5th metatarsal bone

3rd (lateral) cuneiform bone

Cuboid bone

Head of talus
Calcaneus
Trochlea of talus (articulates with tibia)
Lateral (malleolar) process of talus

Calcaneus

Fig. 358: The Bones of the Right Foot, Dorsal View

NOTE: 1) the skeleton of the foot consists of 7 tarsal bones, 5 metatarsal bones and 14 phalanges. The toes are numbered in order from medial to lateral so that the large toe is the 1st digit while the small toe is the 5th digit.

2) the weight of the body is transmitted by the tibia to the talus which then redistributes this weight to the calcaneus inferiorly (the "heel" of the foot) and the navicular bone distally (toward the heads of the metatarsals and the "ball" of the foot).

3) distal to the navicular and calcaneus are the three cuneiform bones and the cuboid; these then articulate with the individual metatarsal bones of the digits. Observe the similarity of the anatomy of the skeleton of the human foot and the hand, but appreciate their marked differences in function.

Extensor hallucis longus

Extensor hallucis brevis

Dorsal interossei

Cuneiform bones

NAVICULAR

CUBOID

TALUS

CALCANEUS

Exte digit long

Extenso digitoru brevis

Peroneus tertiu

Peroneus brevis

Extensor digitorum brevis

Calcaneal tendon

Fig. 359: Dorsal Aspect of the Bones of the Right Foot Showing the Attachments of Muscles

Red = origin; Blue = insertion

NOTE: 1) the insertion of the calcaneal tendon (of Achilles) on the posterior surface of the calcaneus. This tendon is the strongest in the body and a bursa is interposed between the bone and the tendon proximal to this insertion. The only other muscle which attaches to the tarsal bones on this dorsal aspect is the extensor digitorum brevis which arises from the dorsolateral surface of the calcaneus, distal to its articulation with the talus. The medial portion of this muscle (extensor hallucis brevis) inserts on the proximal phalanx of the large toe while three other tendons insert onto the middle phalanx of the 2nd, 3rd and 4th toes.

2) the insertions of the peroneus brevis and tertius onto the base of the 5th metatarsal.

3) the 1st and 2nd dorsal interosseus muscles inserting onto the 2nd toe, while the 3rd and 4th insert onto the dorsolateral aspect of the 3rd and 4th digits. These muscles serve as abductors.

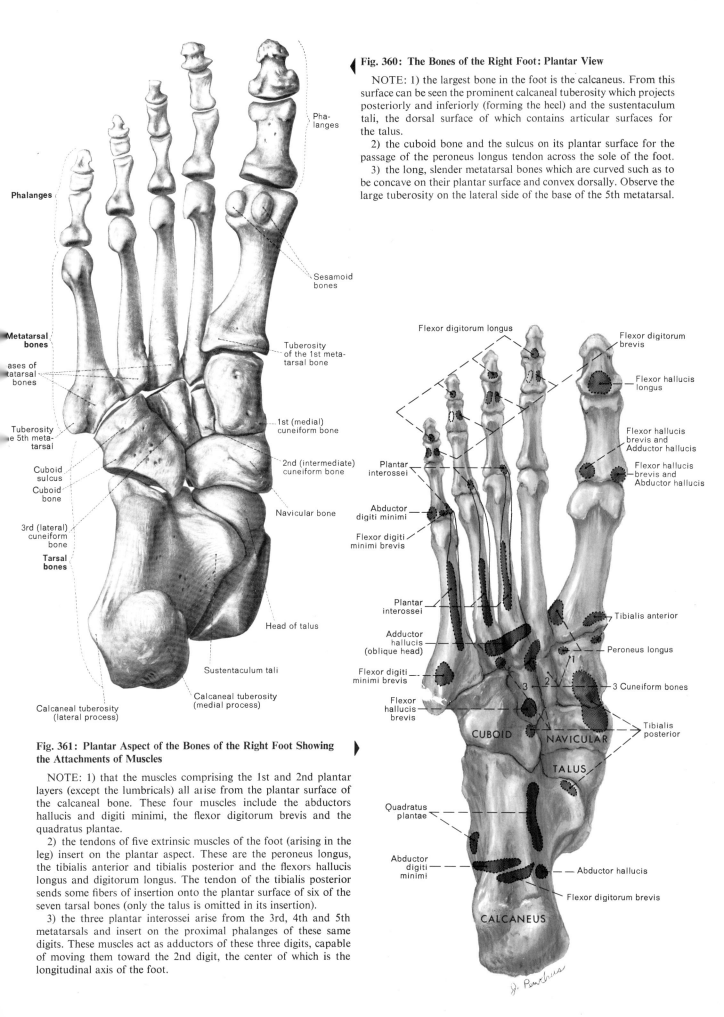

Phalanges

Pha-langes

Sesamoid bones

Metatarsal bones

ases of tatarsal bones

Tuberosity of the 1st meta-tarsal bone

Tuberosity e 5th meta-tarsal

1st (medial) cuneiform bone

Cuboid sulcus

2nd (intermediate) cuneiform bone

Cuboid bone

Navicular bone

3rd (lateral) cuneiform bone

Tarsal bones

Head of talus

Sustentaculum tali

Calcaneal tuberosity (lateral process)

Calcaneal tuberosity (medial process)

Fig. 360: The Bones of the Right Foot: Plantar View

NOTE: 1) the largest bone in the foot is the calcaneus. From this surface can be seen the prominent calcaneal tuberosity which projects posteriorly and inferiorly (forming the heel) and the sustentaculum tali, the dorsal surface of which contains articular surfaces for the talus.

2) the cuboid bone and the sulcus on its plantar surface for the passage of the peroneus longus tendon across the sole of the foot.

3) the long, slender metatarsal bones which are curved such as to be concave on their plantar surface and convex dorsally. Observe the large tuberosity on the lateral side of the base of the 5th metatarsal.

Flexor digitorum longus

Flexor digitorum brevis

Flexor hallucis longus

Flexor hallucis brevis and Adductor hallucis

Flexor hallucis brevis and Abductor hallucis

Plantar interossei

Abductor digiti minimi

Flexor digiti minimi brevis

Plantar interossei

Tibialis anterior

Peroneus longus

Adductor hallucis (oblique head)

Flexor digiti minimi brevis

3 Cuneiform bones

Flexor hallucis brevis

Tibialis posterior

CUBOID

NAVICULAR

TALUS

Quadratus plantae

Abductor digiti minimi

Abductor hallucis

Flexor digitorum brevis

CALCANEUS

J. Penthus

Fig. 361: Plantar Aspect of the Bones of the Right Foot Showing the Attachments of Muscles

NOTE: 1) that the muscles comprising the 1st and 2nd plantar layers (except the lumbricals) all arise from the plantar surface of the calcaneal bone. These four muscles include the abductors hallucis and digiti minimi, the flexor digitorum brevis and the quadratus plantae.

2) the tendons of five extrinsic muscles of the foot (arising in the leg) insert on the plantar aspect. These are the peroneus longus, the tibialis anterior and tibialis posterior and the flexors hallucis longus and digitorum longus. The tendon of the tibialis posterior sends some fibers of insertion onto the plantar surface of six of the seven tarsal bones (only the talus is omitted in its insertion).

3) the three plantar interossei arise from the 3rd, 4th and 5th metatarsals and insert on the proximal phalanges of these same digits. These muscles act as adductors of these three digits, capable of moving them toward the 2nd digit, the center of which is the longitudinal axis of the foot.

Fig. 362: Tendons at the Ankle Region: Dorsolateral View (Right Foot)

NOTE: 1) similar to what is observed at the wrist, tendons at the ankle region passing from the leg into the foot are bound by closely investing retinacula. The tendons themselves are surrounded by synovial sheaths which are indicated in blue in this figure and in Fig. 364.

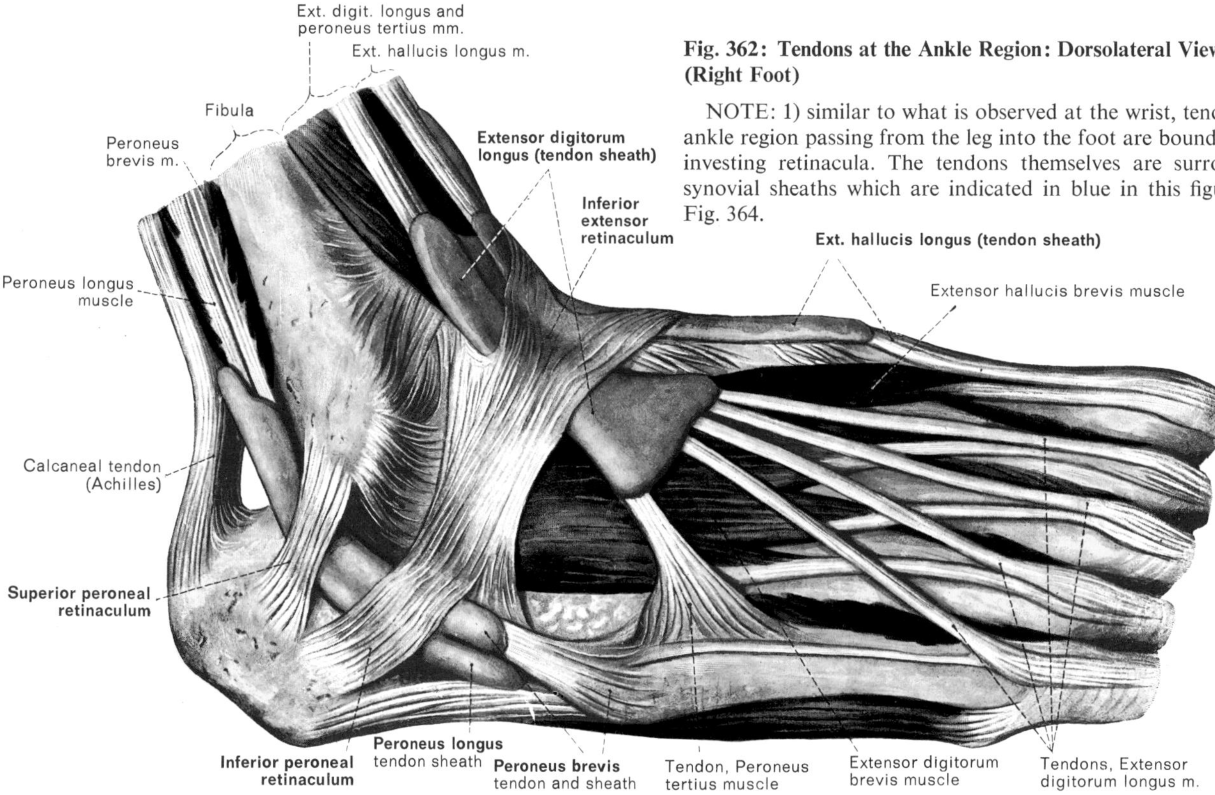

Ext. digit. longus and peroneus tertius mm.
Ext. hallucis longus m.
Fibula
Peroneus brevis m.
Extensor digitorum longus (tendon sheath)
Inferior extensor retinaculum
Ext. hallucis longus (tendon sheath)
Extensor hallucis brevis muscle
Peroneus longus muscle
Calcaneal tendon (Achilles)
Superior peroneal retinaculum
Inferior peroneal retinaculum
Peroneus longus tendon sheath
Peroneus brevis tendon and sheath
Tendon, Peroneus tertius muscle
Extensor digitorum brevis muscle
Tendons, Extensor digitorum longus m.

2) anterior to the ankle joint and on the dorsum of the foot are three separate synovial sheaths. One is for the extensor digitorum longus and peroneus tertius, a second is for the extensor hallucis longus and the third surrounds the tibialis anterior (see Fig. 364). Behind the lateral malleolus is a single tendon sheath for the peroneus longus and brevis which then splits distally to continue along each individual tendon for some distance.

3) the inferior extensor retinaculum and the superior and inferior peroneal retinacula which bind the tendons and their sheaths close to bone.

Fig. 363: The Tendons of the Peroneus Longus and Tibialis Anterior Muscles

Note that the tendons of the tibialis anterior and peroneus longus muscles insert on the medial aspect of the plantar surface of the foot. The peroneus longus muscle achieves this insertion by traversing the sole of the foot from lateral to medial. In this manner, the two muscles form a tendinous sling under the foot which serves to support the transverse arch. Also assisting in this support is the tendon of the tibialis posterior muscle.

Fig. 364: Tendons at the Ankle Region: Medial View (Right Foot)

NOTE: 1) from this medial view can be seen the synovial sheaths and tendons of the tibialis anterior and extensor hallucis longus on the dorsum of the foot, as well as the three tendons which course beneath the medial malleolus from the posterior compartment of the leg into the plantar foot: tibialis posterior, flexor digitorum longus and flexor hallucis longus.

2) the bifurcating nature of the inferior extensor retinaculum and the manner in which the flexor retinaculum secures the structures beneath the medial malleolus.

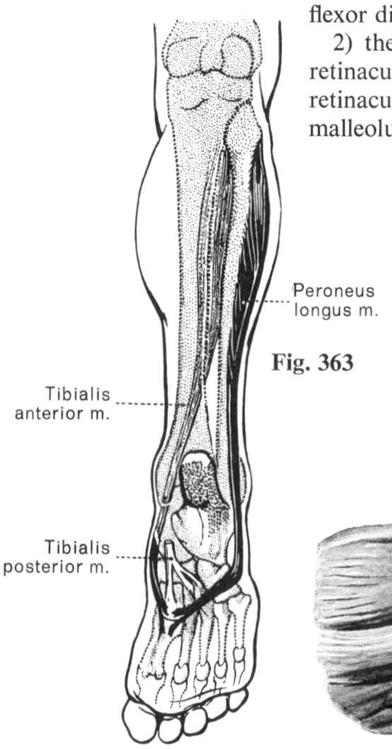

Peroneus longus m.
Tibialis anterior m.
Tibialis posterior m.

Fig. 363

Fig. 364

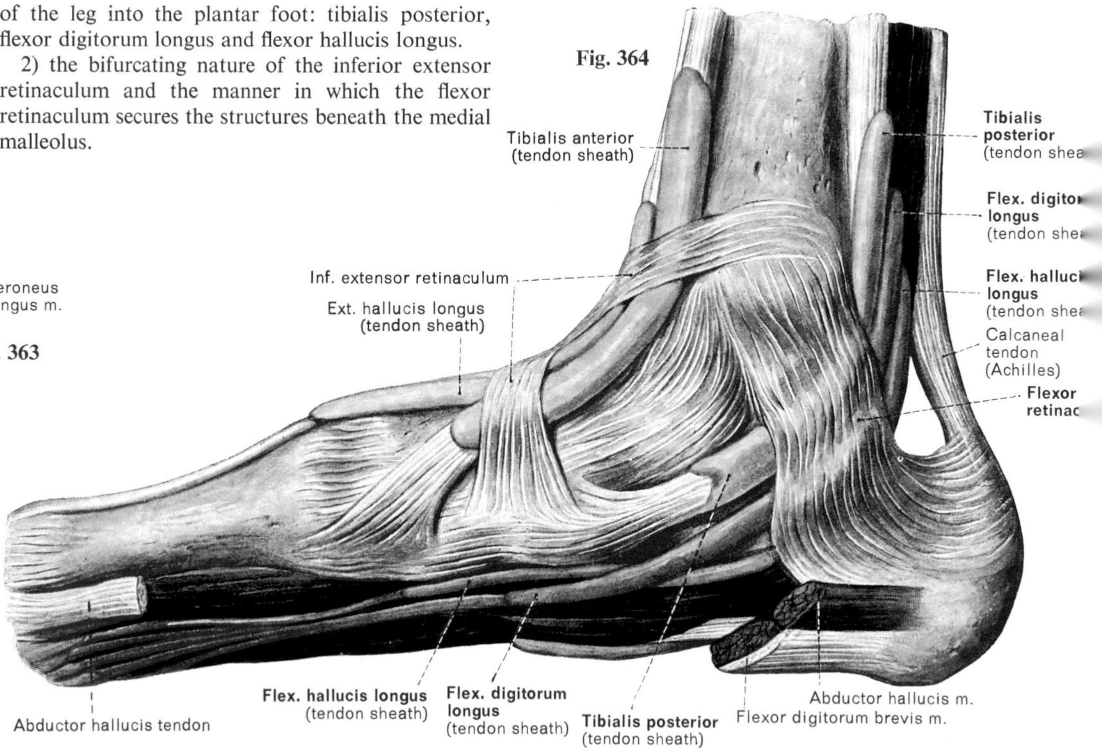

Tibialis anterior (tendon sheath)
Tibialis posterior
Flex. digito
longus
Flex. halluc
longus
Calcaneal tendon (Achilles)
Flexor
Inf. extensor retinaculum
Ext. hallucis longus (tendon sheath)
Flex. hallucis longus (tendon sheath)
Flex. digitorum longus (tendon sheath)
Tibialis posterior (tendon sheath)
Abductor hallucis tendon
Abductor hallucis m.
Flexor digitorum brevis m.

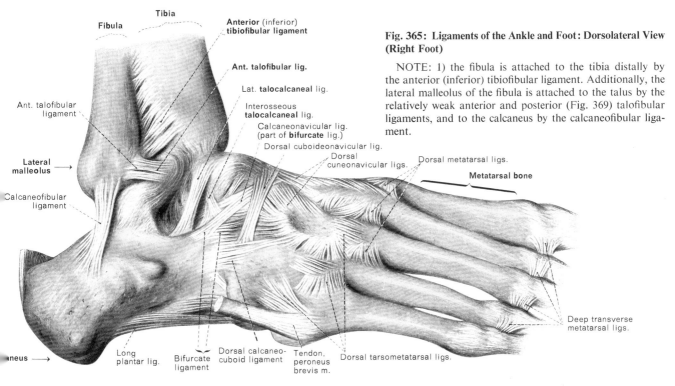

Fig. 365: Ligaments of the Ankle and Foot: Dorsolateral View (Right Foot)

NOTE: 1) the fibula is attached to the tibia distally by the anterior (inferior) tibiofibular ligament. Additionally, the lateral malleolus of the fibula is attached to the talus by the relatively weak anterior and posterior (Fig. 369) talofibular ligaments, and to the calcaneus by the calcaneofibular ligament.

2) the joint between the talus and calcaneus (subtalar joint) is principally strengthened by the interosseous talocalcaneal ligament. The talocalcaneo-navicular joint more anteriorly is of important clinical significance since the weight of the body tends to push the head of the talus down between the navicular and calcaneus. The stability of this joint is assisted dorsolaterally by the calcaneo-navicular ligament (a part of the bifurcate ligament); however, the thick plantar calcaneonavicular or spring ligament (Figs. 366, 368, 370, 371) is the principal support for this joint in the maintenance of the longitudinal arch of the foot.

3) the bifurcate ligament consists of the calcaneonavicular ligament and the calcaneocuboid ligament.

Fig. 366: Ligaments of the Ankle and Foot: Medial View (Right Foot)

NOTE: 1) the medial aspect of the ankle joint is protected by the deltoid ligament which is triangular in shape and which connects the tibia (medial malleolus) to the navicular, calcaneus and talus. The deltoid ligament consists of 4 parts: a) an anterior part which attaches the medial malleolus to the navicular (tibionavicular part), b) a superficial part attaching the malleolus to the sustentaculum tali of the calcaneus (tibiocalcaneal part), and c) and d) the anterior and posterior tibiotalar parts which lie more deeply and attach the malleolus to the adjacent talus.

2) the insertions of the tendons of the tibialis anterior and tibialis posterior muscles which attach on this medial aspect of the foot. Observe also the long plantar and plantar calcaneonavicular ligaments on the plantar surface. These are shown more clearly in Figures 368, 370 and 371.

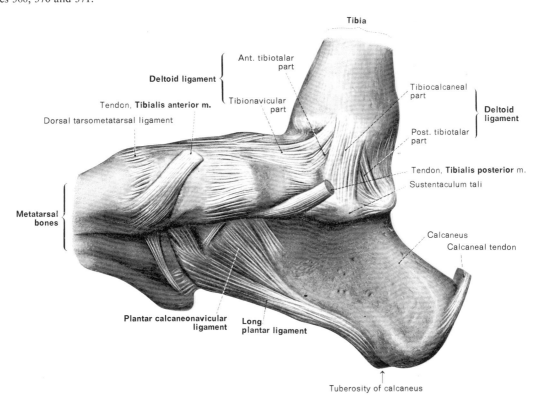

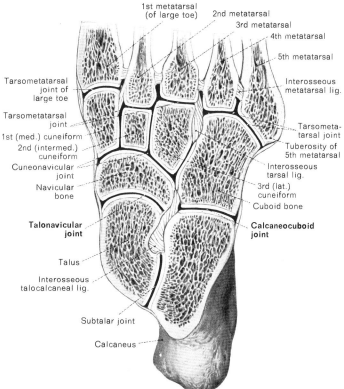

1st metatarsal (of large toe)
2nd metatarsal
3rd metatarsal
4th metatarsal
5th metatarsal

Tarsometatarsal joint of large toe
Tarsometatarsal joint
1st (med.) cuneiform
2nd (intermed.) cuneiform
Cuneonavicular joint
Navicular bone
Talonavicular joint
Talus
Interosseous talocalcaneal lig.
Subtalar joint
Calcaneus

Interosseous metatarsal lig.
Tarsometatarsal joint
Tuberosity of 5th metatarsal
Interosseous tarsal lig.
3rd (lat.) cuneiform
Cuboid bone
Calcaneocuboid joint

Fig. 368: The Talocalcaneonavicular Joint (Viewed from Above), Right

Note that the talus has been removed. This reveals the three articulations it makes with the calcaneus and the anterior articulation it makes with the navicular bone. Observe the plantar calcaneonavicular ("spring") ligament stretching across the plantar aspect of the talocalcaneonavicular joint.

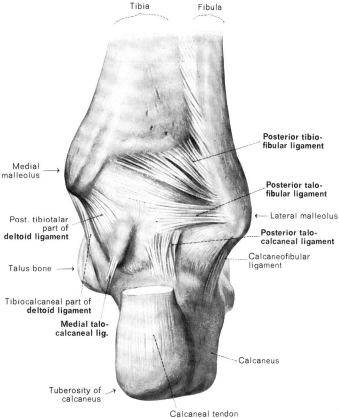

Tibia
Fibula
Posterior tibio-fibular ligament
Posterior talo-fibular ligament
Medial malleolus
Post. tibiotalar part of **deltoid ligament**
Lateral malleolus
Posterior talo-calcaneal ligament
Talus bone
Calcaneofibular ligament
Tibiocalcaneal part of **deltoid ligament**
Medial talo-calcaneal lig.
Calcaneus
Tuberosity of calcaneus
Calcaneal tendon

Fig. 367: The Intertarsal and Tarsometatarsal Joints (Horizontal Section of Right Foot)

NOTE: 1) a transverse intertarsal joint extending across the foot and formed by two separate joint cavities, the calcaneocuboid joint and the talonavicular portion of the talocalcaneonavicular joint. These two joints allow some dorsi and plantarflexion of the anterior part of the foot with respect to the posterior foot.

2) that the joints in the foot form a natural division of the bones into a medial group (talus, navicular, the 3 cuneiform and the medial three metatarsals and phalanges) and a lateral group (calcaneus, cuboid and the lateral two metatarsals and phalanges).

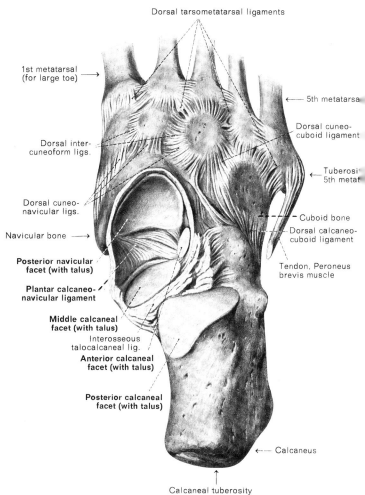

Dorsal tarsometatarsal ligaments
1st metatarsal (for large toe)
5th metatarsal
Dorsal cuneo-cuboid ligament
Dorsal inter-cuneoform ligs.
Tuberosity 5th metatarsal
Dorsal cuneo-navicular ligs.
Navicular bone
Cuboid bone
Dorsal calcaneo-cuboid ligament
Posterior navicular facet (with talus)
Tendon, Peroneus brevis muscle
Plantar calcaneo-navicular ligament
Middle calcaneal facet (with talus)
Interosseous talocalcaneal lig.
Anterior calcaneal facet (with talus)
Posterior calcaneal facet (with talus)
Calcaneus
Calcaneal tuberosity

Fig. 369: The Ankle Joint (Talocrural) Viewed from Behind (Right Foot)

NOTE: 1) the ankle joint is a ginglymus or hinge joint. The bony structures participating in this joint superiorly are the distal end of the tibia and its medial malleolus, and the distal fibula and its lateral malleolus. Together these structures form a concave receptacle for the convex proximal surface of the talus.

2) the posterior aspect of the articular capsule is somewhat strengthened by the posterior talofibular and posterior tibiofibular ligaments. Laterally the calcaneofibular ligament and medially the strong deltoid ligament assist in protecting this joint.

3) the ligamentous bands which help to stabilize the talocalcaneal articulation posteriorly: the posterior and medial talocalcaneal ligaments.

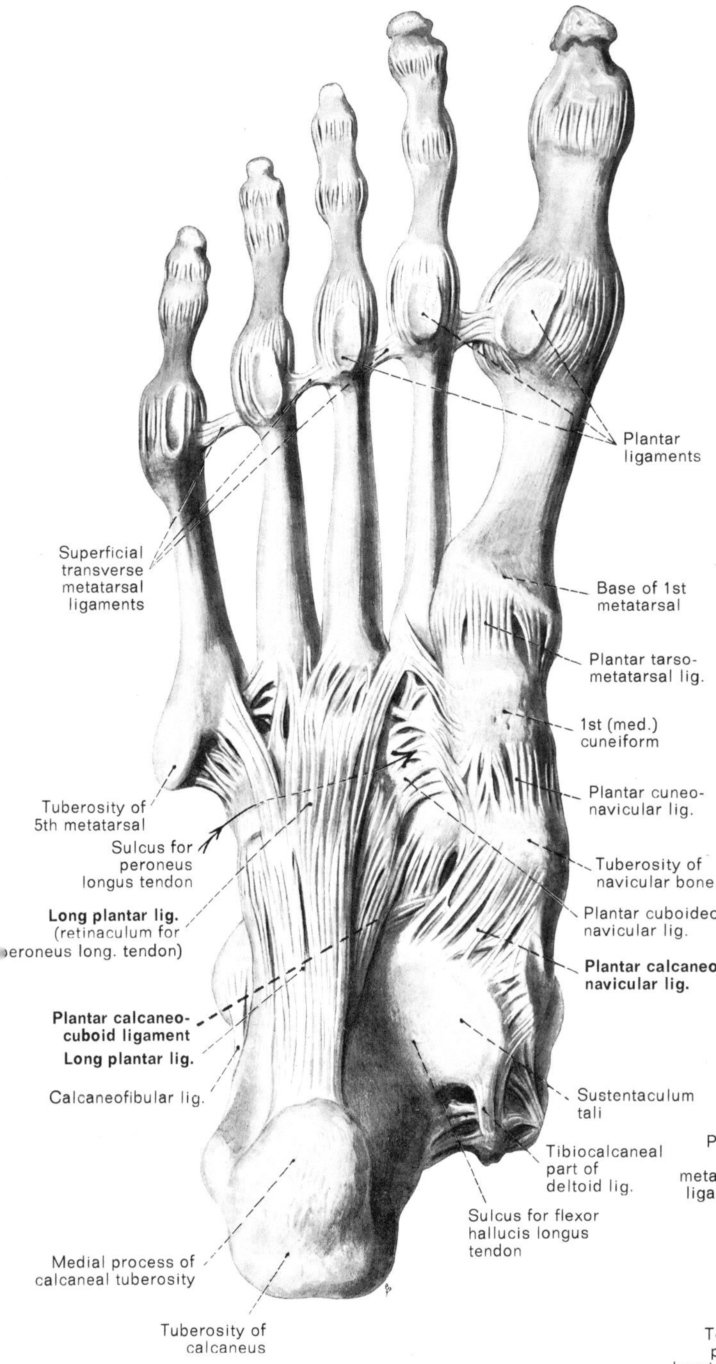
Plantar ligaments
Superficial transverse metatarsal ligaments
Base of 1st metatarsal
Plantar tarso-metatarsal lig.
1st (med.) cuneiform
Tuberosity of 5th metatarsal
Plantar cuneo-navicular lig.
Sulcus for peroneus longus tendon
Tuberosity of navicular bone
Long plantar lig. (retinaculum for peroneus long. tendon)
Plantar cuboideo-navicular lig.
Plantar calcaneo-navicular lig.
Plantar calcaneo-cuboid ligament
Long plantar lig.
Calcaneofibular lig.
Sustentaculum tali
Tibiocalcaneal part of deltoid lig.
Sulcus for flexor hallucis longus tendon
Medial process of calcaneal tuberosity
Tuberosity of calcaneus

Fig. 370: Ligaments on the Plantar Surface of the Right Foot (Superficial)

NOTE: 1) that the long plantar ligament is the longest and most superficial of the plantar tarsal ligaments. It stretchesfrom the calcaneus posteriorly to an oblique ridge on the plantar surface of the cuboid where most of its deeper fibers terminate. A number of the more superficial fibers pass over the cuboid to insert on the bases of the lateral three metatarsal bones, thereby forming a tunnel or retinaculum for the peroneus longus tendon.

2) the plantar calcaneocuboid or short plantar ligament is very strong and lies deeper to the long plantar ligament and closer to the bones. More medially, identify the fibroelastic plantar calcaneonavicular (spring) ligament. It is attached to the sustentaculum tali of the calcaneus and extends along the entire inferior surface of the navicular bone.

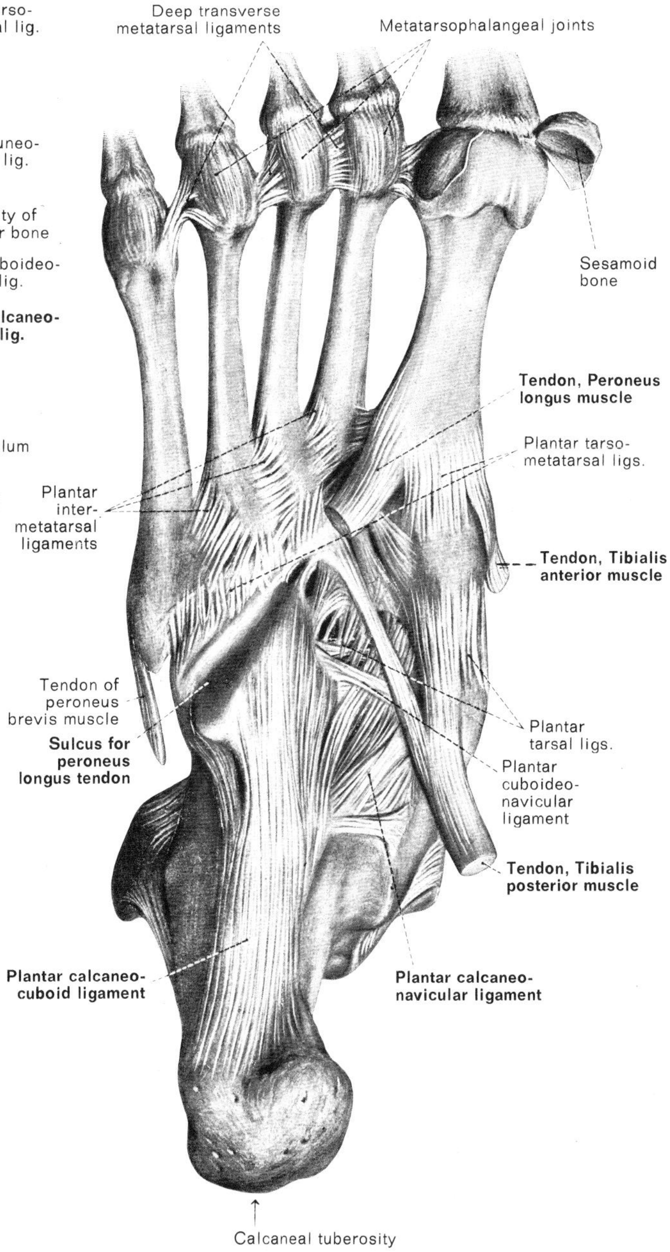
Deep transverse metatarsal ligaments
Metatarsophalangeal joints
Sesamoid bone
Tendon, Peroneus longus muscle
Plantar tarso-metatarsal ligs.
Plantar inter-metatarsal ligaments
Tendon, Tibialis anterior muscle
Tendon of peroneus brevis muscle
Sulcus for peroneus longus tendon
Plantar tarsal ligs.
Plantar cuboideo-navicular ligament
Tendon, Tibialis posterior muscle
Plantar calcaneo-cuboid ligament
Plantar calcaneo-navicular ligament
Calcaneal tuberosity

Fig. 371: The Plantar Calcaneonavicular Ligament and the Insertions of Three Tendons (Right Foot)

NOTE: 1) the metatarsal extensions of the long plantar ligament have been cut away to reveal the groove for the tendon of the peroneus longus muscle. This tendon is seen inserting onto the base of the 1st metatarsal bone. It also sends a small slip of insertion to the 1st cuneiform. Two other long tendons inserting on the medial side of the plantar surface are those of the tibialis anterior and tibialis posterior muscles.

2) that the fibers of the calcaneocuboid (short plantar) and calcaneonavicular (spring) ligaments all stem from the calcaneus and then diverge in a radial manner toward the medial side of the foot. Observe that the course and insertion of the tibialis posterior tendon also lends some support to the short tendon and spring ligaments.

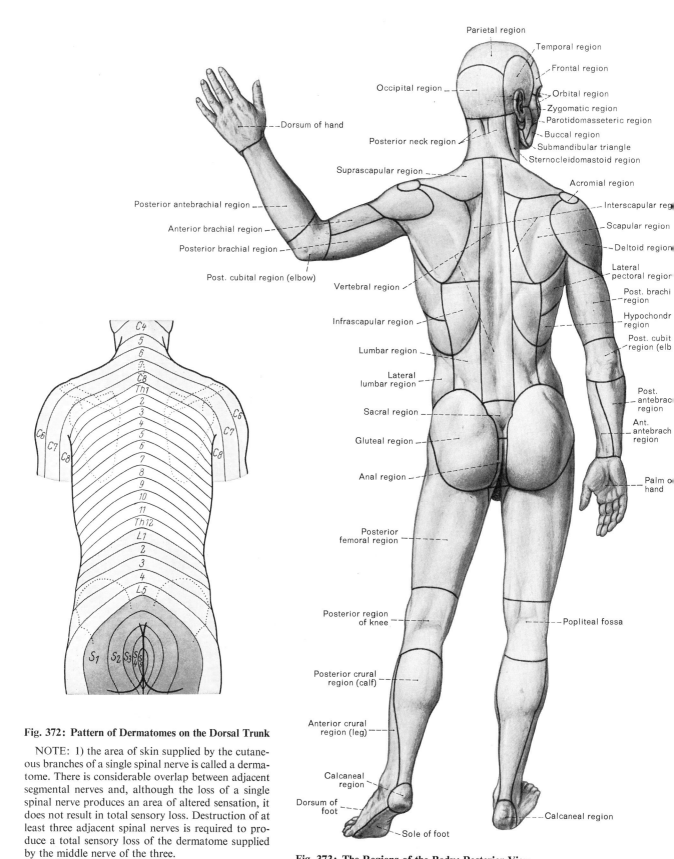

Fig. 372: Pattern of Dermatomes on the Dorsal Trunk

NOTE: 1) the area of skin supplied by the cutaneous branches of a single spinal nerve is called a dermatome. There is considerable overlap between adjacent segmental nerves and, although the loss of a single spinal nerve produces an area of altered sensation, it does not result in total sensory loss. Destruction of at least three adjacent spinal nerves is required to produce a total sensory loss of the dermatome supplied by the middle nerve of the three.

2) mapping of skin areas affected by herpes zoster (shingles) has also allowed the mapping of dermatomes. Another method is the method of "remaining sensibility". In the latter, dermatome areas are established after the destruction of several roots above and below the intact root whose dermatome is being studied.

Fig. 373: The Regions of the Body: Posterior View

NOTE: the posterior aspect of the head, trunk and limbs is subdivided into many topographic regions to allow more exact anatomical localization and communication. Although the boundaries between the regions are somewhat arbitrary, it can be observed that the regions assume the names of bony structures, muscles, organs, joints and orifices comparable to those observed on the anterior aspect of the body (Figure 1).

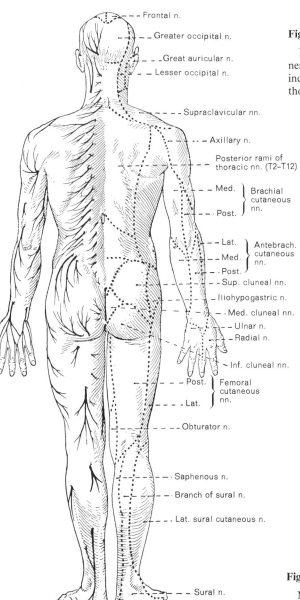

Frontal n.

Greater occipital n.

Great auricular n.

Lesser occipital n.

Supraclavicular nn.

Axillary n.

Posterior rami of thoracic nn. (T2–T12)

Med. } Brachial
Post. } cutaneous nn.

Lat. } Antebrach.
Med. } cutaneous
Post. } nn.

Sup. cluneal nn.

Iliohypogastric n.

Med. cluneal nn.

Ulnar n.

Radial n.

Inf. cluneal nn.

Post. } Femoral
Lat. } cutaneous nn.

Obturator n.

Saphenous n.

Branch of sural n.

Lat. sural cutaneous n.

Sural n.

Fig. 374: The Cutaneous Nerve Surface Areas, Posterior Aspect of the Body

Note that on the left side the position and course of the spinal cutaneous nerves are shown while on the right side the surface areas of distribution are indicated. Demonstrated are the posterior surface zones for the cervical, thoracic, lumbar and sacral segmental nerves.

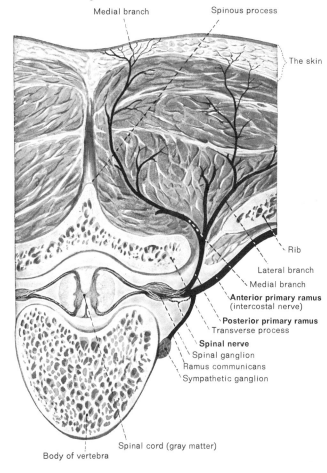

Medial branch

Spinous process

The skin

Rib

Lateral branch

Medial branch

Anterior primary ramus (intercostal nerve)

Posterior primary ramus

Transverse process

Spinal nerve

Spinal ganglion

Ramus communicans

Sympathetic ganglion

Spinal cord (gray matter)

Body of vertebra

Fig. 375: The Branching of a Typical Spinal Nerve

NOTE: Fibers from both dorsal and motor roots join to form a spinal nerve which soon divides into a posterior and an anterior primary ramus. The posterior primary ramus courses dorsally to innervate the muscles and skin of the back. The anterior primary ramus becomes the intercostal nerve, coursing laterally and anteriorly around the body, to innervate the remainder of the segment.

Fig. 376: Cross Section of Back, Lumbar Region

NOTE: the sacrospinalis muscle is ensheathed by the thick lumbar part of the thoracolumbar fascia which attaches medially to the spinous and transverse processes of the lumbar vertebrae and which becomes continuous laterally with the aponeuroses and fasciae of the latissimus dorsi and anterior abdominal muscles.

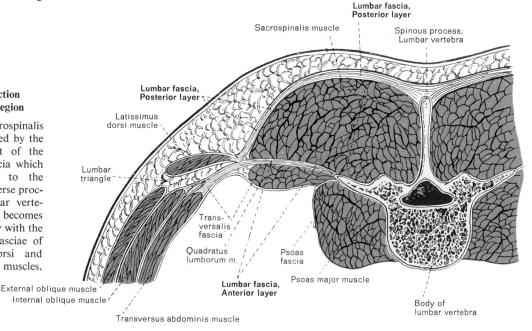

Lumbar fascia, Posterior layer

Sacrospinalis muscle

Spinous process, Lumbar vertebra

Lumbar fascia, Posterior layer

Latissimus dorsi muscle

Lumbar triangle

Transversalis fascia

Quadratus lumborum m.

Psoas fascia

Lumbar fascia, Anterior layer

Psoas major muscle

External oblique muscle

Internal oblique muscle

Transversus abdominis muscle

Body of lumbar vertebra

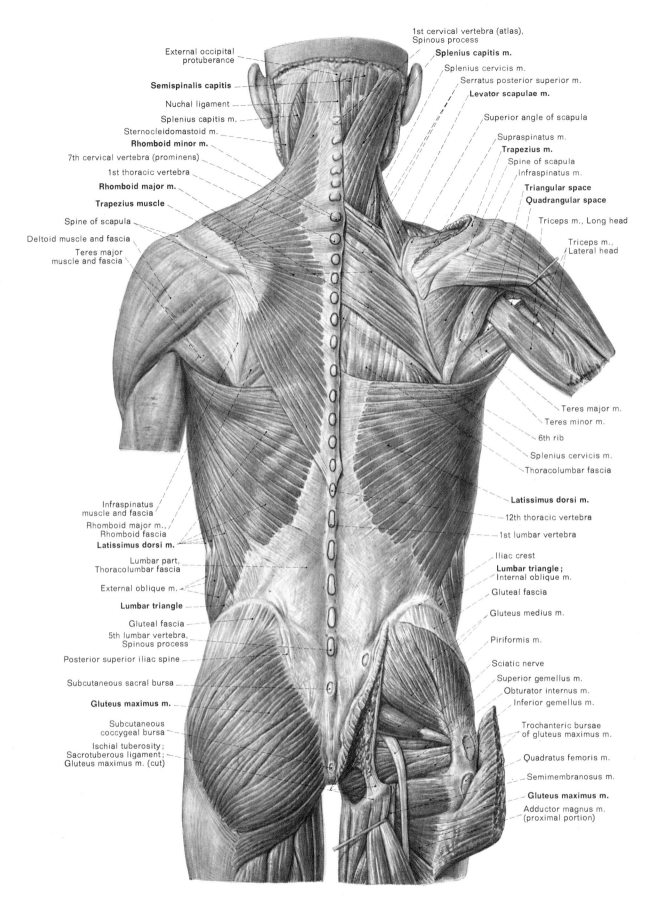

External occipital protuberance

Semispinalis capitis

Nuchal ligament

Splenius capitis m.

Sternocleidomastoid m.

Rhomboid minor m.

7th cervical vertebra (prominens)

1st thoracic vertebra

Rhomboid major m.

Trapezius muscle

Spine of scapula

Deltoid muscle and fascia

Teres major muscle and fascia

Infraspinatus muscle and fascia

Rhomboid major m., Rhomboid fascia

Latissimus dorsi m.

Lumbar part, Thoracolumbar fascia

External oblique m.

Lumbar triangle

Gluteal fascia

5th lumbar vertebra, Spinous process

Posterior superior iliac spine

Subcutaneous sacral bursa

Gluteus maximus m.

Subcutaneous coccygeal bursa

Ischial tuberosity; Sacrotuberous ligament; Gluteus maximus m. (cut)

1st cervical vertebra (atlas), Spinous process

Splenius capitis m.

Splenius cervicis m.

Serratus posterior superior m.

Levator scapulae m.

Superior angle of scapula

Supraspinatus m.

Trapezius m.

Spine of scapula

Infraspinatus m.

Triangular space

Quadrangular space

Triceps m., Long head

Triceps m., Lateral head

Teres major m.

Teres minor m.

6th rib

Splenius cervicis m.

Thoracolumbar fascia

Latissimus dorsi m.

12th thoracic vertebra

1st lumbar vertebra

Iliac crest

Lumbar triangle; Internal oblique m.

Gluteal fascia

Gluteus medius m.

Piriformis m.

Sciatic nerve

Superior gemellus m.

Obturator internus m.

Inferior gemellus m.

Trochanteric bursae of gluteus maximus m.

Quadratus femoris m.

Semimembranosus m.

Gluteus maximus m.

Adductor magnus m. (proximal portion)

Fig. 377: Muscles of the Posterior Neck, Shoulder, Back and Gluteal Region

Note that the most superficial layer of back muscles includes the latissimus dorsi and trapezius. Beneath the trapezius, observe the levator scapulae and rhomboid major and minor muscles attaching along the vertebral border of the scapula. In the neck, the splenius capitis and semispinalis capitis muscles lie directly under the trapezius.

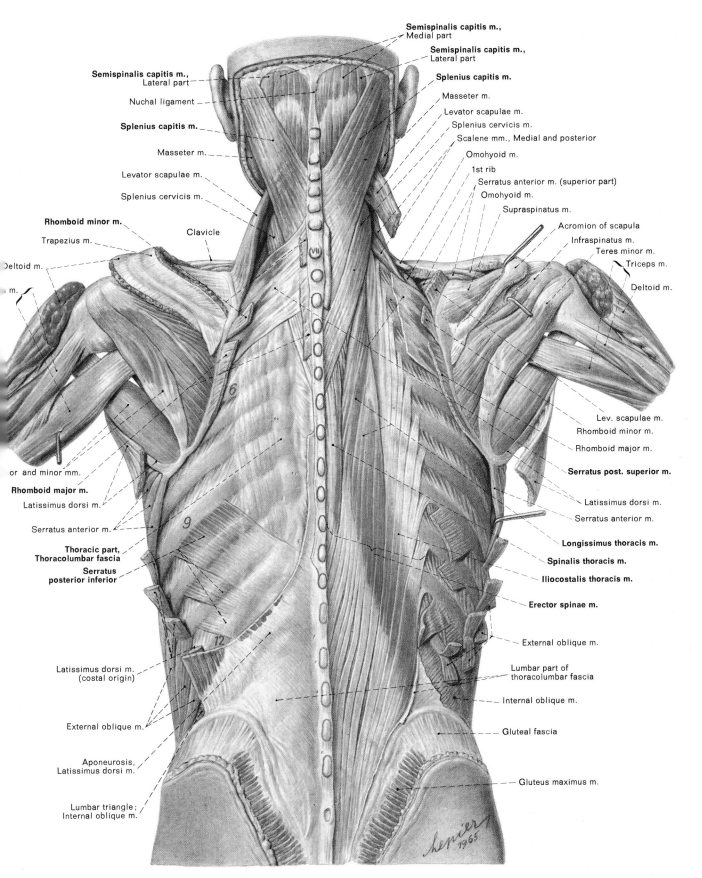

Semispinalis capitis m., Medial part
Semispinalis capitis m., Lateral part
Splenius capitis m.
Masseter m.
Levator scapulae m.
Splenius cervicis m.
Scalene mm., Medial and posterior
Omohyoid m.
1st rib
Serratus anterior m. (superior part)
Omohyoid m.
Supraspinatus m.
Acromion of scapula
Infraspinatus m.
Teres minor m.
Triceps m.
Deltoid m.

Semispinalis capitis m., Lateral part
Nuchal ligament
Splenius capitis m.
Masseter m.
Levator scapulae m.
Splenius cervicis m.
Rhomboid minor m.
Trapezius m.
Clavicle
Deltoid m.
m.

Lev. scapulae m.
Rhomboid minor m.
Rhomboid major m.
Serratus post. superior m.
Latissimus dorsi m.
Serratus anterior m.
Longissimus thoracis m.
Spinalis thoracis m.
Iliocostalis thoracis m.
Erector spinae m.
External oblique m.
Lumbar part of thoracolumbar fascia
Internal oblique m.
Gluteal fascia
Gluteus maximus m.

or and minor mm.
Rhomboid major m.
Latissimus dorsi m.
Serratus anterior m.
Thoracic part, Thoracolumbar fascia
Serratus posterior inferior
Latissimus dorsi m. (costal origin)
External oblique m.
Aponeurosis, Latissimus dorsi m.
Lumbar triangle; Internal oblique m.

Fig. 378: Muscles of the Back: Intermediate Layer (left), Deep Layer (right)

NOTE: 1) *on the left side* the superficial back muscles (trapezius and latissimus dorsi) have been cut, as have the rhomboid major and minor which attach the vertebral border of the scapula to the vertebral column. Observe the underlying serratus posterior superior and serratus posterior inferior muscles.

2) *on the right side* the serratus posterior muscles and the thoracolumbar fascia have been removed revealing the erector spinae muscle (formerly called the sacrospinalis muscle).

3) *in the neck* the splenius cervicis, splenius capitis and semispinalis capitis underlie the trapezius.

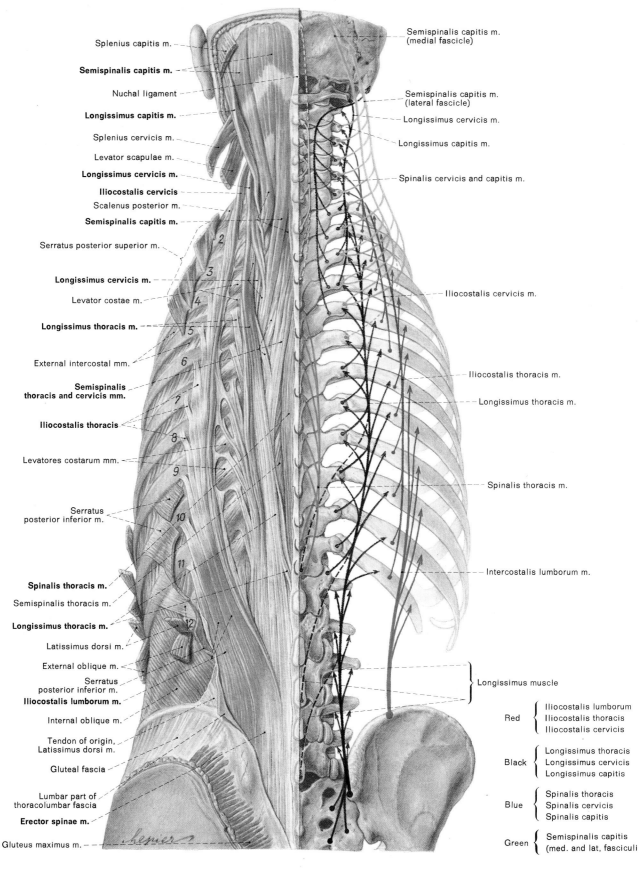

Splenius capitis m.

Semispinalis capitis m.

Nuchal ligament

Longissimus capitis m.

Splenius cervicis m.

Levator scapulae m.

Longissimus cervicis m.

Iliocostalis cervicis

Scalenus posterior m.

Semispinalis capitis m.

Serratus posterior superior m.

Longissimus cervicis m.

Levator costae m.

Longissimus thoracis m.

External intercostal mm.

Semispinalis thoracis and cervicis mm.

Iliocostalis thoracis

Levatores costarum mm.

Serratus posterior inferior m.

Spinalis thoracis m.

Semispinalis thoracis m.

Longissimus thoracis m.

Latissimus dorsi m.

External oblique m.

Serratus posterior inferior m.

Iliocostalis lumborum m.

Internal oblique m.

Tendon of origin, Latissimus dorsi m.

Gluteal fascia

Lumbar part of thoracolumbar fascia

Erector spinae m.

Gluteus maximus m.

Semispinalis capitis m. (medial fascicle)

Semispinalis capitis m. (lateral fascicle)

Longissimus cervicis m.

Longissimus capitis m.

Spinalis cervicis and capitis m.

Iliocostalis cervicis m.

Iliocostalis thoracis m.

Longissimus thoracis m.

Spinalis thoracis m.

Intercostalis lumborum m.

Longissimus muscle

Red	Iliocostalis lumborum Iliocostalis thoracis Iliocostalis cervicis
Black	Longissimus thoracis Longissimus cervicis Longissimus capitis
Blue	Spinalis thoracis Spinalis cervicis Spinalis capitis
Green	Semispinalis capitis (med. and lat, fasciculi

Fig. 379: Deep Muscles of the Back and Neck: the Erector Spinae Muscle

NOTE: 1) *on the left,* the erector spinae (sacrospinalis) muscle is separated into its iliocostalis, longissimus and spinalis portions. In the neck observe the semispinalis capitis which has both medial and lateral fascicles. The semispinalis cervicis and thoracis extend inferiorly from above and lie deep to the sacrospinalis layer of musculature.

2) *on the right,* all of the muscles have been removed and their attachments have been diagrammed by means of colored lines.

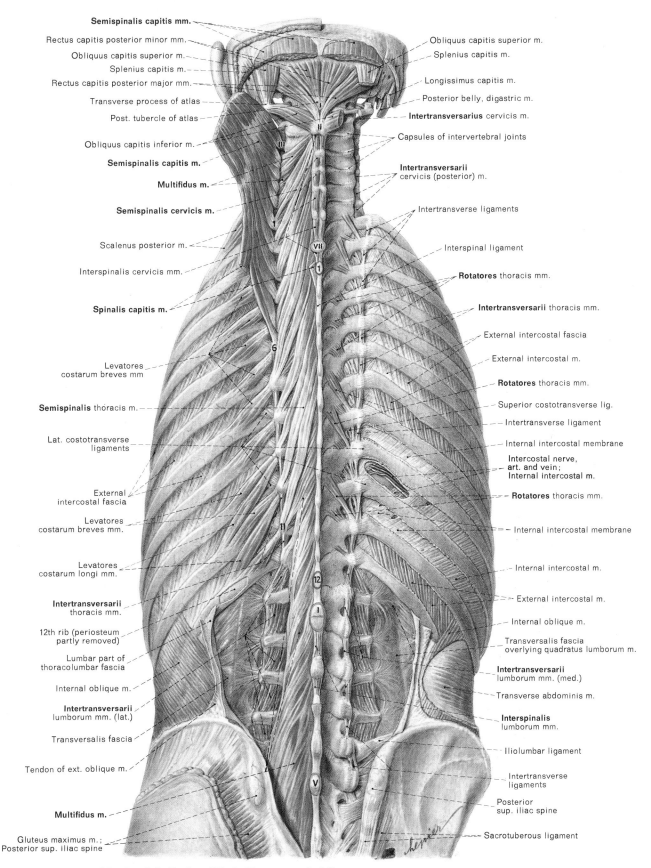

Fig. 380: Deep Muscles of the Back and Neck: Transversospinal Group

NOTE: 1) the transversospinal groups of muscles lie deep to the erector spinae muscles and generally extend between the transverse processes of the vertebrae to the spinous processes of more superior vertebrae. Their actions extend the vertebral column, or upon acting individually and on one side, they bend and rotate the vertebrae.

2) within this group of muscles are the semispinalis (thoracis, cervicis, and capitis), the multifidus, the rotatores (lumborum, thoracis, cervicis), the interspinales (lumborum, thoracis, cervicis) and the intertransversarii.

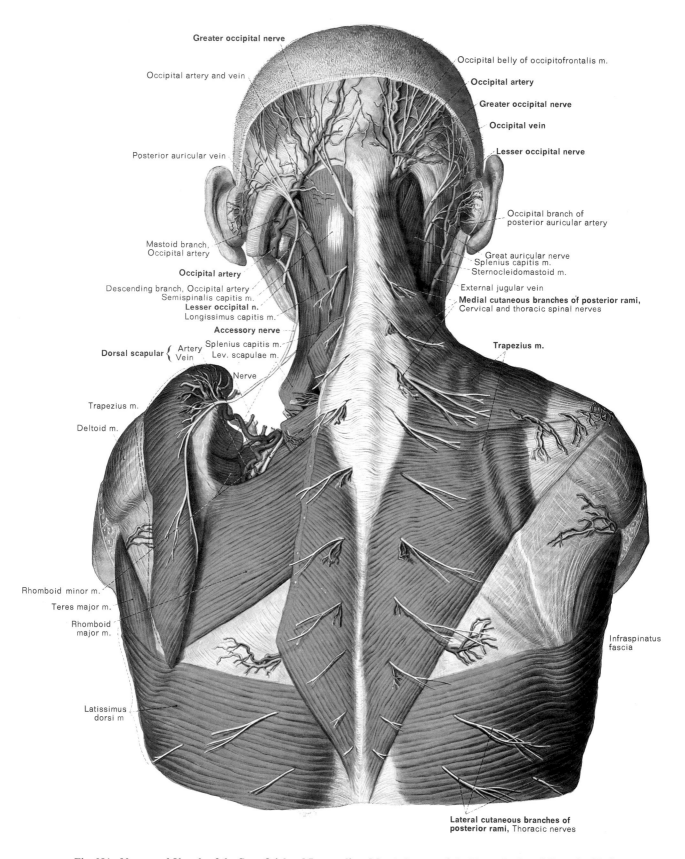

Fig. 381: Nerves and Vessels of the Superficial and Intermediate Muscle Layers of the Upper Back and Posterior Neck

NOTE: 1) the segmental distribution of the cutaneous branches of the posterior primary rami of the cervical and thoracic nerves over the posterior neck and back. Observe the accessory nerve (XI) as it descends to innervate the trapezius and sternocleidomastoid muscles.

2) the greater occipital nerve which is a sensory nerve ascending to the posterior scalp. It derives from the posterior primary ramus of the C-2 spinal nerve and is accompanied in its course by the occipital artery and vein. Observe also the lesser occipital nerve which courses to the lateral posterior scalp and which arises from the anterior primary ramus of C-2.

2) the dorsal scapular nerve, artery and vein which course beneath the levator scapulae and the rhomboid muscles.

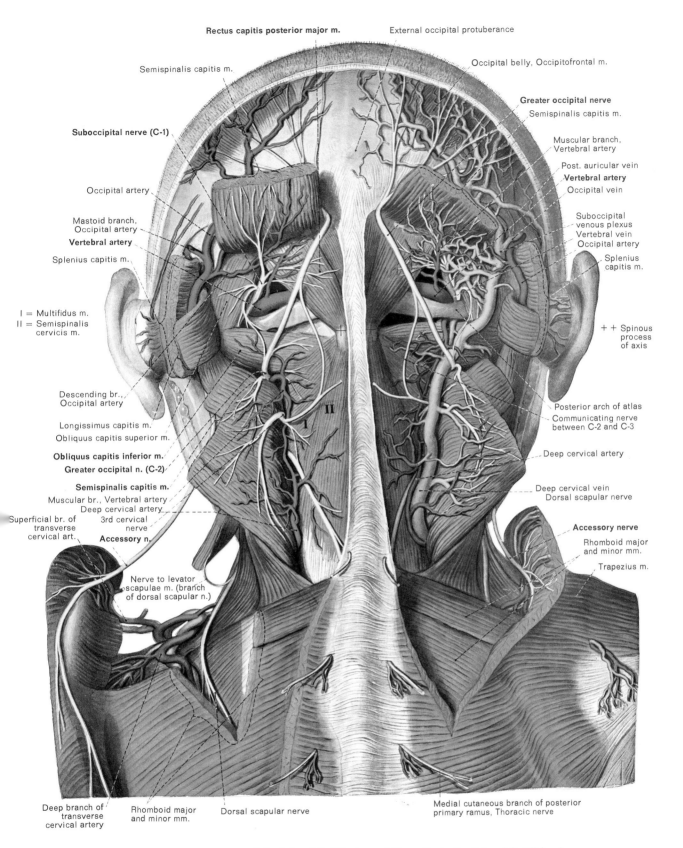

Rectus capitis posterior major m.

External occipital protuberance

Semispinalis capitis m.

Occipital belly, Occipitofrontal m.

Greater occipital nerve

Semispinalis capitis m.

Suboccipital nerve (C-1)

Muscular branch, Vertebral artery

Post. auricular vein

Vertebral artery

Occipital vein

Occipital artery

Mastoid branch, Occipital artery

Suboccipital venous plexus
Vertebral vein
Occipital artery

Vertebral artery

Splenius capitis m.

Splenius capitis m.

I = Multifidus m.
II = Semispinalis cervicis m.

+ + Spinous process of axis

Descending br., Occipital artery

Posterior arch of atlas

Communicating nerve between C-2 and C-3

Longissimus capitis m.
Obliquus capitis superior m.

Deep cervical artery

Obliquus capitis inferior m.
Greater occipital n. (C-2)

Semispinalis capitis m.
Muscular br., Vertebral artery
Deep cervical artery   3rd cervical
                           nerve
Superficial br. of
transverse
cervical art.   Accessory n.

Deep cervical vein
Dorsal scapular nerve

Accessory nerve

Rhomboid major
and minor mm.

Trapezius m.

Nerve to levator
scapulae m. (branch
of dorsal scapular n.)

Deep branch of
transverse
cervical artery

Rhomboid major
and minor mm.

Dorsal scapular nerve

Medial cutaneous branch of posterior
primary ramus, Thoracic nerve

Fig. 382: The Deep Vessels and Nerves of the Suboccipital Region and Upper Back; the Suboccipital Triangle

NOTE: 1) the suboccipital triangle lies directly beneath the semispinalis capitis muscle and is bounded by the rectus capitis posterior major, obliquus capitis superior and the obliquus capitis inferior.

2) the vertebral artery crosses (from lateral to medial) the suboccipital triangle while the suboccipital nerve (posterior primary ramus of C-1) emerges through the triangle to distribute motor innervation to the three muscles which bound the triangle as well as the rectus capitis posterior minor and the overlying semispinalis capitis muscle.

3) the greater occipital nerve (posterior primary ramus of C-2) is a sensory nerve which makes its appearance caudal to the obliquus capitis inferior and then courses medially and superiorly to become subcutaneous just lateral and below the external occipital protuberance.

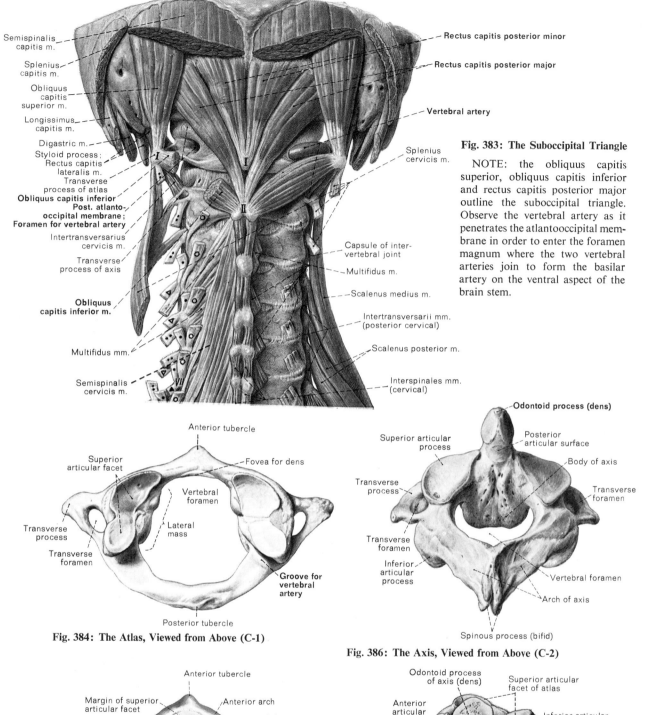

Semispinalis capitis m.

Splenius capitis m.

Obliquus capitis superior m.

Longissimus capitis m.

Digastric m.

Styloid process; Rectus capitis lateralis m.

Transverse process of atlas

Obliquus capitis inferior Post. atlanto-occipital membrane; Foramen for vertebral artery

Intertransversarius cervicis m.

Transverse process of axis

Obliquus capitis inferior m.

Multifidus mm.

Semispinalis cervicis m.

Rectus capitis posterior minor

Rectus capitis posterior major

Vertebral artery

Splenius cervicis m.

Capsule of intervertebral joint

Multifidus m.

Scalenus medius m.

Intertransversarii mm. (posterior cervical)

Scalenus posterior m.

Interspinales mm. (cervical)

Fig. 383: The Suboccipital Triangle

NOTE: the obliquus capitis superior, obliquus capitis inferior and rectus capitis posterior major outline the suboccipital triangle. Observe the vertebral artery as it penetrates the atlantooccipital membrane in order to enter the foramen magnum where the two vertebral arteries join to form the basilar artery on the ventral aspect of the brain stem.

Anterior tubercle

Superior articular facet

Fovea for dens

Vertebral foramen

Lateral mass

Transverse process

Transverse foramen

Groove for vertebral artery

Posterior tubercle

Fig. 384: The Atlas, Viewed from Above (C-1)

Odontoid process (dens)

Superior articular process

Posterior articular surface

Body of axis

Transverse process

Transverse foramen

Transverse foramen

Inferior articular process

Vertebral foramen

Arch of axis

Spinous process (bifid)

Fig. 386: The Axis, Viewed from Above (C-2)

Anterior tubercle

Margin of superior articular facet

Anterior arch

Inferior articular facet

Vertebral foramen

Lateral mass

Transverse foramen

Transverse process

Posterior arch

Posterior tubercle

Fig. 385: The Atlas, Caudal View (C-1)

Odontoid process of axis (dens)

Superior articular facet of atlas

Anterior articular surface of dens

Inferior articular facet of atlas

Posterior arch of atlas

Fovea for dens

Superior process and superior articular surface of axis

Body of axis

Transverse foramen

Spinous process of axis

Arch of axis

Transverse process

Inferior articular process

Fig. 387: Articulated Atlas and Axis, Median Sagittal Section

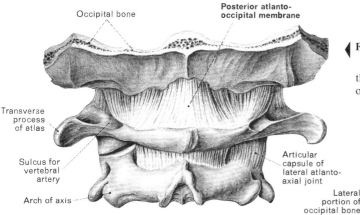

Occipital bone

Posterior atlanto-
occipital membrane

Transverse
process
of atlas

Sulcus for
vertebral
artery

Arch of axis

Articular
capsule of
lateral atlanto-
axial joint

Fig. 388: Atlantooccipital and Atlantoaxial Joints (Posterior View)

NOTE: the posterior atlantooccipital membrane extends from the posterior margin of the foramen magnum to the upper border of the posterior arch of the atlas.

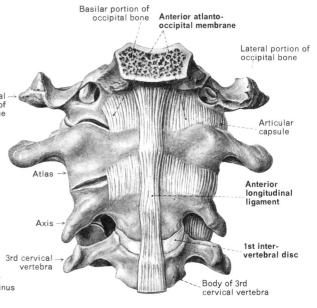

Basilar portion of
occipital bone

Anterior atlanto-
occipital membrane

Lateral portion of
occipital bone

Lateral
portion of
occipital bone

Atlas

Axis

3rd cervical
vertebra

Articular
capsule

Anterior
longitudinal
ligament

1st inter-
vertebral disc

Body of 3rd
cervical vertebra

Fig. 389: Articulations of Occipital Bone and First Three Cervical Vertebrae (Anterior)

NOTE: the anterior atlantooccipital membrane extending between the occipital bone and the anterior arch of the atlas and continuing laterally to join the articular capsules. Also observe the anterior longitudinal ligament.

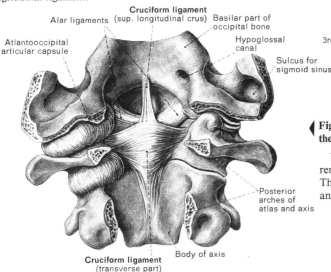

Cruciform ligament
(sup. longitudinal crus)

Alar ligaments

Basilar part of
occipital bone

Atlantooccipital
articular capsule

Hypoglossal
canal

Sulcus for
sigmoid sinus

Posterior
arches of
atlas and axis

Cruciform ligament
(transverse part)

Body of axis

Fig. 391: Median Atlantoaxial Joint (from Above)

NOTE: that the odontoid process (dens) of the axis articulates with the anterior arch of the atlas thereby forming the median atlantoaxial joint, and that the thick strong transverse ligament (part of the cruciform ligament) of the atlas retains the dens on its posterior surface.

Fig. 390: The Atlantooccipital and Atlantoaxial Joints Showing the Cruciform Ligament

NOTE: the posterior arches of the atlas and axis have been removed and the cruciform ligament is seen from this posterior view. This ligament consists of the transverse ligament (see Figure 391) and the longitudinal fascicles extending superiorly and inferiorly.

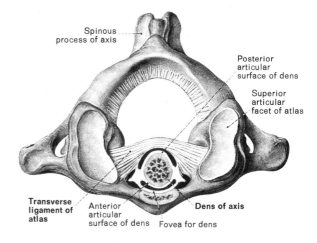

Spinous
process of axis

Posterior
articular
surface of dens

Superior
articular
facet of atlas

Transverse
ligament of
atlas

Anterior
articular
surface of dens

Dens of axis

Fovea for dens

Fig. 392: The Alar and Apical Ligaments

NOTE: this figure's orientation is similar to Figure 390. The posterior arches of the atlas and axis have been removed as well as the cruciform ligament (both transverse and longitudinal parts). This reveals the odontoid process of the axis which is attached superiorly to the occipital bone by the two alar ligaments and the apical ligament of the dens. These ligaments tend to limit lateral rotation of the skull.

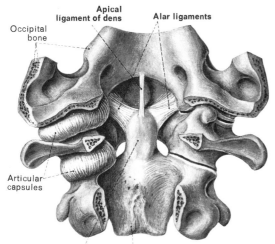

Apical
ligament of dens

Alar ligaments

Occipital
bone

Articular
capsules

Dens of axis

Body of axis

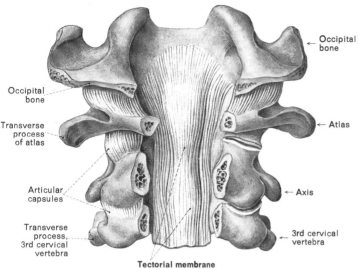

Occipital bone

Occipital bone

Transverse process of atlas

Articular capsules

Transverse process, 3rd cervical vertebra

Tectorial membrane

← Atlas

← Axis

3rd cervical vertebra

Fig. 394: Median section of Atlantooccipital Region

NOTE: the relationships from anterior to posterior of the following structures: the anterior arch of the atlas, the joint between it and the dens, the dens, the "joint" between the dens and the transverse ligament of the atlas, the tectorial membrane and finally, the dura mater covering the spinal cord.

Fig. 393: The Tectorial Membrane, Dorsal View

NOTE: the tectorial membrane is a broadened upward extension of the posterior longitudinal ligament and attaches the axis to the occipital bone (see also Figure 394). This membrane is seen to cover the posterior surface of the odontoid process and lies dorsal to the cruciform ligament, covering it as well.

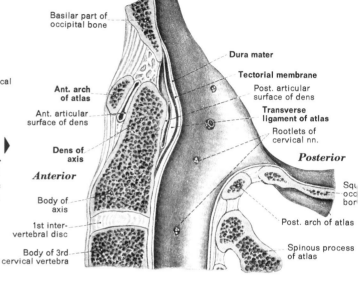

Basilar part of occipital bone

Dura mater

Tectorial membrane

Ant. arch of atlas

Post. articular surface of dens

Ant. articular surface of dens

Transverse ligament of atlas

Rootlets of cervical nn.

Dens of axis

Posterior

Anterior

Body of axis

Squ occ bor

1st intervertebral disc

Post. arch of atlas

Body of 3rd cervical vertebra

Spinous process of atlas

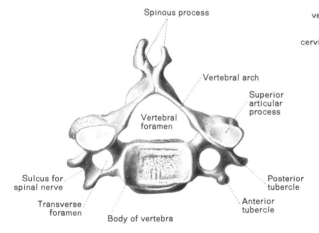

Spinous process

Vertebral arch

Superior articular process

Vertebral foramen

Sulcus for spinal nerve

Posterior tubercle

Transverse foramen

Anterior tubercle

Body of vertebra

Fig. 395: Fifth Cervical Vertebra (from Above)

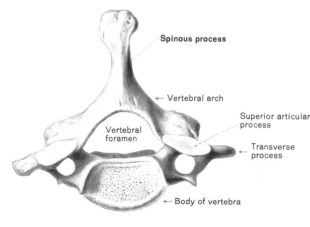

Spinous process

Vertebral arch

Superior articular process

Vertebral foramen

Transverse process

Body of vertebra

Fig. 396: Seventh Cervical Vertebra (from Above)

NOTE: the 7th cervical vertebra, being transitional between the cervical and thoracic vertebrae, has a transverse foramen similar to the cervical and a large spinous process similar to the thoracic. The latter gives it the name vertebra prominens.

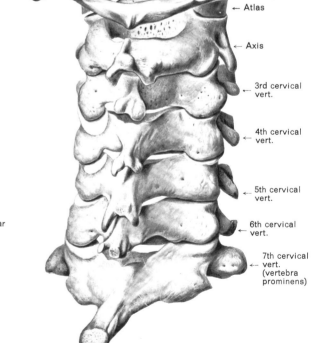

Dens of axis

Groove for vertebral artery

← Atlas

← Axis

3rd cervical vert.

4th cervical vert.

5th cervical vert.

6th cervical vert.

7th cervical vert. (vertebra prominens)

Fig. 397: The Cervical Spinal Column (Dorsal)

NOTE: while flexion and extension of the head are performed at the atlantooccipital joint, rotation of the head is the result of rotation of the atlas on the axis.

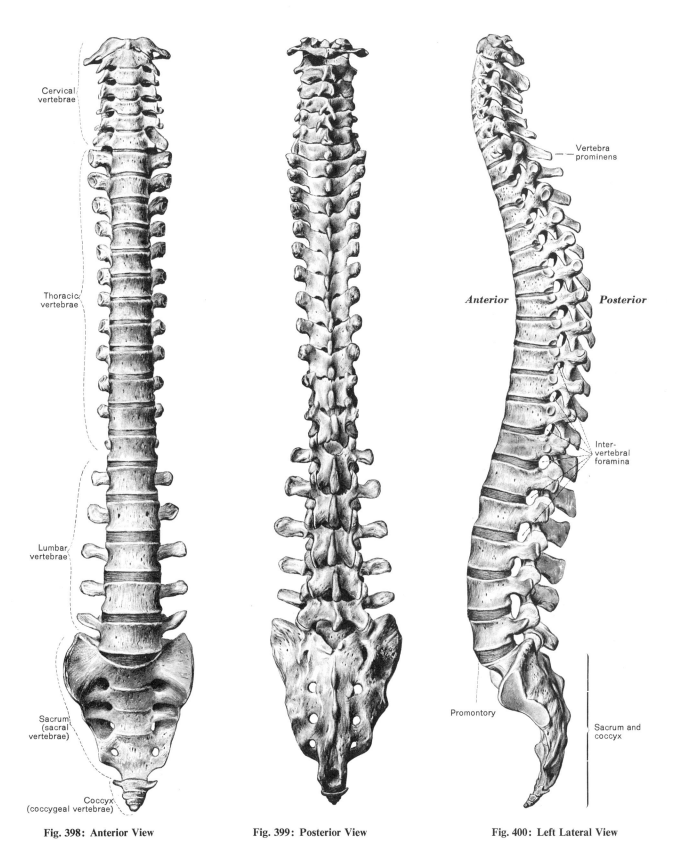

Fig. 398: Anterior View   **Fig. 399: Posterior View**   **Fig. 400: Left Lateral View**

Figs. 398, 399 and 400: The Vertebral Column, Including the Sacrum and Coccyx

NOTE: 1) the vertebral column generally consists of 7 cervical, 12 thoracic and 5 lumbar vertebrae and the sacrum and coccyx, thus, 26 bones in all. Its principal functions are to assist in the maintenance of the erect posture in man, to encase and protect the spinal cord and to allow attachments of the musculature important for movements of the head and trunk.

2) from a dorsal or ventral view, the normal spinal column is straight. When viewed from the side, the spinal column presents two ventrally convex curvatures (cervical and lumbar) and two dorsally convex curvatures (thoracic and sacral).

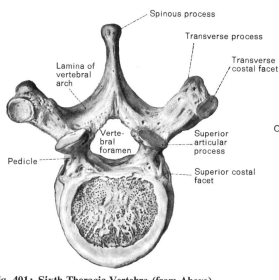

Fig. 401: Sixth Thoracic Vertebra (from Above)

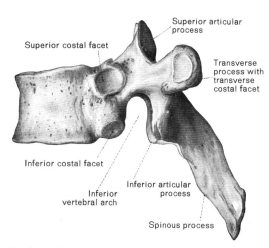

Fig. 402: Sixth Thoracic Vertebra (from Left Lateral Side)

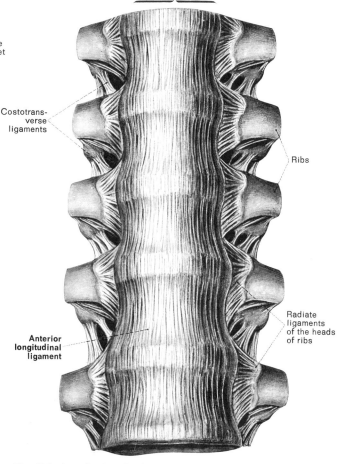

Fig. 404: Anterior Longitudinal Ligament (Ventral View)

NOTE: the anterior longitudinal ligament extends from the axis to the sacrum along the anterior aspect of the bodies of the vertebrae and the intervertebral discs to which it is firmly attached. Its longitudinal fibers are white and glistening.

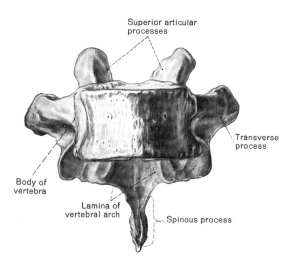

Fig. 403: Tenth Thoracic Vertebra (Ventral View)

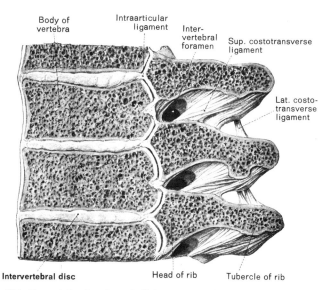

Fig. 405: Frontal Section through Spinal Column Showing Costovertebral Articulations

NOTE: the intervertebral discs, the intraarticular and costotransverse ligaments, and the intervertebral foramina which transmit the spinal nerves.

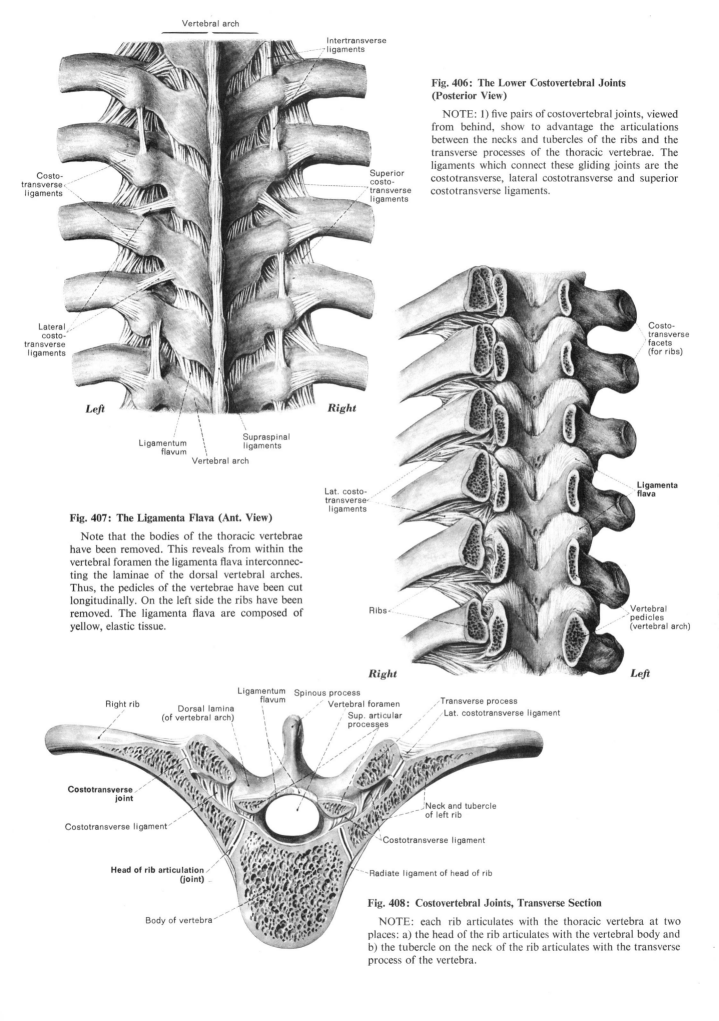

Vertebral arch

Intertransverse ligaments

Costo-transverse ligaments

Superior costo-transverse ligaments

Lateral costo-transverse ligaments

Left

Right

Ligamentum flavum

Supraspinal ligaments

Vertebral arch

Fig. 406: The Lower Costovertebral Joints (Posterior View)

NOTE: 1) five pairs of costovertebral joints, viewed from behind, show to advantage the articulations between the necks and tubercles of the ribs and the transverse processes of the thoracic vertebrae. The ligaments which connect these gliding joints are the costotransverse, lateral costotransverse and superior costotransverse ligaments.

Costo-transverse facets (for ribs)

Lat. costo-transverse ligaments

Ligamenta flava

Ribs

Vertebral pedicles (vertebral arch)

Right

Left

Fig. 407: The Ligamenta Flava (Ant. View)

Note that the bodies of the thoracic vertebrae have been removed. This reveals from within the vertebral foramen the ligamenta flava interconnecting the laminae of the dorsal vertebral arches. Thus, the pedicles of the vertebrae have been cut longitudinally. On the left side the ribs have been removed. The ligamenta flava are composed of yellow, elastic tissue.

Right rib

Dorsal lamina (of vertebral arch)

Ligamentum flavum

Spinous process

Vertebral foramen

Sup. articular processes

Transverse process

Lat. costotransverse ligament

Costotransverse joint

Costotransverse ligament

Neck and tubercle of left rib

Costotransverse ligament

Head of rib articulation (joint)

Radiate ligament of head of rib

Body of vertebra

Fig. 408: Costovertebral Joints, Transverse Section

NOTE: each rib articulates with the thoracic vertebra at two places: a) the head of the rib articulates with the vertebral body and b) the tubercle on the neck of the rib articulates with the transverse process of the vertebra.

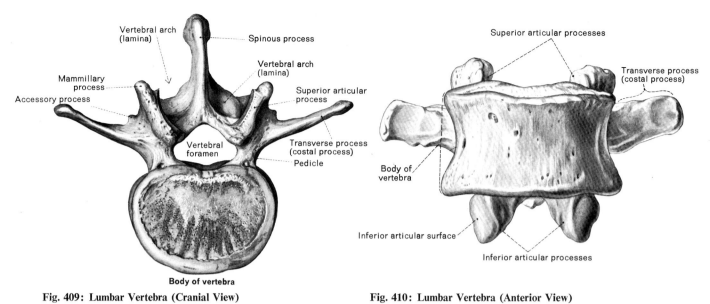

Fig. 409: Lumbar Vertebra (Cranial View)

Fig. 410: Lumbar Vertebra (Anterior View)

NOTE: the large bodies characteristic of the lumbar vertebrae.

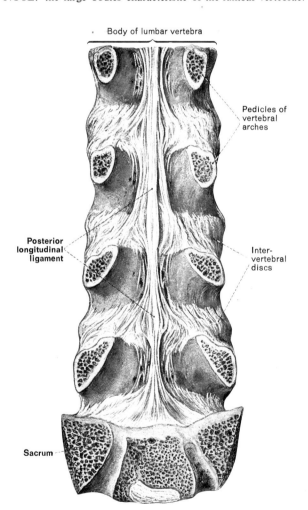

Fig. 411: Posterior Longitudinal Ligament and Intervertebral Discs, Lumbosacral Region

NOTE: this dorsal view of the spinal column shows the pedicles of the vertebral arches of the lumbar vertebrae severed to expose the posterior longitudinal ligament coursing along the posterior aspect of the bodies of the lumbar vertebrae within the vertebral canal. This ligament extends from the axis (where it joins the tectorial membrane) to the sacrum which is shown in this figure.

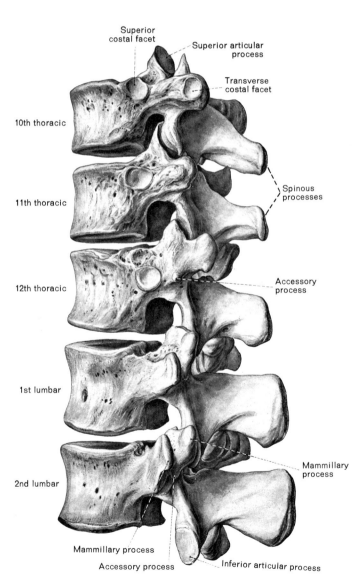

Fig. 412: Last Three Thoracic and First Two Lumbar Vertebrae (Lateral View)

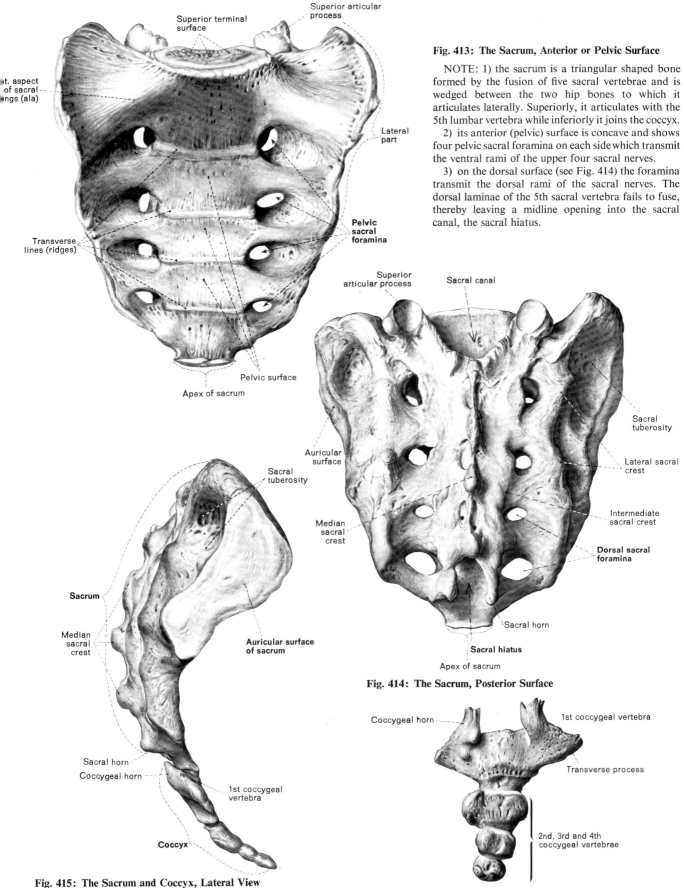

Superior terminal surface

Superior articular process

t. aspect of sacral ings (ala)

Lateral part

Transverse lines (ridges)

Pelvic sacral foramina

Pelvic surface

Apex of sacrum

Fig. 413: The Sacrum, Anterior or Pelvic Surface

NOTE: 1) the sacrum is a triangular shaped bone formed by the fusion of five sacral vertebrae and is wedged between the two hip bones to which it articulates laterally. Superiorly, it articulates with the 5th lumbar vertebra while inferiorly it joins the coccyx.

2) its anterior (pelvic) surface is concave and shows four pelvic sacral foramina on each side which transmit the ventral rami of the upper four sacral nerves.

3) on the dorsal surface (see Fig. 414) the foramina transmit the dorsal rami of the sacral nerves. The dorsal laminae of the 5th sacral vertebra fails to fuse, thereby leaving a midline opening into the sacral canal, the sacral hiatus.

Superior articular process

Sacral canal

Sacral tuberosity

Lateral sacral crest

Auricular surface

Median sacral crest

Intermediate sacral crest

Dorsal sacral foramina

Sacral horn

Sacral hiatus

Apex of sacrum

Fig. 414: The Sacrum, Posterior Surface

Sacral tuberosity

Sacrum

Median sacral crest

Auricular surface of sacrum

Sacral horn

Coccygeal horn

1st coccygeal vertebra

Coccyx

Fig. 415: The Sacrum and Coccyx, Lateral View

NOTE: the auricular (ear-like) surface of the sacrum articulates with the iliac portion of the pelvis. Inferiorly, the sacral apex joins the coccyx.

Coccygeal horn

1st coccygeal vertebra

Transverse process

2nd, 3rd and 4th coccygeal vertebrae

Fig. 416: The Coccyx, Dorsal View

NOTE: this coccyx has 4 segments, but in many instances there are 3 or 5.

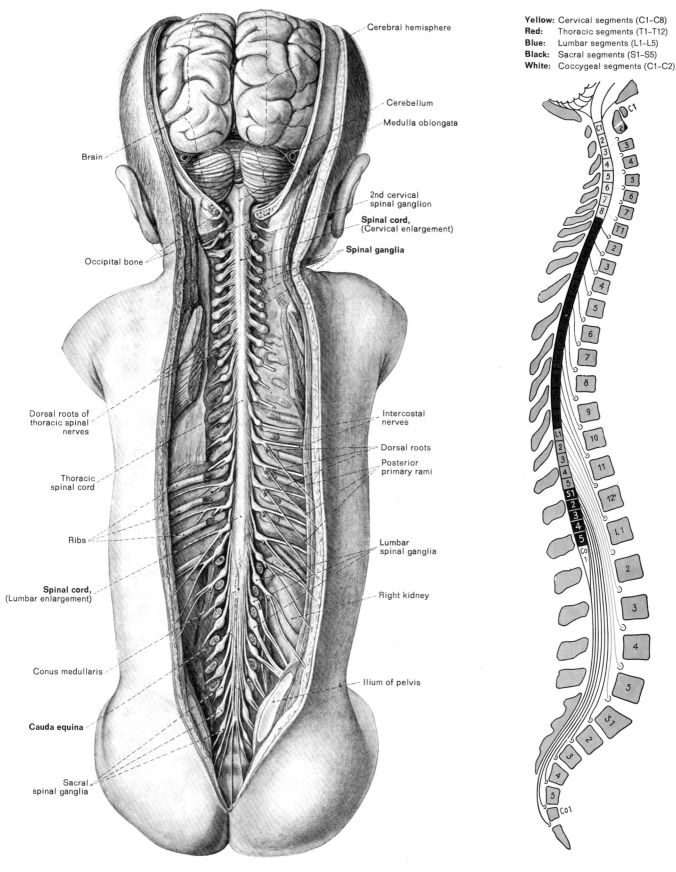

Cerebral hemisphere

Cerebellum

Medulla oblongata

Brain

2nd cervical
spinal ganglion

Spinal cord,
(Cervical enlargement)

Spinal ganglia

Occipital bone

Dorsal roots of
thoracic spinal
nerves

Thoracic
spinal cord

Ribs

Spinal cord,
(Lumbar enlargement)

Conus medullaris

Cauda equina

Sacral
spinal ganglia

Intercostal
nerves

Dorsal roots

Posterior
primary rami

Lumbar
spinal ganglia

Right kidney

Ilium of pelvis

Yellow: Cervical segments (C1–C8)
Red: Thoracic segments (T1–T12)
Blue: Lumbar segments (L1–L5)
Black: Sacral segments (S1–S5)
White: Coccygeal segments (C1–C2)

Fig. 417: The Spinal Cord and Brain of a Newborn Child (Posterior View)

NOTE: 1) the central nervous system has been exposed by removal of the spinal column and dorsal cranium. The spinal ganglia have been dissected as well as their corresponding spinal nerves.

2) although in this dissection it appears as though the substance of the spinal cord terminates at about L-1, it is more usual in the newborn for the cord to end at about L-3 or L-4, thereby filling the spinal canal more completely than in the adult.

Fig. 418: The Emerging Spinal Nerves and their Segments in the Adult

NOTE: many spinal nerves travel considerable distances before leaving the vertebral canal in the adult.

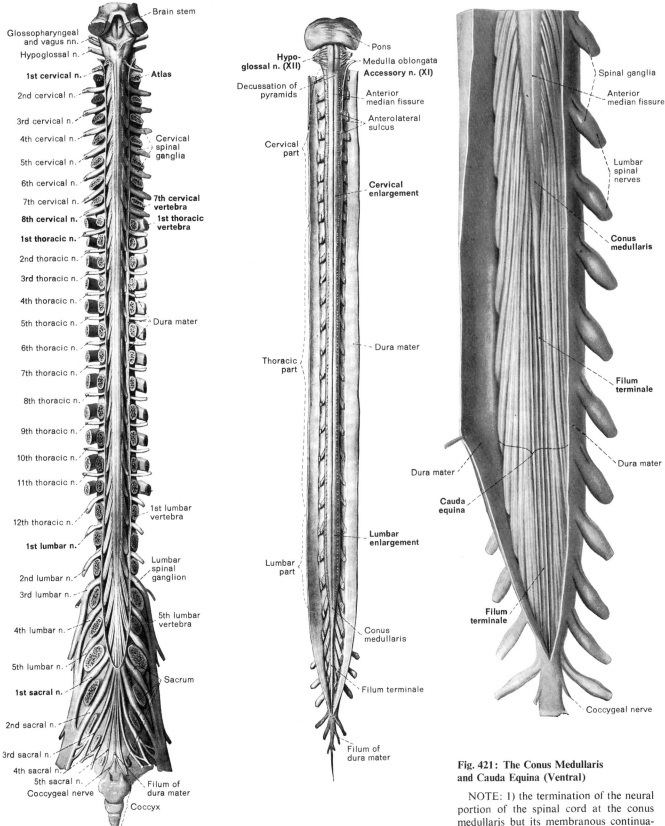

Fig. 419: The Spinal Cord within the Vertebral Canal (Dorsal View)

NOTE: 1) the 1st cervical nerve emerges above the first vertebra and the 8th cervical nerve emerges below the 7th vertebra.

2) the cervical spinal cord is continuous above with the medulla oblongata of the brain stem.

Fig. 420: The Spinal Cord (Ventral View)

NOTE: 1) the origin of the spinal portion of the accessory nerve (Cranial XI) arising from the cervical spinal cord and ascending to join the bulbar portion of that nerve.

2) the alignment of the rootlets of the hypoglossal nerve (Cranial XII) with the ventral roots of the spinal cord.

Fig. 421: The Conus Medullaris and Cauda Equina (Ventral)

NOTE: 1) the termination of the neural portion of the spinal cord at the conus medullaris but its membranous continuation as the filum terminalis which consists principally of pia mater.

2) the long (approx. 8 inches) cauda equina (horse's tail) consisting of the intravertebral portions of the lower spinal nerves.

3) prolongations of the dura mater continue to cover the spinal nerves for some distance as they enter the intervertebral foramina.

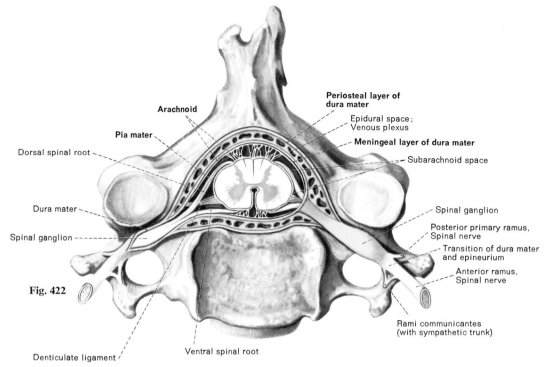

Periosteal layer of dura mater

Epidural space; Venous plexus

Meningeal layer of dura mater

Subarachnoid space

Arachnoid

Pia mater

Dorsal spinal root

Spinal ganglion

Posterior primary ramus, Spinal nerve

Dura mater

Spinal ganglion

Transition of dura mater and epineurium

Anterior ramus, Spinal nerve

Rami communicantes (with sympathetic trunk)

Fig. 422

Denticulate ligament

Ventral spinal root

Fig. 422: Meninges of Spinal Cord shown at Cervical Level (Transverse Section)

NOTE: 1) the meningeal dura mater (inner layer of yellow) surrounds the spinal cord and continues along the spinal nerve through the intervertebral foramen. Its outer periosteal layer (outer layer of yellow) is formed of connective tissue which closely adheres to the bone of the vertebrae which forms the vertebral canal.

2) the delicate, film-like arachnoid which lies between the meningeal layer of dura mater and the vascularized pia mater which is closely applied to the cord.

Posterior median sulcus

Anterior median fissure

Denticulate ligaments

Dura mater

Posterolateral sulcus

Dorsal root filaments

Arachnoid

Fig. 424

Spinal ganglia

Dura mater (meningeal)

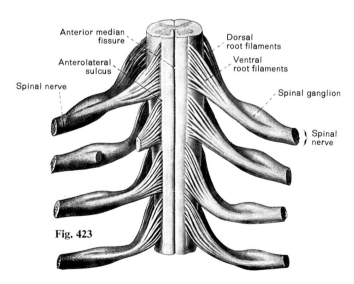

Anterior median fissure

Anterolateral sulcus

Spinal nerve

Dorsal root filaments

Ventral root filaments

Spinal ganglion

Spinal nerve

Fig. 423

Fig. 423: Spinal Cord with Nerve Roots

NOTE: the many filaments which form the dorsal and ventral roots of a spinal nerve enter into and emerge from the cord in a straight line.

◄ **Fig. 424: Spinal Cord with Dura Mater Dissected Open (Dorsal View)**

Note that extensions of the pia mater to the meningeal dura mater between the roots of the spinal nerves are called denticulate ligaments. The arachnoid sends fine attachments to both the pia and dura.

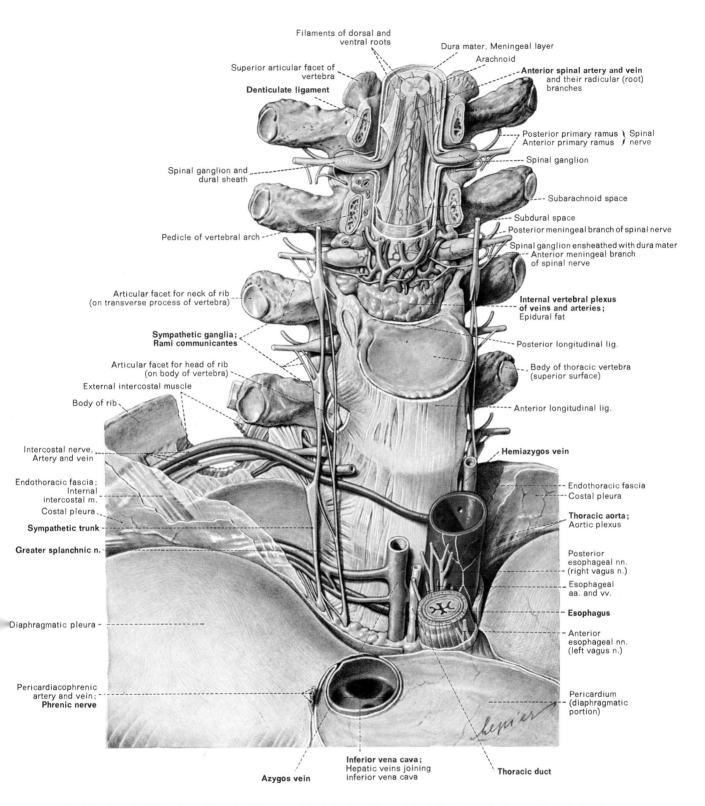

Filaments of dorsal and ventral roots

Dura mater, Meningeal layer

Arachnoid

Superior articular facet of vertebra

Denticulate ligament

Anterior spinal artery and vein
and their radicular (root) branches

Posterior primary ramus ⎱ Spinal
Anterior primary ramus ⎰ nerve

Spinal ganglion

Spinal ganglion and dural sheath

Subarachnoid space

Subdural space

Posterior meningeal branch of spinal nerve

Pedicle of vertebral arch

Spinal ganglion ensheathed with dura mater

Anterior meningeal branch of spinal nerve

Articular facet for neck of rib (on transverse process of vertebra)

Internal vertebral plexus of veins and arteries;
Epidural fat

Sympathetic ganglia; Rami communicantes

Posterior longitudinal lig.

Articular facet for head of rib (on body of vertebra)

Body of thoracic vertebra (superior surface)

External intercostal muscle

Body of rib

Anterior longitudinal lig.

Intercostal nerve, Artery and vein

Hemiazygos vein

Endothoracic fascia; Internal intercostal m.

Endothoracic fascia

Costal pleura

Costal pleura

Thoracic aorta; Aortic plexus

Sympathetic trunk

Posterior esophageal nn. (right vagus n.)

Greater splanchnic n.

Esophageal aa. and vv.

Esophagus

Anterior esophageal nn. (left vagus n.)

Diaphragmatic pleura

Pericardiacophrenic artery and vein; **Phrenic nerve**

Pericardium (diaphragmatic portion)

Azygos vein

Inferior vena cava; Hepatic veins joining inferior vena cava

Thoracic duct

Fig. 425: Anterior Dissection of Vertebral Column, Spinal Cord and Prevertebral Structures at a Lower Thoracic Level

NOTE: 1) the internal vertebral plexus of veins and arteries which lie in the epidural space which also contains the epidural fat. These should not be confused with the spinal vessels which are situated in the pia mater and which are seen to be intimately applied to the spinal cord tissue.

2) the ganglionated sympathetic chain observable here in the thoracic region receiving and giving communicating rami with the spinal nerves. Note also the formation of the greater splanchnic nerve and its descent prevertebrally into the abdomen.

3) the aorta, inferior vena cava, azygos and hemiazygos veins, esophagus and thoracic duct all lying anterior or somewhat to the left of the vertebral column and passing through the diaphragm.

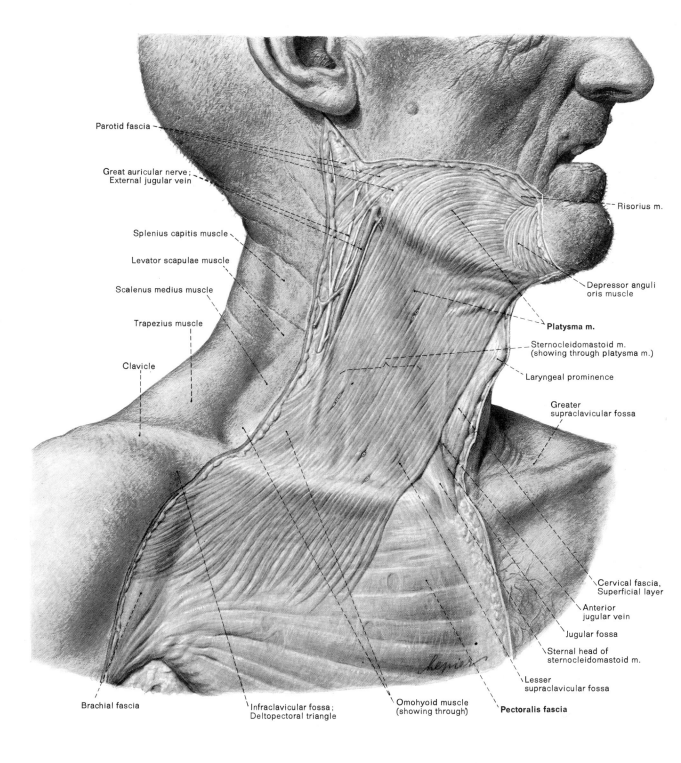

Parotid fascia

Great auricular nerve;
External jugular vein

Splenius capitis muscle

Levator scapulae muscle

Scalenus medius muscle

Trapezius muscle

Clavicle

Brachial fascia

Infraclavicular fossa;
Deltopectoral triangle

Omohyoid muscle
(showing through)

Pectoralis fascia

Risorius m.

Depressor anguli
oris muscle

Platysma m.

Sternocleidomastoid m.
(showing through platysma m.)

Laryngeal prominence

Greater
supraclavicular fossa

Cervical fascia,
Superficial layer

Anterior
jugular vein

Jugular fossa

Sternal head of
sternocleidomastoid m.

Lesser
supraclavicular fossa

Fig. 426: The Right Platysma Muscle and Pectoral Fascia

NOTE: 1) the platysma muscle is a broad, thin quadrangular muscle located in the superficial fascia on the anterolateral aspect of the neck, extending from the angle of the mouth and chin across the clavicle to the upper part of the thorax and anterior shoulder.

2) the platysma muscle can be considered as one of the muscles of facial expression which characteristically do not arise and insert on bony structures but within superficial fascia instead. Upon contraction, the platysma tends to depress the angle of the mouth and wrinkle the skin of the neck, thereby participating in the formation of facial expressions of anxiety, sadness, dissatisfaction and suffering.

3) similar to the other muscles of facial expression, the platysma is innervated by the cervical branch of the facial or VIIth cranial nerve.

4) overlying the pectoralis major is the well developed pectoralis fascia which extends from the midline in the thorax laterally to the axilla. Observe the external jugular vein and great auricular nerve exposed in the upper lateral aspect of the neck.

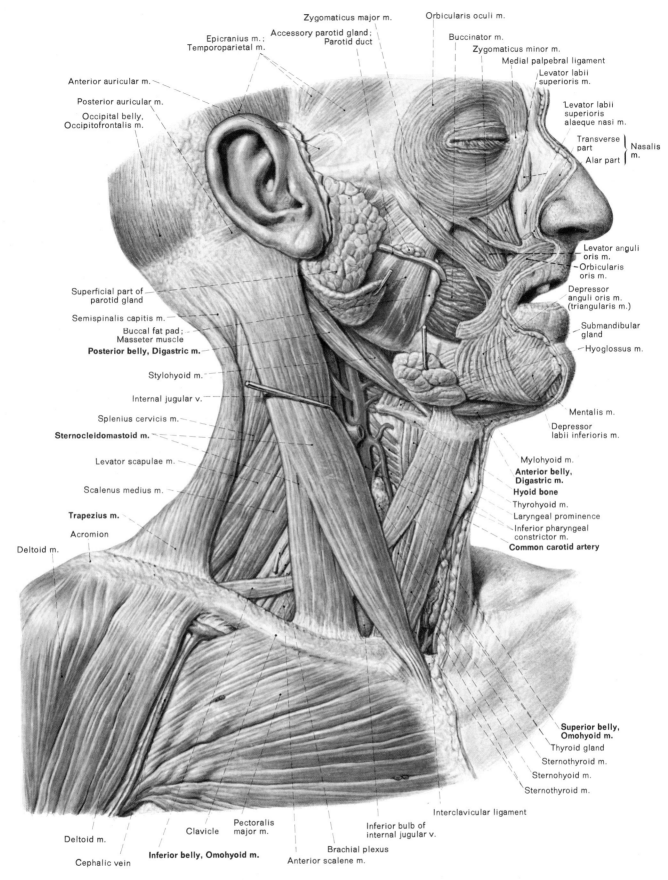

Anterior auricular m.

Posterior auricular m.

Occipital belly, Occipitofrontalis m.

Epicranius m.; Temporoparietal m.

Accessory parotid gland; Parotid duct

Zygomaticus major m.

Orbicularis oculi m.

Buccinator m.

Zygomaticus minor m.

Medial palpebral ligament

Levator labii superioris m.

Levator labii superioris alaeque nasi m.

Transverse part

Alar part

Nasalis m.

Superficial part of parotid gland

Semispinalis capitis m.

Buccal fat pad; Masseter muscle

Posterior belly, Digastric m.

Stylohyoid m.

Internal jugular v.

Splenius cervicis m.

Sternocleidomastoid m.

Levator scapulae m.

Scalenus medius m.

Trapezius m.

Acromion

Deltoid m.

Levator anguli oris m.

Orbicularis oris m.

Depressor anguli oris m. (triangularis m.)

Submandibular gland

Hyoglossus m.

Mentalis m.

Depressor labii inferioris m.

Mylohyoid m.

Anterior belly, Digastric m.

Hyoid bone

Thyrohyoid m.

Laryngeal prominence

Inferior pharyngeal constrictor m.

Common carotid artery

Superior belly, Omohyoid m.

Thyroid gland

Sternothyroid m.

Sternohyoid m.

Sternothyroid m.

Interclavicular ligament

Deltoid m.

Cephalic vein

Clavicle

Inferior belly, Omohyoid m.

Pectoralis major m.

Anterior scalene m.

Brachial plexus

Inferior bulb of internal jugular v.

Fig. 427: The Anterior and Posterior Triangles of the Neck

NOTE: 1) the *anterior triangle* of the neck is bounded by the midline of the neck, the anterior border of the sternocleidomastoid and the mandible. This area is further subdivided by the superior belly of the omohyoid and the two bellies of the digastric into the following: a) *muscular triangle* (midline, superior belly of omohyoid, sternocleidomastoid), b) *carotid triangle* (superior belly of omohyoid, sternocleido-mastoid and posterior belly of digastric), c) *submandibular triangle* (anterior and posterior bellies of digastric and the inferior margin of the mandible), and d) *suprahyoid triangle* (midline, anterior belly of digastric and hyoid bone).

2) the *posterior triangle* of the neck is bounded by the posterior border of the sternocleidomastoid, the trapezius and the clavicle. This area is subdivided into the *occipital triangle* and *subclavian triangle* by the inferior belly of the omohyoid muscle.

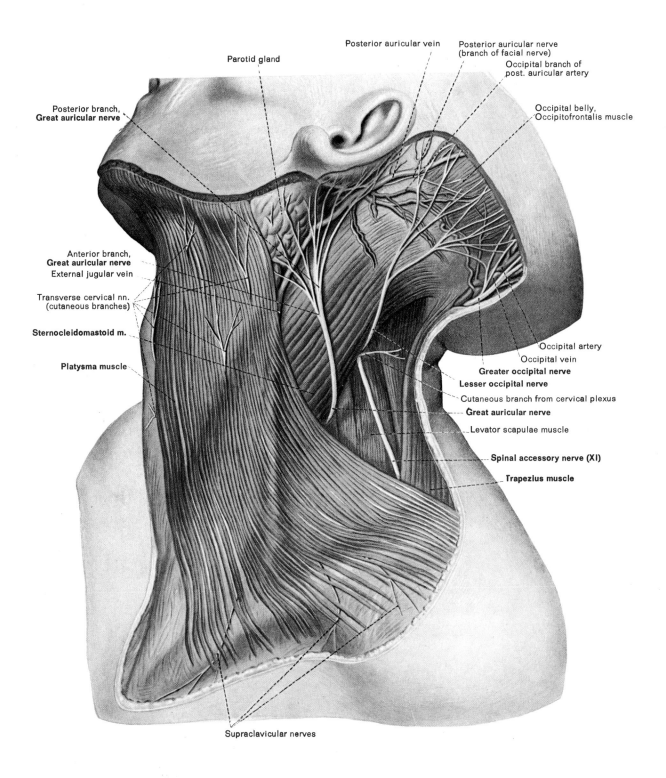

Parotid gland

Posterior auricular vein

Posterior auricular nerve
(branch of facial nerve)

Occipital branch of
post. auricular artery

Posterior branch,
Great auricular nerve

Occipital belly,
Occipitofrontalis muscle

Anterior branch,
Great auricular nerve

External jugular vein

Transverse cervical nn.
(cutaneous branches)

Sternocleidomastoid m.

Platysma muscle

Occipital artery

Occipital vein

Greater occipital nerve

Lesser occipital nerve

Cutaneous branch from cervical plexus

Great auricular nerve

Levator scapulae muscle

Spinal accessory nerve (XI)

Trapezius muscle

Supraclavicular nerves

Fig. 428: Nerves and Blood Vessels of the Neck, Stage 1: Platysma Layer

NOTE: 1) the skin has been removed from both anterior and posterior triangles of the neck to reveal the platysma muscle. Observe the cutaneous branches of the transverse cervical nerves emanating from the cervical plexus and penetrating through the platysma (and superficial fascia) to reach the skin of the anterolateral aspect of the neck.

2) four other nerves: a) the great auricular (C-2, C-3), b) the lesser occipital (C-2), c) the greater occipital (C-2) and d) the spinal accessory (XI).

3) after it has supplied the sternocleidomastoid muscle, the spinal accessory nerve (XI) descends in the posterior triangle to reach the trapezius muscle which it also supplies with motor innervation.

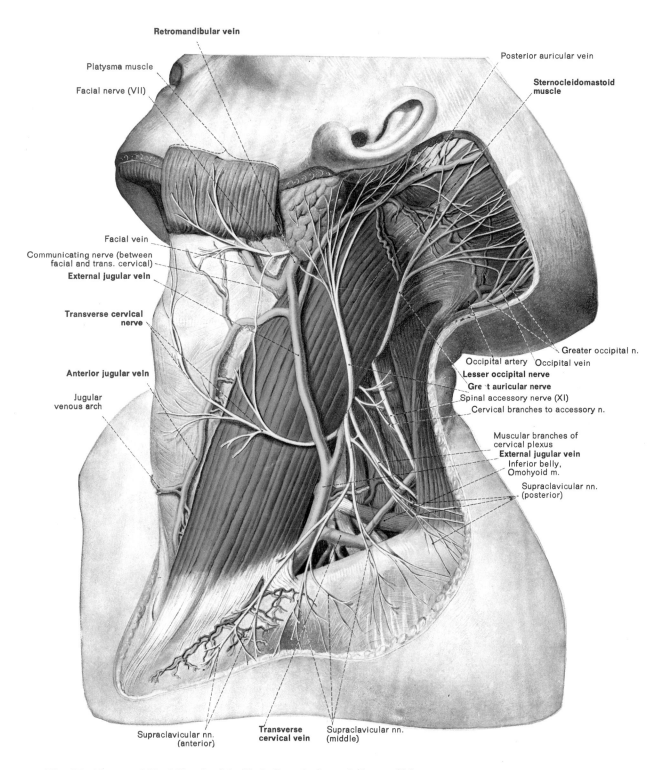

Retromandibular vein

Platysma muscle

Facial nerve (VII)

Posterior auricular vein

Sternocleidomastoid muscle

Facial vein

Communicating nerve (between facial and trans. cervical)

External jugular vein

Transverse cervical nerve

Anterior jugular vein

Jugular venous arch

Greater occipital n.

Occipital artery Occipital vein

Lesser occipital nerve

Gre t auricular nerve

Spinal accessory nerve (XI)

Cervical branches to accessory n.

Muscular branches of cervical plexus

External jugular vein

Inferior belly, Omohyoid m.

Supraclavicular nn. (posterior)

Supraclavicular nn. (anterior)

Transverse cervical vein

Supraclavicular nn. (middle)

Fig. 429: Nerves and Blood Vessels of the Neck, Stage 2: Sternocleidomastoid Layer

NOTE: 1) with the platysma reflected upward, the full extent of the sternocleidomastoid muscle is exposed. Observe that the nerves of the cervical plexus diverge at the posterior border of the sternocleidomastoid muscle: the great auricular and lesser occipital ascend to the head, the transverse colli course across the neck toward the midline while the supraclavicular descend over the clavicle.

2) the external jugular vein formed by the junction of the retromandibular and posterior auricular veins. The external jugular crosses the sternocleidomastoid muscle obliquely and receives tributaries from the anterior jugular, posterior external jugular, transverse cervical and suprascapular veins before terminating into the subclavian vein.

3) the cervical branch of the facial (VII) nerve supplying the inner surface of the platysma muscle with motor innervation.

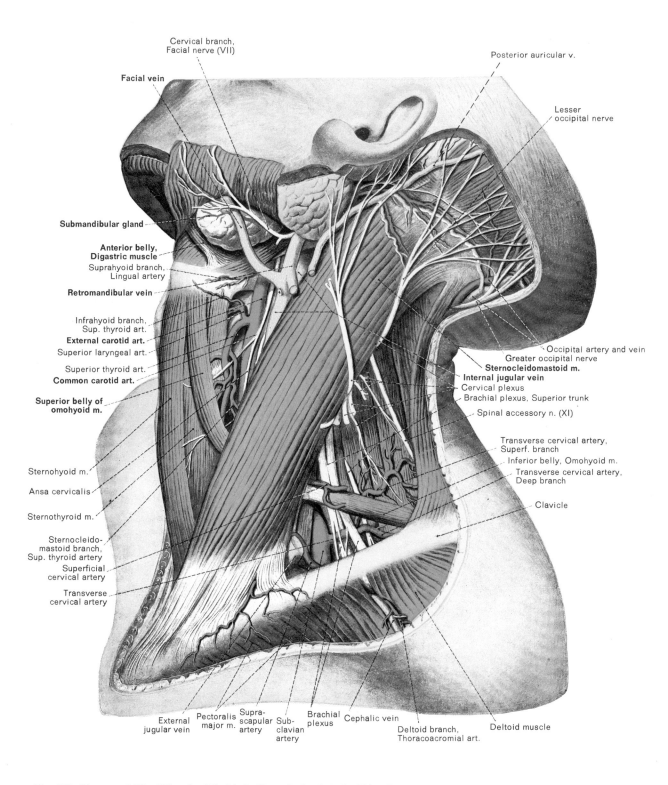

Labels on figure:

Cervical branch, Facial nerve (VII)
Facial vein
Posterior auricular v.
Lesser occipital nerve
Submandibular gland
Anterior belly, Digastric muscle
Suprahyoid branch, Lingual artery
Retromandibular vein
Infrahyoid branch, Sup. thyroid art.
External carotid art.
Superior laryngeal art.
Superior thyroid art.
Common carotid art.
Superior belly of omohyoid m.
Occipital artery and vein
Greater occipital nerve
Sternocleidomastoid m.
Internal jugular vein
Cervical plexus
Brachial plexus, Superior trunk
Spinal accessory n. (XI)
Sternohyoid m.
Ansa cervicalis
Sternothyroid m.
Sternocleido-mastoid branch, Sup. thyroid artery
Superficial cervical artery
Transverse cervical artery
Transverse cervical artery, Superf. branch
Inferior belly, Omohyoid m.
Transverse cervical artery, Deep branch
Clavicle
External jugular vein
Pectoralis major m.
Supra-scapular artery
Sub-clavian artery
Brachial plexus
Cephalic vein
Deltoid branch, Thoracoacromial art.
Deltoid muscle

Fig. 430: Nerves and Blood Vessels of the Neck, Stage 3: the Anterior Triangle

NOTE: 1) with the investing fascia removed, the outlines of the muscular, carotid and submandibular triangles which subdivide the anterior neck region are revealed.

2) the infrahyoid (strap) muscles which cover the thyroid gland in the *muscular triangle* (bounded by sternocleidomastoid, midline and superior belly of omohyoid).

3) the carotid vessels and jugular vein in the *carotid triangle* (bounded by superior belly of omohyoid, posterior belly of digastric and sternocleidomastoid).

4) the submandibular gland in the *submandibular triangle* (bounded by anterior and posterior bellies of digastric and the inferior border of the mandible).

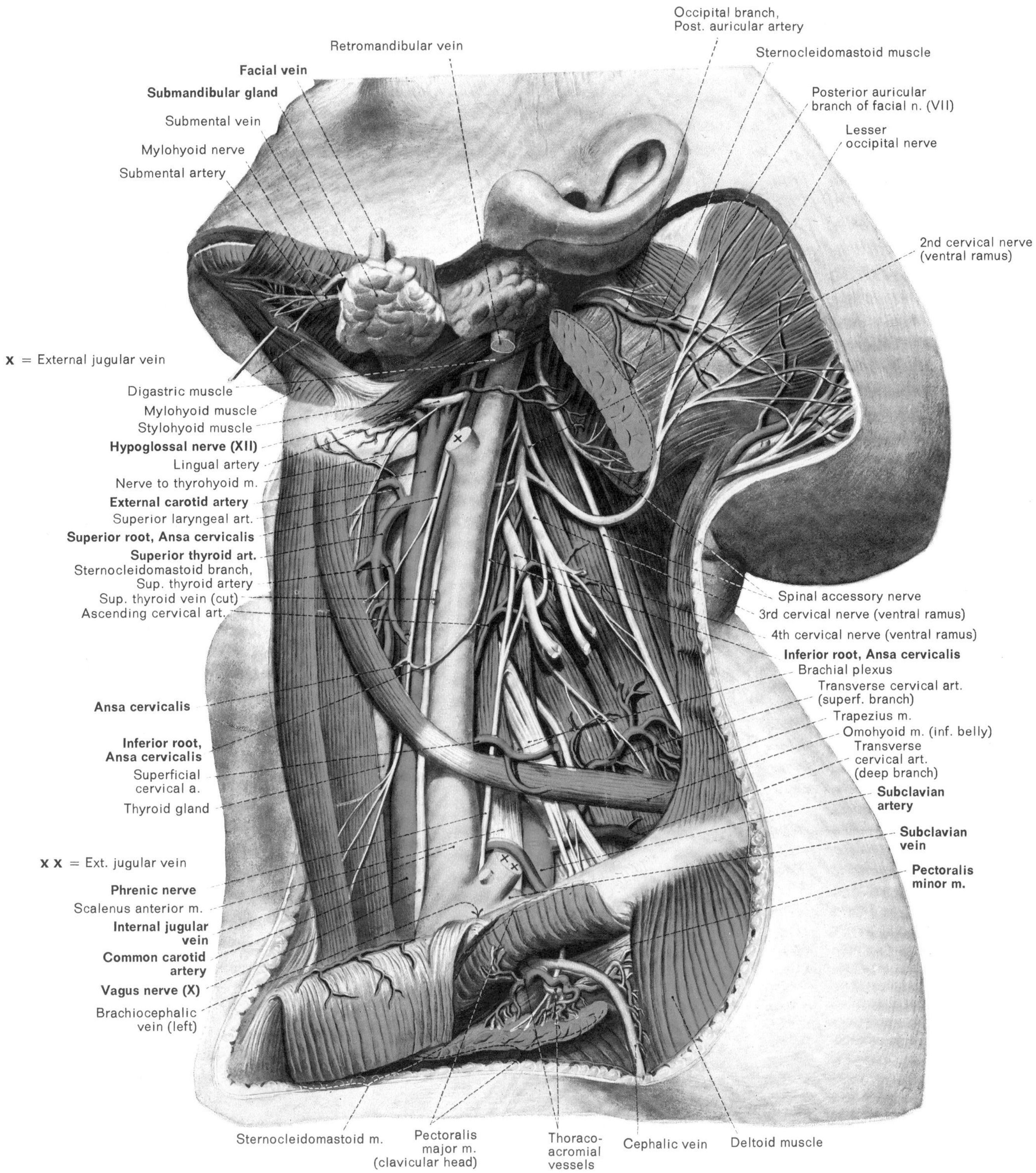

Retromandibular vein

Occipital branch,
Post. auricular artery

Sternocleidomastoid muscle

Facial vein

Submandibular gland

Posterior auricular
branch of facial n. (VII)

Submental vein

Mylohyoid nerve

Lesser
occipital nerve

Submental artery

2nd cervical nerve
(ventral ramus)

x = External jugular vein

Digastric muscle

Mylohyoid muscle

Stylohyoid muscle

Hypoglossal nerve (XII)

Lingual artery

Nerve to thyrohyoid m.

External carotid artery

Superior laryngeal art.

Superior root, Ansa cervicalis

Superior thyroid art.

Sternocleidomastoid branch,
Sup. thyroid artery

Sup. thyroid vein (cut)

Ascending cervical art.

Spinal accessory nerve

3rd cervical nerve (ventral ramus)

4th cervical nerve (ventral ramus)

Inferior root, Ansa cervicalis

Brachial plexus

Transverse cervical art.
(superf. branch)

Trapezius m.

Omohyoid m. (inf. belly)

Transverse
cervical art.
(deep branch)

**Subclavian
artery**

Ansa cervicalis

**Inferior root,
Ansa cervicalis**

Superficial
cervical a.

Thyroid gland

**Subclavian
vein**

**Pectoralis
minor m.**

x x = Ext. jugular vein

Phrenic nerve

Scalenus anterior m.

**Internal jugular
vein**

**Common carotid
artery**

Vagus nerve (X)

Brachiocephalic
vein (left)

Sternocleidomastoid m.

Pectoralis
major m.
(clavicular head)

Thoraco-
acromial
vessels

Cephalic vein

Deltoid muscle

Fig. 431: Nerves and Blood Vessels of the Neck, Stage 4: the Large Vessels

NOTE: 1) the sternocleidomastoid muscle and the superficial veins and nerves have been removed to expose the internal and external carotid arteries, the internal jugular vein, both bellies of the omohyoid muscle, the vagus nerve and the ansa cervicalis.

2) superiorly, the facial vein has been cut and the submandibular gland elevated, thereby exposing the hypoglossal nerve (XII). Observe that nerve fibers (originating from C-1 and travelling for a short distance) leave the hypoglossal nerve to descend in the neck. These form the superior root of the ansa cervicalis and are joined by other descending fibers from C-2 and C-3 which are called the inferior root of the ansa cervicalis. These two roots form the ansa cervicalis, from which innervation for a number of the strap muscles is derived.

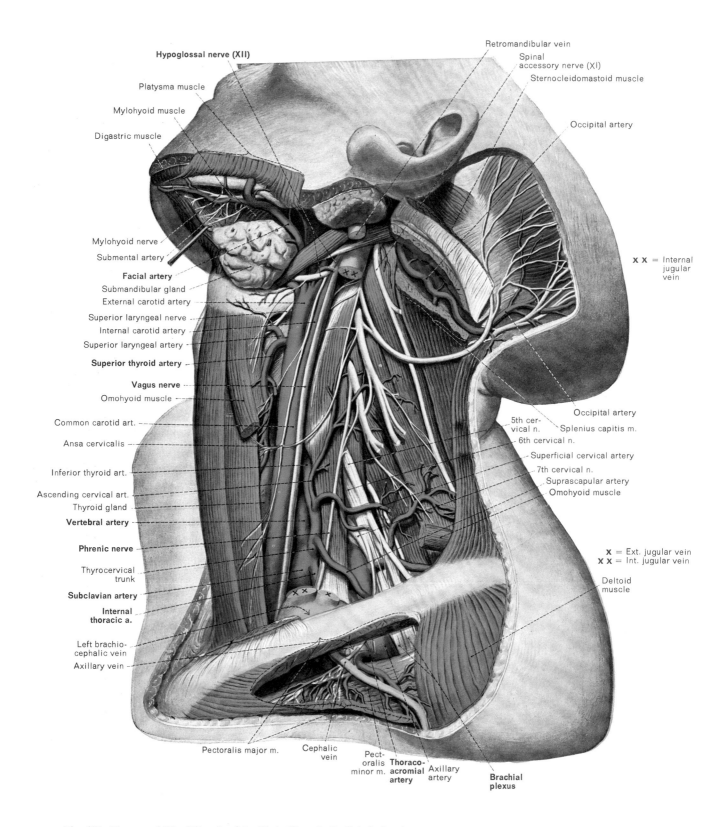

Hypoglossal nerve (XII)

Platysma muscle

Mylohyoid muscle

Digastric muscle

Mylohyoid nerve

Submental artery

Facial artery

Submandibular gland

External carotid artery

Superior laryngeal nerve

Internal carotid artery

Superior laryngeal artery

Superior thyroid artery

Vagus nerve

Omohyoid muscle

Common carotid art.

Ansa cervicalis

Inferior thyroid art.

Ascending cervical art.

Thyroid gland

Vertebral artery

Phrenic nerve

Thyrocervical trunk

Subclavian artery

Internal thoracic a.

Left brachio-cephalic vein

Axillary vein

Retromandibular vein

Spinal accessory nerve (XI)

Sternocleidomastoid muscle

Occipital artery

X X = Internal jugular vein

Occipital artery

5th cervical n.

Splenius capitis m.

6th cervical n.

Superficial cervical artery

7th cervical n.

Suprascapular artery

Omohyoid muscle

X = Ext. jugular vein
X X = Int. jugular vein

Deltoid muscle

Pectoralis major m.

Cephalic vein

Pectoralis minor m.

Thoracoacromial artery

Axillary artery

Brachial plexus

Fig. 432: Nerves and Blood Vessels of the Neck, Stage 5: the Subclavian Artery

NOTE: 1) with the internal and external jugular veins removed, the subclavian artery becomes exposed as it ascends from the thorax and loops in the subclavian triangle of the neck to descend beneath the clavicle into the axilla. Observe the vertebral, thyrocervical and internal thoracic branches and the transverse cervical artery which comes off separately in this dissection and which divides into an ascending superficial branch and a descending deep branch (not labelled).

2) the vagus nerve coursing with the internal and common carotid arteries and the phrenic nerve descending in the neck along the surface of the anterior scalene muscle toward the thorax.

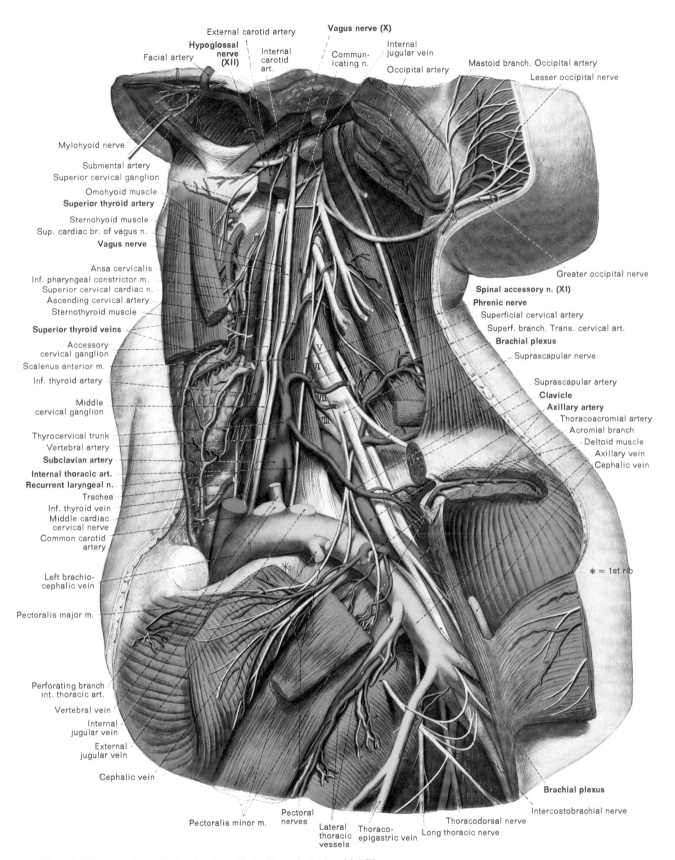

Fig. 433: Nerves and Blood Vessels of the Neck, Stage 6: the brachial Plexus

NOTE: 1) with the carotid arteries, jugular vein and clavicle removed, the roots forming the trunks of the brachial plexus are exposed as they divide and descend into the axilla to surround the axillary artery.

2) the sympathetic trunk lying deep to the carotid arteries and coursing with the vagus nerve and the superior cardiac branch of the vagus nerve.

3) the thyroid gland receiving the superior and inferior thyroid arteries and being drained by the thyroid veins. Observe also the proximity of the recurrent laryngeal nerve to the thyroid gland.

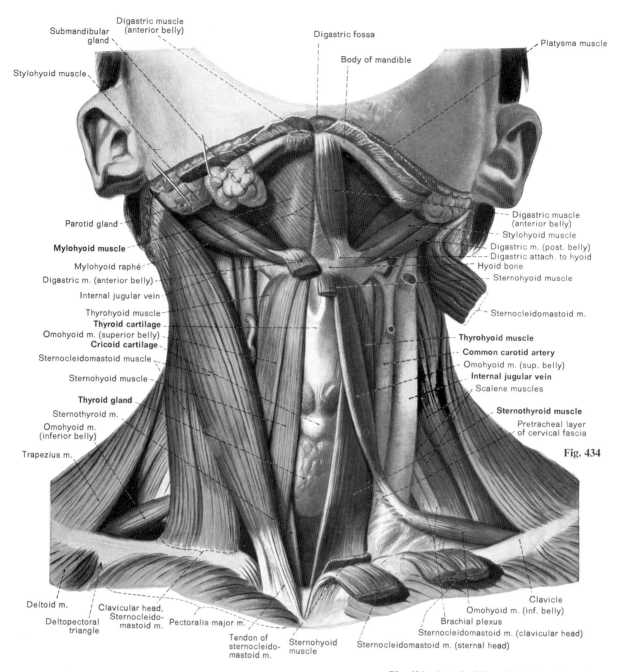

Submandibular gland

Stylohyoid muscle

Digastric muscle (anterior belly)

Digastric fossa

Body of mandible

Platysma muscle

Parotid gland

Mylohyoid muscle

Mylohyoid raphé

Digastric m. (anterior belly)

Internal jugular vein

Thyrohyoid muscle

Thyroid cartilage

Omohyoid m. (superior belly)

Cricoid cartilage

Sternocleidomastoid muscle

Sternohyoid muscle

Thyroid gland

Sternothyroid m.

Omohyoid m. (inferior belly)

Trapezius m.

Digastric muscle (anterior belly)

Stylohyoid muscle

Digastric m. (post. belly)

Digastric attach. to hyoid

Hyoid bone

Sternohyoid muscle

Sternocleidomastoid m.

Thyrohyoid muscle

Common carotid artery

Omohyoid m. (sup. belly)

Internal jugular vein

Scalene muscles

Sternothyroid muscle

Pretracheal layer of cervical fascia

Fig. 434

Deltoid m.

Deltopectoral triangle

Clavicular head, Sternocleidomastoid m.

Pectoralis major m.

Tendon of sternocleidomastoid m.

Sternohyoid muscle

Sternocleidomastoid m. (sternal head)

Brachial plexus

Sternocleidomastoid m. (clavicular head)

Omohyoid m. (inf. belly)

Clavicle

Fig. 434: Anterior View of the Musculature in the Neck

NOTE: 1) the right superior belly of the digastric muscle was removed and submandibular gland elevated in order to show the mylohyoid muscle. On the left side, the sternocleidomastoid and sternohyoid muscles have been transected and the submandibular gland removed.

2) the relationship of the strap muscles to the thyroid gland and realize that inferior to the thyroid and above the suprasternal notch, the trachea lies immediately under the skin.

Fig. 435

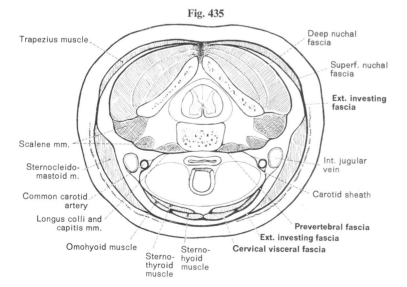

Trapezius muscle

Scalene mm.

Sternocleidomastoid m.

Common carotid artery

Longus colli and capitis mm.

Omohyoid muscle

Sternothyroid muscle

Sternohyoid muscle

Deep nuchal fascia

Superf. nuchal fascia

Ext. investing fascia

Int. jugular vein

Carotid sheath

Prevertebral fascia

Ext. investing fascia

Cervical visceral fascia

Fig. 435: Fascial Planes of the Neck in a Newborn Child (Cross Section)

NOTE: the external investing fascia splits to encase the sternocleidomastoid and trapezius muscles. The prevertebral fascia encloses the vertebral column and its muscles, while the cervical visceral fascia encloses the esophagus, trachea, thyroid gland and strap muscles.

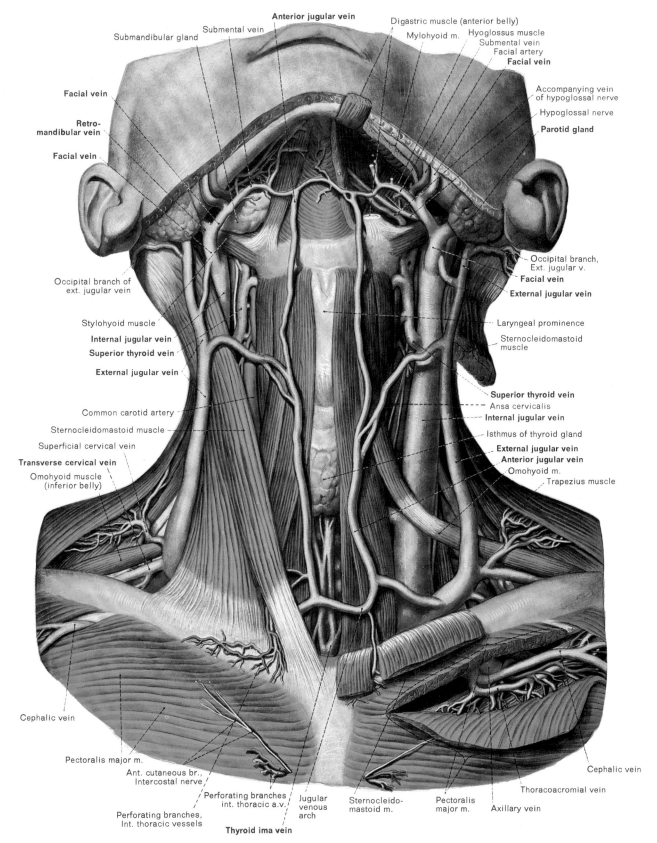

Fig. 436: **Veins of the Neck and Infraclavicular Region**

NOTE: 1) the jugular system of veins, although somewhat variable, generally consists of an anterior jugular, external jugular and internal jugular vein, all of which are shown on the left side where the sternocleidomastoid muscle has been removed.

2) the anterior jugular descends close to the midline, is frequently small and drains laterally through several tributaries into the external jugular vein. The external jugular courses along the surface of the sternocleidomastoid muscle. It commences usually within the parotid gland and enlarges through the junction of occipital, retromandibular and facial branches. It flows into the subclavian vein with the internal jugular after it receives branches from the shoulder and clavicular regions.

3) the internal jugular is large and collects blood from the brain, face and neck. At its junction with the subclavian, the brachiocephalic vein is formed.

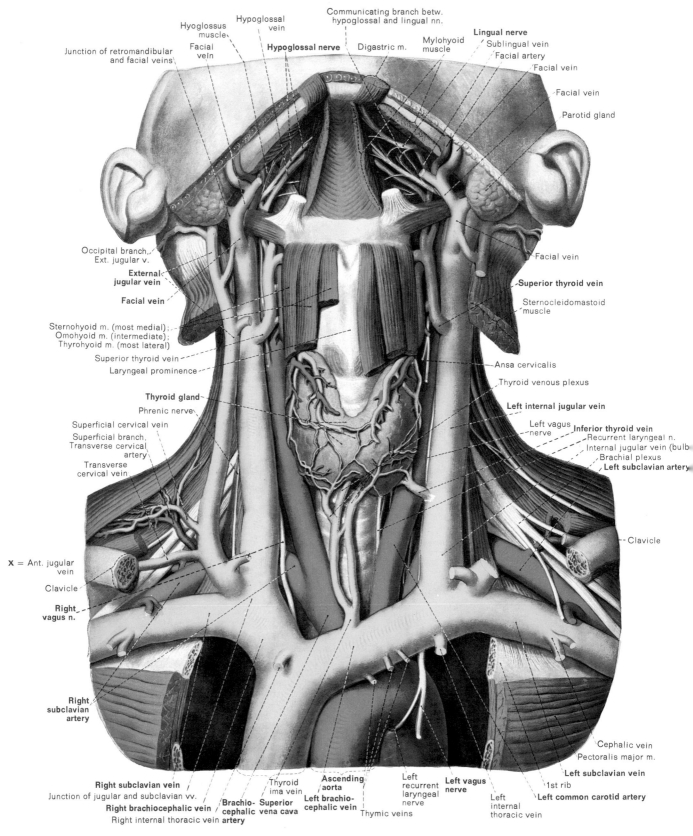

Fig. 437: Deep Arteries and Veins of the Neck and Great Vessels of the Thorax

NOTE: 1) in the neck, the sternocleidomastoid and strap muscles have been removed, thereby exposing the carotid arteries, internal jugular veins and thyroid gland.

2) the middle portion of the anterior thoracic wall has been resected in order to show the aortic arch and its branches, the brachiocephalic veins, the superior vena cava and the vagus nerves.

3) in the submandibular region, the mylohyoid and anterior digastric muscles have been cut revealing the lingual and hypoglossal nerves.

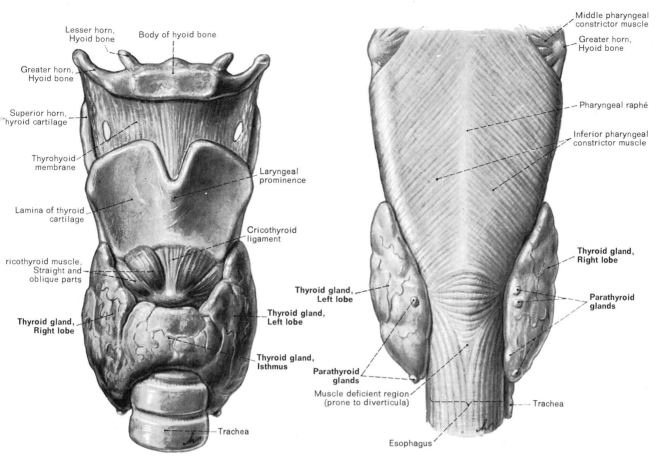

Fig. 438: Lesser horn, Hyoid bone — Body of hyoid bone — Greater horn, Hyoid bone — Superior horn, hyroid cartilage — Thyrohyoid membrane — Lamina of thyroid cartilage — Laryngeal prominence — Cricothyroid ligament — ricothyroid muscle, Straight and oblique parts — **Thyroid gland, Right lobe** — **Thyroid gland, Left lobe** — **Thyroid gland, Isthmus** — Trachea

Fig. 439: Middle pharyngeal constrictor muscle — Greater horn, Hyoid bone — Pharyngeal raphé — Inferior pharyngeal constrictor muscle — **Thyroid gland, Right lobe** — **Parathyroid glands** — **Thyroid gland, Left lobe** — **Parathyroid glands** — Muscle deficient region (prone to diverticula) — Trachea — Esophagus

Fig. 438: Ventral View of Thyroid Gland Showing Relation to Larynx and Trachea

Fig. 439: Dorsal View of Thyroid Gland Showing Relation to Pharynx and Parathyroids

Fig. 440: Cross Section of Cervical Viscera Showing Relation of Thyroid Gland to Trachea, Esophagus, Parathyroid Glands and Cervical Vessels and Nerves

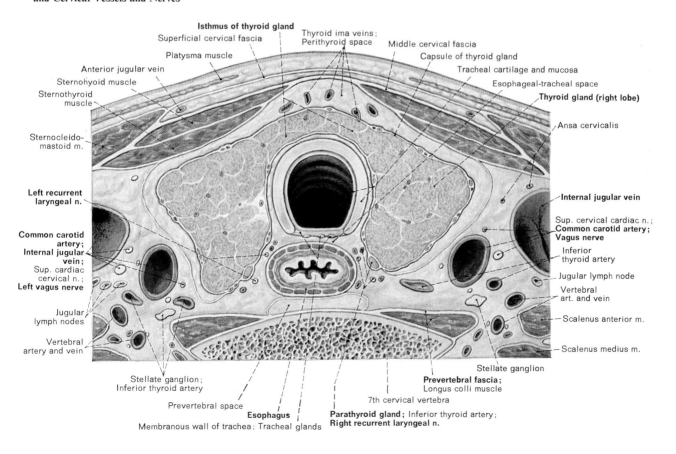

Isthmus of thyroid gland — Superficial cervical fascia — Platysma muscle — Thyroid ima veins; Perithyroid space — Middle cervical fascia — Capsule of thyroid gland — Tracheal cartilage and mucosa — Esophageal-tracheal space — **Thyroid gland (right lobe)** — Anterior jugular vein — Sternohyoid muscle — Sternothyroid muscle — Sternocleido-mastoid m. — Ansa cervicalis — **Left recurrent laryngeal n.** — **Internal jugular vein** — Sup. cervical cardiac n.; **Common carotid artery; Vagus nerve** — **Common carotid artery; Internal jugular vein; Sup. cardiac cervical n.; Left vagus nerve** — Inferior thyroid artery — Jugular lymph node — Vertebral art. and vein — Jugular lymph nodes — Vertebral artery and vein — Scalenus anterior m. — Scalenus medius m. — Stellate ganglion; Inferior thyroid artery — Stellate ganglion — **Prevertebral fascia**; Longus colli muscle — Prevertebral space — 7th cervical vertebra — **Esophagus** — **Parathyroid gland**; Inferior thyroid artery; **Right recurrent laryngeal n.** — Membranous wall of trachea; Tracheal glands

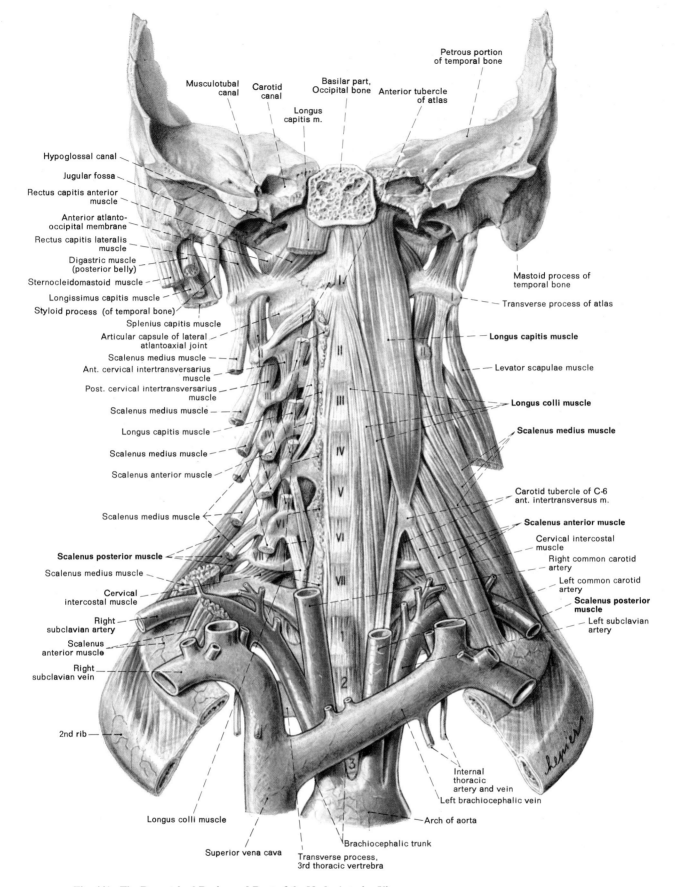

Fig. 441: The Prevertebral Region and Root of the Neck, Anterior View

NOTE: 1) on the specimen's right side, the longus capitis, longus colli and scalene muscles have been removed, exposing the transverse processes of the cervical vertebrae onto which these muscles are seen to attach.

2) the scalenus posterior muscle inserts on the 2nd rib, whereas both the scalenus anterior and medius insert onto the 1st rib. Thus, when these muscles are fixed superiorly, they would act as inspiratory muscles by elevating the first two ribs. Fixed inferiorly, they assist in bending the cervical vertebral column to one or the other side. Between the scalenus anterior and medius emerge the roots which form the trunks of the brachial plexus (see Fig. 443).

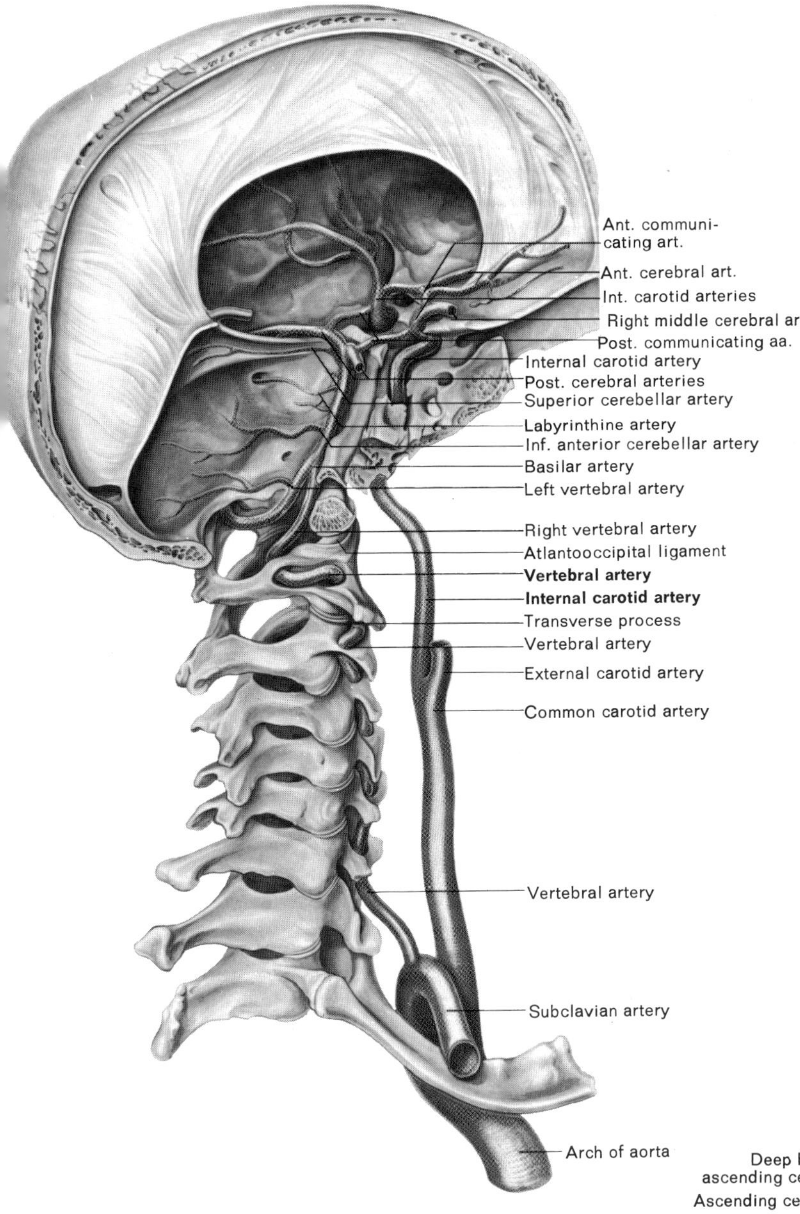

Labels (Fig. 442):
- Ant. communicating art.
- Ant. cerebral art.
- Int. carotid arteries
- Right middle cerebral art.
- Post. communicating aa.
- Internal carotid artery
- Post. cerebral arteries
- Superior cerebellar artery
- Labyrinthine artery
- Inf. anterior cerebellar artery
- Basilar artery
- Left vertebral artery
- Right vertebral artery
- Atlantooccipital ligament
- **Vertebral artery**
- **Internal carotid artery**
- Transverse process
- Vertebral artery
- External carotid artery
- Common carotid artery
- Vertebral artery
- Subclavian artery
- Arch of aorta

Fig. 442: The Vertebral and Internal Carotid Arteries

NOTE: 1) both the internal carotid and vertebral arteries ascend in the neck to enter the cranial cavity in order to supply blood to the substance of the brain. Although the vertebral arteries do give off certain spinal and muscular branches in the neck prior to entering the skull, the internal carotid arteries do not branch until they have entered the cranial cavity at the base of the brain.

2) the origin of the vertebral artery from the subclavian and its ascent in the neck through the intervertebral foramina of the transverse processes of the cervical vertebrae. The two vertebral arteries join to form the basilar artery which courses along the ventral aspect of the brainstem to supply the brainstem and cerebellum which rest on the floor of the posterior cranial fossa.

3) the internal carotid artery begins at the bifurcation of the common carotid to its entrance into the carotid canal in the petrous portion of the temporal bone. After a somewhat tortuous course, it enters the cranial cavity to supply the orbit (through its ophthalmic branch) and the cerebral hemispheres. At the base of the brain communicating vessels join with others from the basilar to form the cerebral arterial circle of Willis.

Fig. 443: The Right Subclavian Artery and its Branches

NOTE: 1) the right subclavian artery arises from the brachiocephalic trunk, although on the left it branches from the aorta. It ascends into the root of the neck, arches laterally and then descends beneath the 1st rib and clavicle to become the axillary artery.

2) the subclavian artery generally has four major branches and sometimes five. These are the vertebral artery, the thyrocervical trunk, the internal thoracic artery and the costocervical trunk. In about 40% of bodies, there is also a transverse cervical artery arising directly from the subclavian. There is considerable variability in the origin of vessels such as the suprascapular artery, the transverse cervical artery and the superficial and deep cervical branches.

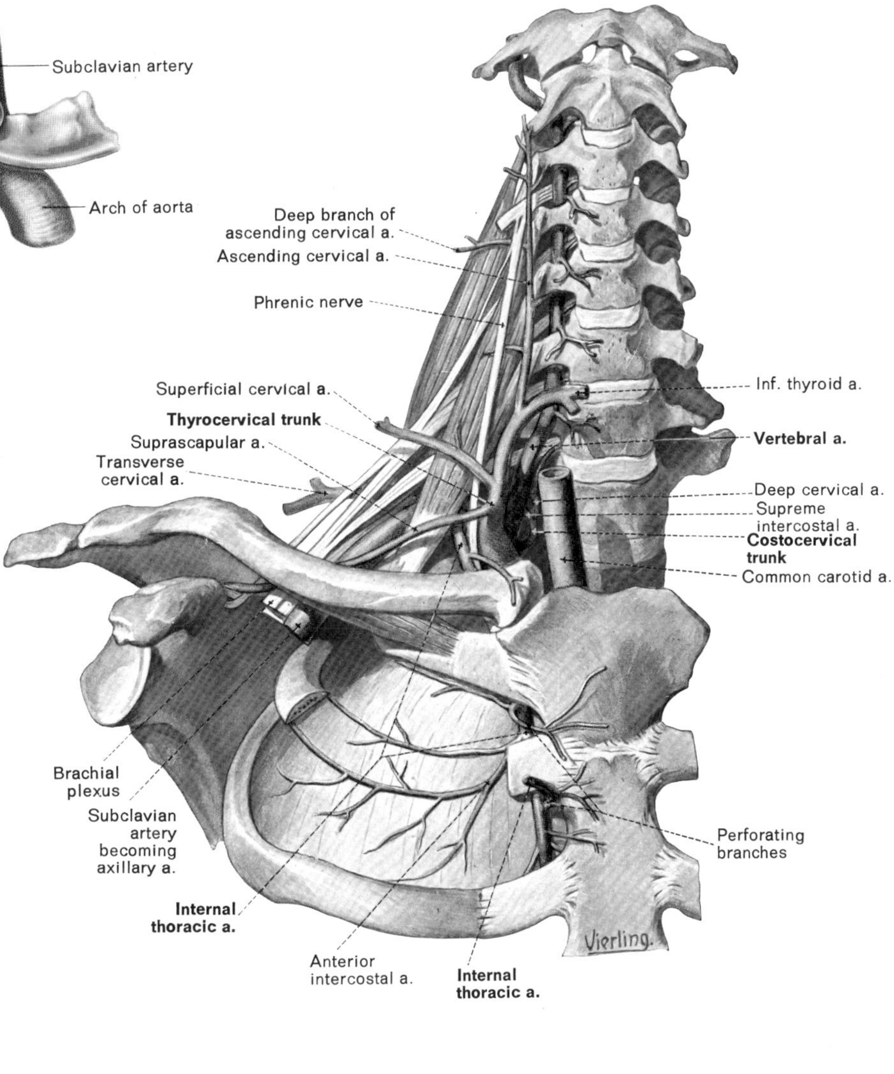

Labels (Fig. 443):
- Deep branch of ascending cervical a.
- Ascending cervical a.
- Phrenic nerve
- Superficial cervical a.
- **Thyrocervical trunk**
- Suprascapular a.
- Transverse cervical a.
- Brachial plexus
- Subclavian artery becoming axillary a.
- **Internal thoracic a.**
- Anterior intercostal a.
- **Internal thoracic a.**
- Inf. thyroid a.
- **Vertebral a.**
- Deep cervical a.
- Supreme intercostal a.
- **Costocervical trunk**
- Common carotid a.
- Perforating branches

Vierling.

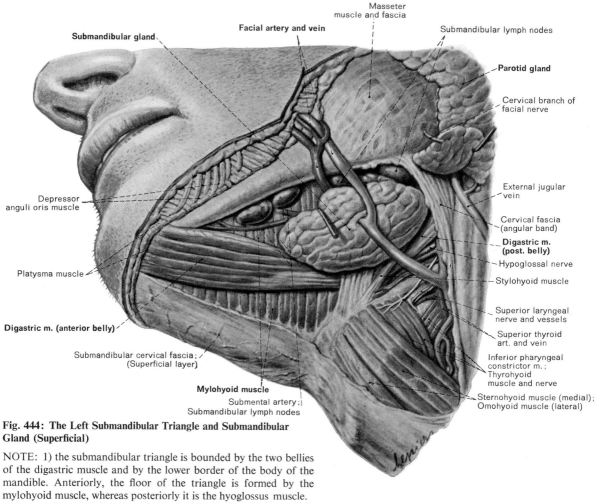

Fig. 444: The Left Submandibular Triangle and Submandibular Gland (Superficial)

NOTE: 1) the submandibular triangle is bounded by the two bellies of the digastric muscle and by the lower border of the body of the mandible. Anteriorly, the floor of the triangle is formed by the mylohyoid muscle, whereas posteriorly it is the hyoglossus muscle.

2) the submandibular gland is situated in the anterior part of the triangle. Crossing obliquely are the anterior facial vein and facial artery. Overlying the posterior part of the triangle is the inferior extension of the parotid gland. Likewise, arranged along the lower border of the body of the mandible are a number of submandibular lymph nodes.

Fig. 445: The Suprahyoid Muscles and Hyoid Bone (Viewed from Below)

Note that indicated on the mandible are the inner attachments of the mylohyoid muscle (broken line) and the anterior belly of the digastric muscle (circle). Observe the attachments of the mylohyoid, digastric and stylohyoid muscles as well as the stylohyoid ligament onto the hyoid bone.

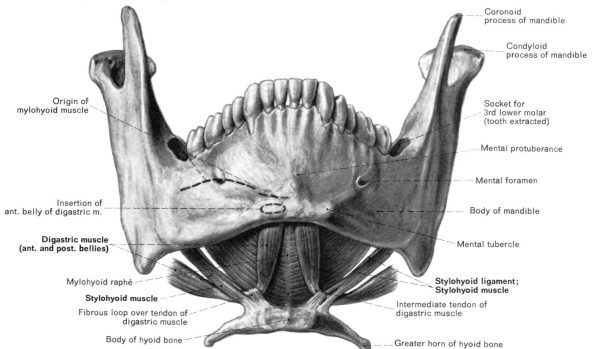

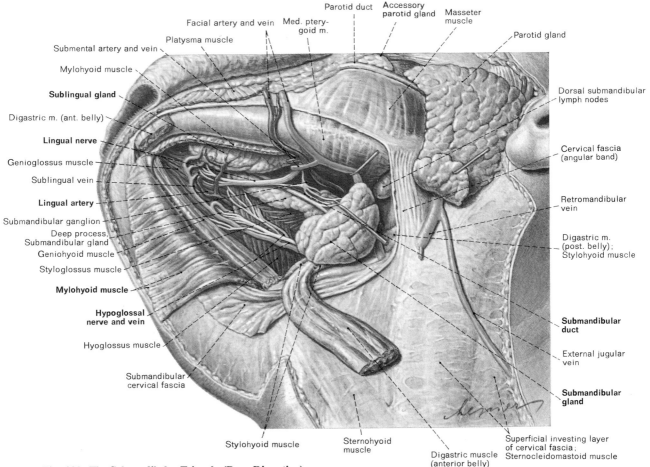

Fig. 446: The Submandibular Triangle (Deep Dissection)

NOTE: 1) the anterior belly of the digastric muscle and the mylohyoid muscle have been reflected in order to reveal the following structures: the sublingual gland, the lingual nerve, the submandibular ganglion and duct, the hypoglossal nerve and vein and the lingual artery.

2) presynaptic parasympathetic fibers (VII) accompany the lingual nerve (V) to reach the submandibular ganglion where they synapse with postganglionic neurons whose fibers innervate both the submandibular and sublingual glands.

3) the hypoglossal (XII) nerve is the motor nerve to all tongue muscles, while the lingual nerve (V) supplies the anterior 2/3rds of the tongue with general sensation.

Fig. 447: The Mylohyoid and Geniohyoid Muscles (Viewed from Above)

Note that the mylohyoid muscles along with the geniohyoid muscles form the muscular floor of the oral cavity. The mylohyoids arise along the mylohyoid lines of the mandible and insert into the median fibrous raphé which extends from the hyoid bone to the symphysis menti. Observe that the genioglossal muscles have been severed near their origin.

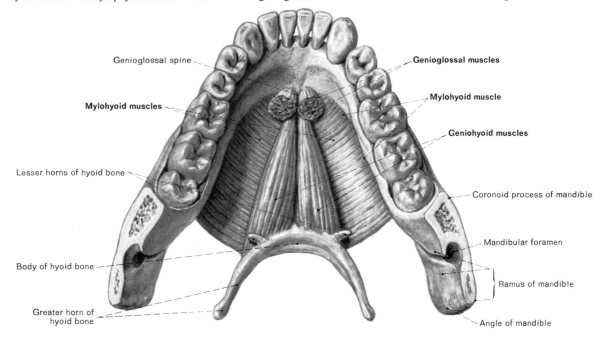

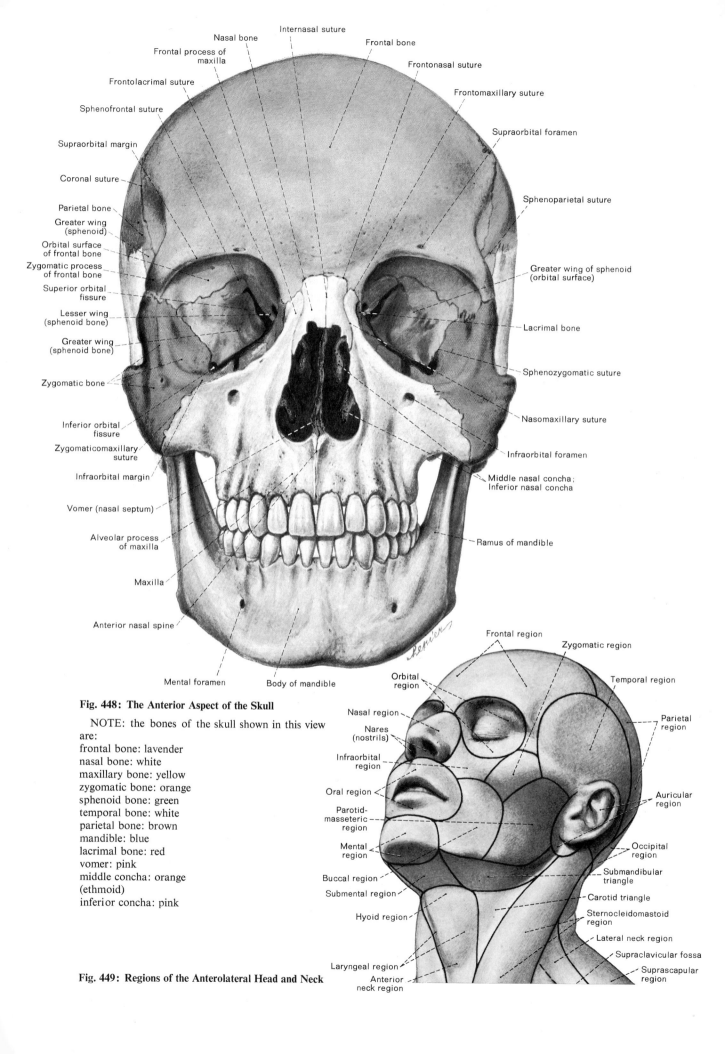

Internasal suture
Nasal bone
Frontal process of maxilla
Frontolacrimal suture
Sphenofrontal suture
Supraorbital margin
Coronal suture
Parietal bone
Greater wing (sphenoid)
Orbital surface of frontal bone
Zygomatic process of frontal bone
Superior orbital fissure
Lesser wing (sphenoid bone)
Greater wing (sphenoid bone)
Zygomatic bone
Inferior orbital fissure
Zygomaticomaxillary suture
Infraorbital margin
Vomer (nasal septum)
Alveolar process of maxilla
Maxilla
Anterior nasal spine
Mental foramen
Body of mandible

Frontal bone
Frontonasal suture
Frontomaxillary suture
Supraorbital foramen
Sphenoparietal suture
Greater wing of sphenoid (orbital surface)
Lacrimal bone
Sphenozygomatic suture
Nasomaxillary suture
Infraorbital foramen
Middle nasal concha; Inferior nasal concha
Ramus of mandible

Fig. 448: The Anterior Aspect of the Skull

NOTE: the bones of the skull shown in this view are:
frontal bone: lavender
nasal bone: white
maxillary bone: yellow
zygomatic bone: orange
sphenoid bone: green
temporal bone: white
parietal bone: brown
mandible: blue
lacrimal bone: red
vomer: pink
middle concha: orange (ethmoid)
inferior concha: pink

Frontal region
Zygomatic region
Orbital region
Temporal region
Nasal region
Parietal region
Nares (nostrils)
Infraorbital region
Oral region
Auricular region
Parotid-masseteric region
Mental region
Occipital region
Buccal region
Submandibular triangle
Submental region
Carotid triangle
Sternocleidomastoid region
Hyoid region
Lateral neck region
Supraclavicular fossa
Laryngeal region
Suprascapular region
Anterior neck region

Fig. 449: Regions of the Anterolateral Head and Neck

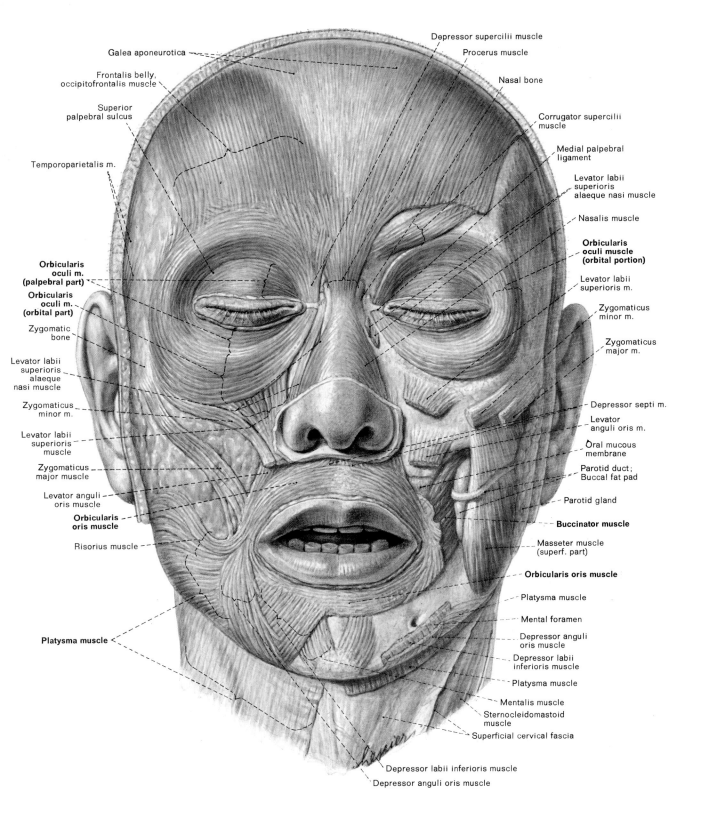

Fig. 450: The Muscles of Facial Expression (Anterior View)

NOTE: 1) the muscles of facial expression are superficial muscles located within the layers of subcutaneous fascia. Having developed from the mesoderm of the 2nd branchial arch, they are all innervated by the nerve of that arch, the seventh cranial or facial nerve.

2) the facial muscles may be grouped into: a) the muscles of the scalp, b) the muscles of external ear, c) the muscles of the eyelid, d) the nasal muscles and e) the oral muscles. Frequently, the limits of the facial muscles are not easily defined and there is a tendency for them to merge. The platysma muscle also belongs in the facial group even though it extends over the neck.

3) the circular muscles surrounding the eyes (orbicularis oculi) and the mouth (orbicularis oris) assist in closure of the orbital and oral apertures and thus contribute to functions such as blinking of the eyelids and the oral ingestion of liquids and food.

4) since facial muscles can respond to thoughts and emotions, they are of assistance in communicative functions. The buccinator muscles are flat and are situated on the lateral aspects of the oral cavity. They assist in mastication by pressing the checks against the teeth and thus prevent food from accumulating in the oral vestibule.

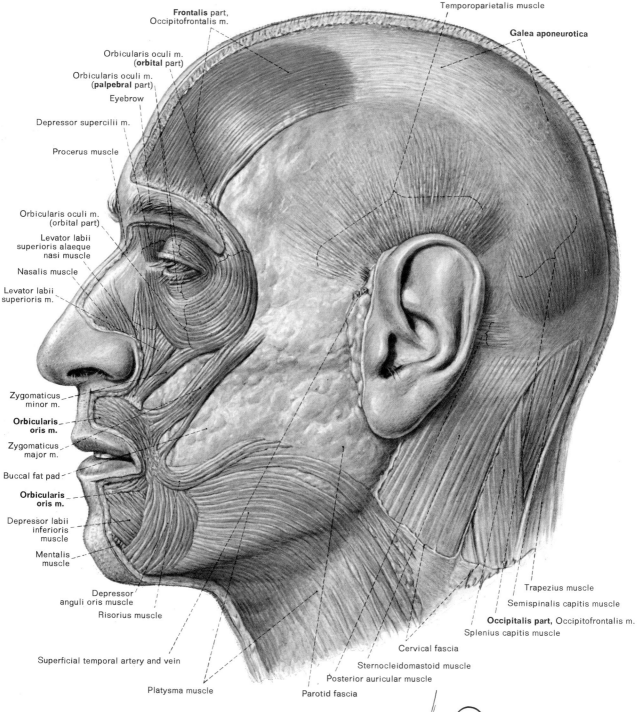

Frontalis part,
Occipitofrontalis m.

Orbicularis oculi m.
(**orbital** part)

Orbicularis oculi m.
(**palpebral** part)

Eyebrow

Depressor supercilii m.

Procerus muscle

Orbicularis oculi m.
(orbital part)

Levator labii
superioris alaeque
nasi muscle

Nasalis muscle

Levator labii
superioris m.

Zygomaticus
minor m.

**Orbicularis
oris m.**

Zygomaticus
major m.

Buccal fat pad

**Orbicularis
oris m.**

Depressor labii
inferioris
muscle

Mentalis
muscle

Depressor
anguli oris muscle

Risorius muscle

Superficial temporal artery and vein

Platysma muscle

Temporoparietalis muscle

Galea aponeurotica

Trapezius muscle

Semispinalis capitis muscle

Occipitalis part, Occipitofrontalis m.

Splenius capitis muscle

Cervical fascia

Sternocleidomastoid muscle

Posterior auricular muscle

Parotid fascia

**Fig. 451: Muscles of Facial Expression and the Superficial Posterior
Cervical Muscles**

Note that the frontalis and occipitalis portions of the occipitofrontalis muscle are continuous with an epicranial aponeurosis
called the galea aponeurotica. The orbicularis oculi consists of
orbital, palpebral and lacrimal (not shown) portions. Into the
orbicularis oris merge a number of facial muscles in a somewhat
radial manner.

**Fig. 452: Branches of the Facial Nerve Supplying the Superficial
Facial Muscles**

Note that all the muscles of facial expression are innervated by
branches of the 7th cranial nerve, the facial nerve. These branches
include the temporal, zygomatic, buccal, mandibular, cervical and
posterior auricular nerves.

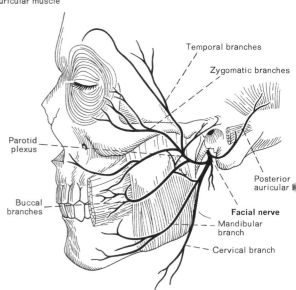

Temporal branches

Zygomatic branches

Parotid
plexus

Buccal
branches

Posterior
auricular

Facial nerve

Mandibular
branch

Cervical branch

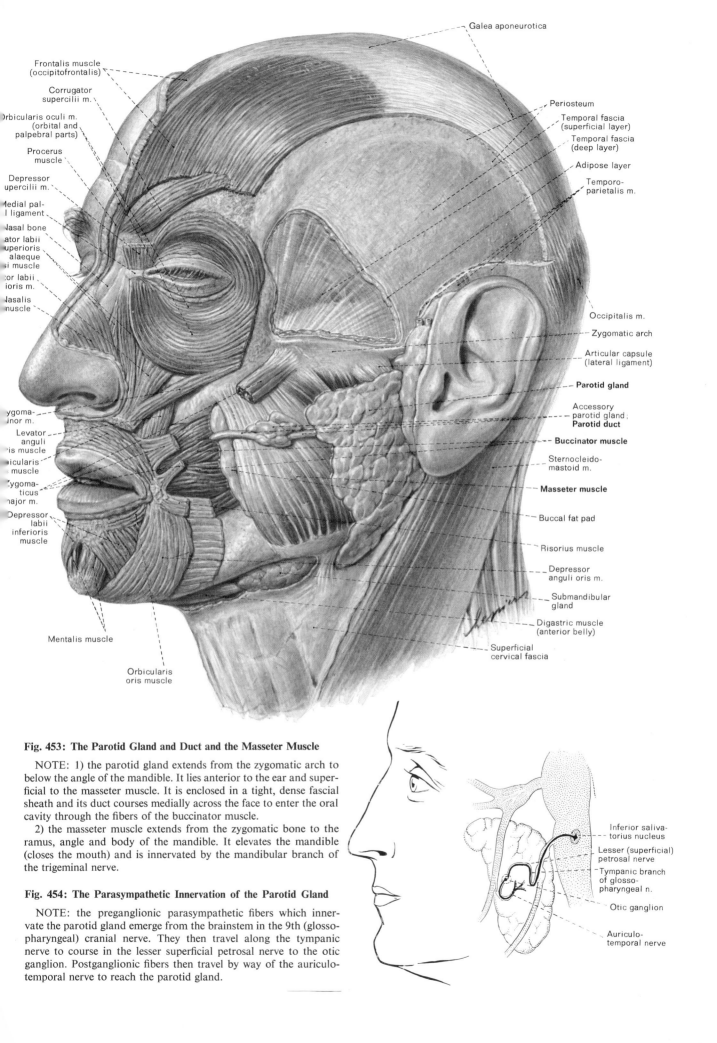

Galea aponeurotica

Frontalis muscle
(occipitofrontalis)

Corrugator
supercilii m.

Orbicularis oculi m.
(orbital and
palpebral parts)

Procerus
muscle

Depressor
supercilii m.

Medial pal-
l ligament

Nasal bone

Levator labii
superioris
alaeque
nasi muscle

Levator labii
superioris m.

Nasalis
muscle

Zygomaticus
minor m.

Levator
anguli
oris muscle

Orbicularis
oris muscle

Zygomaticus
major m.

Depressor
labii
inferioris
muscle

Mentalis muscle

Orbicularis
oris muscle

Periosteum

Temporal fascia
(superficial layer)

Temporal fascia
(deep layer)

Adipose layer

Temporo-
parietalis m.

Occipitalis m.

Zygomatic arch

Articular capsule
(lateral ligament)

Parotid gland

Accessory
parotid gland;
Parotid duct

Buccinator muscle

Sternocleido-
mastoid m.

Masseter muscle

Buccal fat pad

Risorius muscle

Depressor
anguli oris m.

Submandibular
gland

Digastric muscle
(anterior belly)

Superficial
cervical fascia

Inferior saliva-
torius nucleus

Lesser (superficial)
petrosal nerve

Tympanic branch
of glosso-
pharyngeal n.

Otic ganglion

Auriculo-
temporal nerve

Fig. 453: The Parotid Gland and Duct and the Masseter Muscle

NOTE: 1) the parotid gland extends from the zygomatic arch to
below the angle of the mandible. It lies anterior to the ear and superficial to the masseter muscle. It is enclosed in a tight, dense fascial
sheath and its duct courses medially across the face to enter the oral
cavity through the fibers of the buccinator muscle.

2) the masseter muscle extends from the zygomatic bone to the
ramus, angle and body of the mandible. It elevates the mandible
(closes the mouth) and is innervated by the mandibular branch of
the trigeminal nerve.

Fig. 454: The Parasympathetic Innervation of the Parotid Gland

NOTE: the preganglionic parasympathetic fibers which innervate the parotid gland emerge from the brainstem in the 9th (glossopharyngeal) cranial nerve. They then travel along the tympanic
nerve to course in the lesser superficial petrosal nerve to the otic
ganglion. Postganglionic fibers then travel by way of the auriculotemporal nerve to reach the parotid gland.

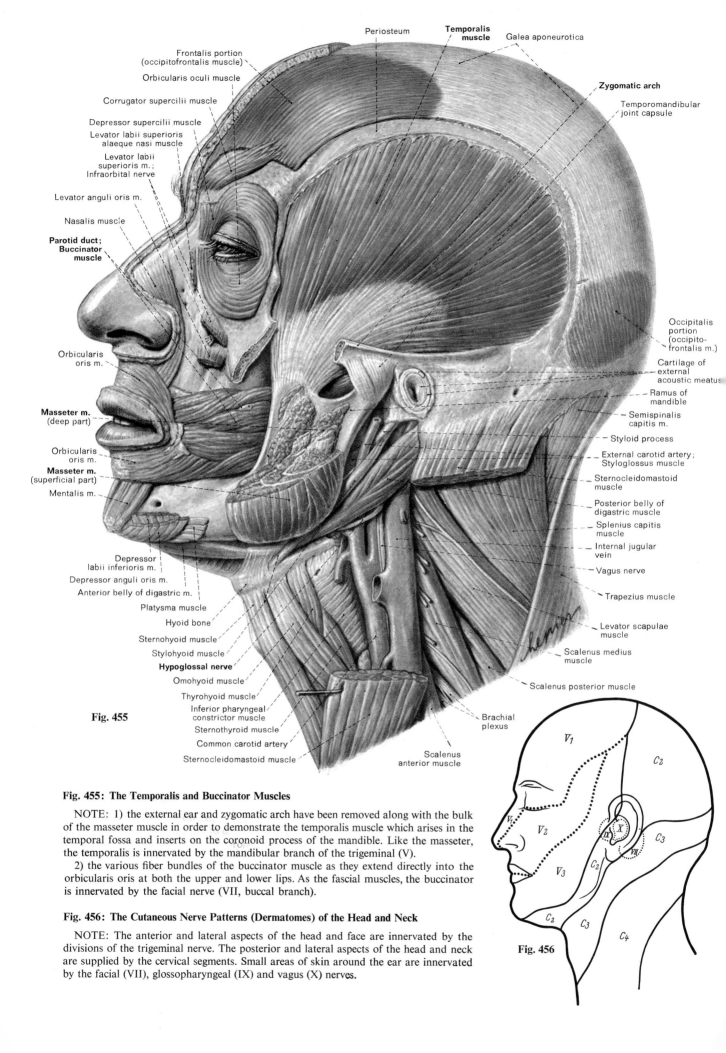

Periosteum — Temporalis muscle — Galea aponeurotica

Frontalis portion (occipitofrontalis muscle)

Orbicularis oculi muscle

Corrugator supercilii muscle

Depressor supercilii muscle

Levator labii superioris alaeque nasi muscle

Levator labii superioris m.; Infraorbital nerve

Levator anguli oris m.

Nasalis muscle

Parotid duct; Buccinator muscle

Orbicularis oris m.

Masseter m. (deep part)

Orbicularis oris m.

Masseter m. (superficial part)

Mentalis m.

Depressor labii inferioris m.

Depressor anguli oris m.

Anterior belly of digastric m.

Platysma muscle

Hyoid bone

Sternohyoid muscle

Stylohyoid muscle

Hypoglossal nerve

Omohyoid muscle

Thyrohyoid muscle

Inferior pharyngeal constrictor muscle

Sternothyroid muscle

Common carotid artery

Sternocleidomastoid muscle

Fig. 455

Zygomatic arch

Temporomandibular joint capsule

Occipitalis portion (occipito-frontalis m.)

Cartilage of external acoustic meatus

Ramus of mandible

Semispinalis capitis m.

Styloid process

External carotid artery; Styloglossus muscle

Sternocleidomastoid muscle

Posterior belly of digastric muscle

Splenius capitis muscle

Internal jugular vein

Vagus nerve

Trapezius muscle

Levator scapulae muscle

Scalenus medius muscle

Scalenus posterior muscle

Brachial plexus

Scalenus anterior muscle

Fig. 455: The Temporalis and Buccinator Muscles

NOTE: 1) the external ear and zygomatic arch have been removed along with the bulk of the masseter muscle in order to demonstrate the temporalis muscle which arises in the temporal fossa and inserts on the coronoid process of the mandible. Like the masseter, the temporalis is innervated by the mandibular branch of the trigeminal (V).

2) the various fiber bundles of the buccinator muscle as they extend directly into the orbicularis oris at both the upper and lower lips. As the fascial muscles, the buccinator is innervated by the facial nerve (VII, buccal branch).

Fig. 456: The Cutaneous Nerve Patterns (Dermatomes) of the Head and Neck

NOTE: The anterior and lateral aspects of the head and face are innervated by the divisions of the trigeminal nerve. The posterior and lateral aspects of the head and neck are supplied by the cervical segments. Small areas of skin around the ear are innervated by the facial (VII), glossopharyngeal (IX) and vagus (X) nerves.

Fig. 456

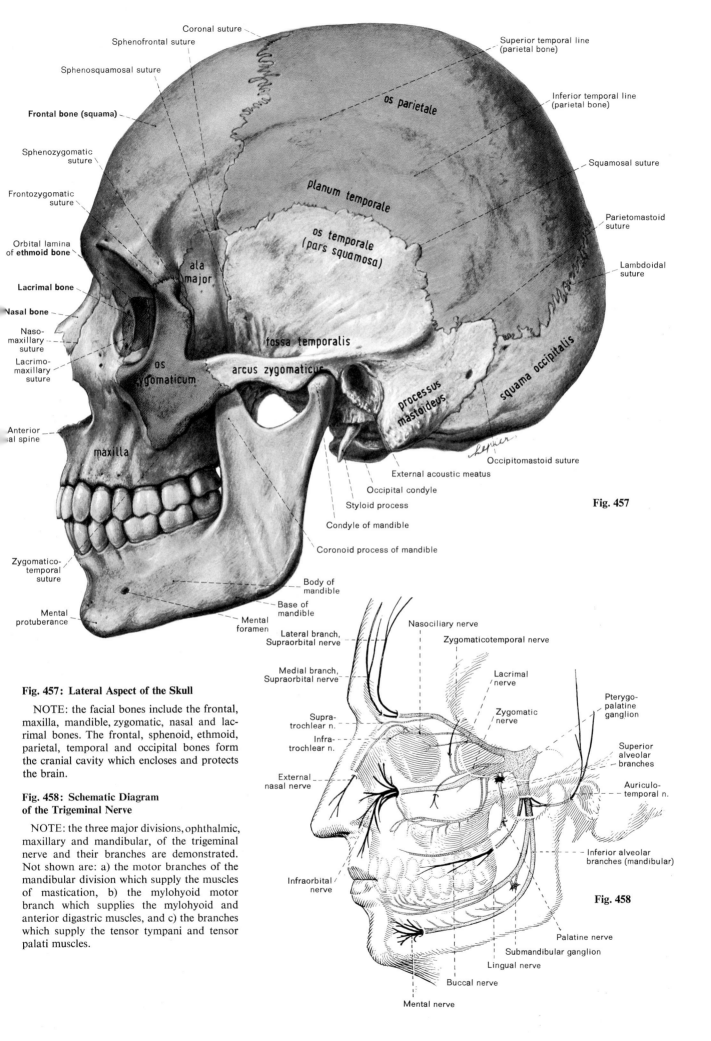

Fig. 457: Lateral Aspect of the Skull

NOTE: the facial bones include the frontal, maxilla, mandible, zygomatic, nasal and lacrimal bones. The frontal, sphenoid, ethmoid, parietal, temporal and occipital bones form the cranial cavity which encloses and protects the brain.

Fig. 458: Schematic Diagram of the Trigeminal Nerve

NOTE: the three major divisions, ophthalmic, maxillary and mandibular, of the trigeminal nerve and their branches are demonstrated. Not shown are: a) the motor branches of the mandibular division which supply the muscles of mastication, b) the mylohyoid motor branch which supplies the mylohyoid and anterior digastric muscles, and c) the branches which supply the tensor tympani and tensor palati muscles.

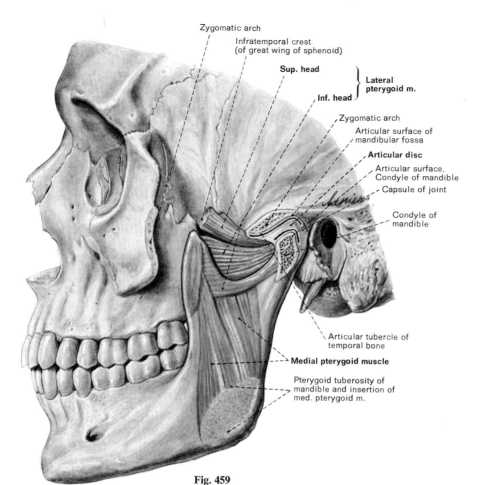

Zygomatic arch

Infratemporal crest
(of great wing of sphenoid)

Sup. head

} **Lateral
pterygoid m.**

Inf. head

Zygomatic arch

Articular surface of
mandibular fossa

Articular disc

Articular surface,
Condyle of mandible

Capsule of joint

Condyle of
mandible

Articular tubercle of
temporal bone

Medial pterygoid muscle

Pterygoid tuberosity of
mandible and insertion of
med. pterygoid m.

Fig. 459

Fig. 459: The Medial and Lateral Pterygoid Muscles (Lateral View)

NOTE: 1) the left zygomatic arch has been removed. Posteriorly, the bone has been cut through the temporomandibular joint revealing the articular disc. The location of the medial pterygoid muscle and part of the lateral pterygoid muscle on the inner aspect of the ramus of the mandible is represented as though the bone were transparent.

2) the lateral pterygoid muscle arises by two heads, a superior from the great wing of the sphenoid bone and an inferior from the lateral surface of the lateral pterygoid plate of the sphenoid. The two heads insert posteriorly on the neck of the condyle of the mandible. The lateral pterygoid muscle opens and protracts the mandible and also moves it from side to side.

3) the medial pterygoid muscle arises from the medial surface of the lateral pterygoid plate of the sphenoid as well as from the palatine bone and inserts on the medial surface of the ramus and angle of the mandible. It assists the masseter and temporalis in closing the jaw.

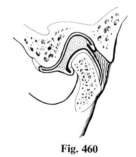

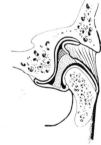

Fig. 460   **Fig. 461**

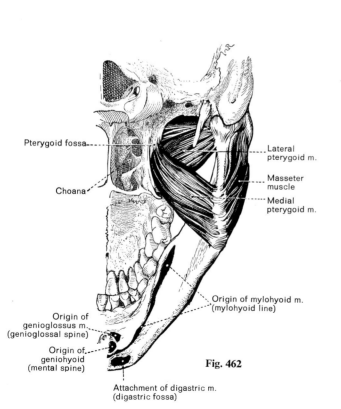

Pterygoid fossa

Choana

Lateral
pterygoid m.

Masseter
muscle

Medial
pterygoid m.

Origin of mylohyoid m.
(mylohyoid line)

Origin of
genioglossus m.
(genioglossal spine)

Origin of
geniohyoid
(mental spine)

Attachment of digastric m.
(digastric fossa)

Fig. 462

Figs. 460 and 461: Sagittal Sections of Temporomandibular Joint

NOTE: 1) the articular disc (stippled structure) is an oval plate interposed between the mandibular fossa of the temporal bone and the condyle of the mandible. Thus, there exists a joint cavity between the disc and the mandibular fossa and another between the disc and the condyle.

2) with the jaw closed (460), the head of the condyle of the mandible and the articular disc lie totally within the mandibular fossa. When the jaw is opened (461), the condyle turns in a hinge-fashion on the disc and both bone and disc glide forward within the joint capsule to lie opposite the articular tubercle of the temporal bone.

Fig. 462: The Pterygoid Muscles as seen from Below

NOTE: 1) the insertion of the medial pterygoid muscle on the medial aspect of the mandible forms a sling with the masseter muscle which inserts on the outer aspect of the jaw. Observe that the lateral pterygoid courses principally in the horizontal plane.

2) the sites of attachment of four muscles on the mandible observable from this inferior view, the mylohyoid, anterior belly of the digastric, geniohyoid and genioglossus.

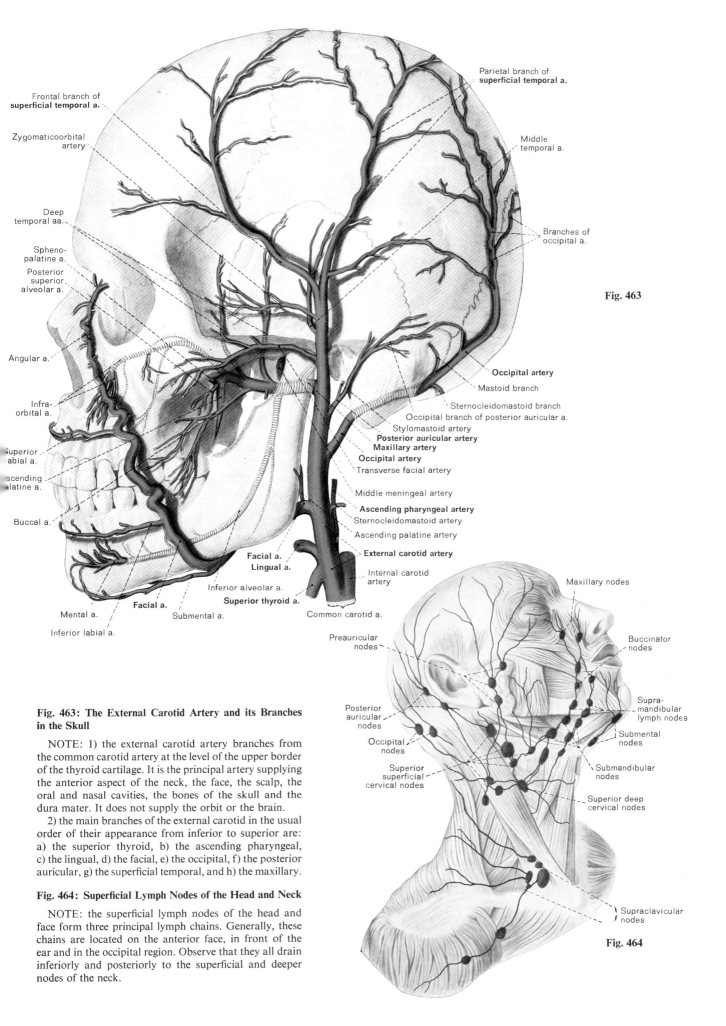

Fig. 463

Frontal branch of **superficial temporal a.**

Zygomaticoorbital artery

Deep temporal aa.

Spheno-palatine a.

Posterior superior alveolar a.

Angular a.

Infra-orbital a.

Superior labial a.

Ascending palatine a.

Buccal a.

Mental a.

Inferior labial a.

Facial a.

Submental a.

Facial a.
Lingual a.

Inferior alveolar a.

Superior thyroid a.

Common carotid a.

Internal carotid artery

External carotid artery

Ascending palatine artery

Sternocleidomastoid artery

Ascending pharyngeal artery

Middle meningeal artery

Transverse facial artery

Occipital artery

Maxillary artery

Posterior auricular artery

Stylomastoid artery

Occipital branch of posterior auricular a.

Sternocleidomastoid branch

Mastoid branch

Occipital artery

Branches of occipital a.

Middle temporal a.

Parietal branch of **superficial temporal a.**

Maxillary nodes

Buccinator nodes

Supra-mandibular lymph nodes

Submental nodes

Submandibular nodes

Superior deep cervical nodes

Supraclavicular nodes

Superior superficial cervical nodes

Occipital nodes

Posterior auricular nodes

Preauricular nodes

Fig. 464

Fig. 463: The External Carotid Artery and its Branches in the Skull

NOTE: 1) the external carotid artery branches from the common carotid artery at the level of the upper border of the thyroid cartilage. It is the principal artery supplying the anterior aspect of the neck, the face, the scalp, the oral and nasal cavities, the bones of the skull and the dura mater. It does not supply the orbit or the brain.

2) the main branches of the external carotid in the usual order of their appearance from inferior to superior are: a) the superior thyroid, b) the ascending pharyngeal, c) the lingual, d) the facial, e) the occipital, f) the posterior auricular, g) the superficial temporal, and h) the maxillary.

Fig. 464: Superficial Lymph Nodes of the Head and Neck

NOTE: the superficial lymph nodes of the head and face form three principal lymph chains. Generally, these chains are located on the anterior face, in front of the ear and in the occipital region. Observe that they all drain inferiorly and posteriorly to the superficial and deeper nodes of the neck.

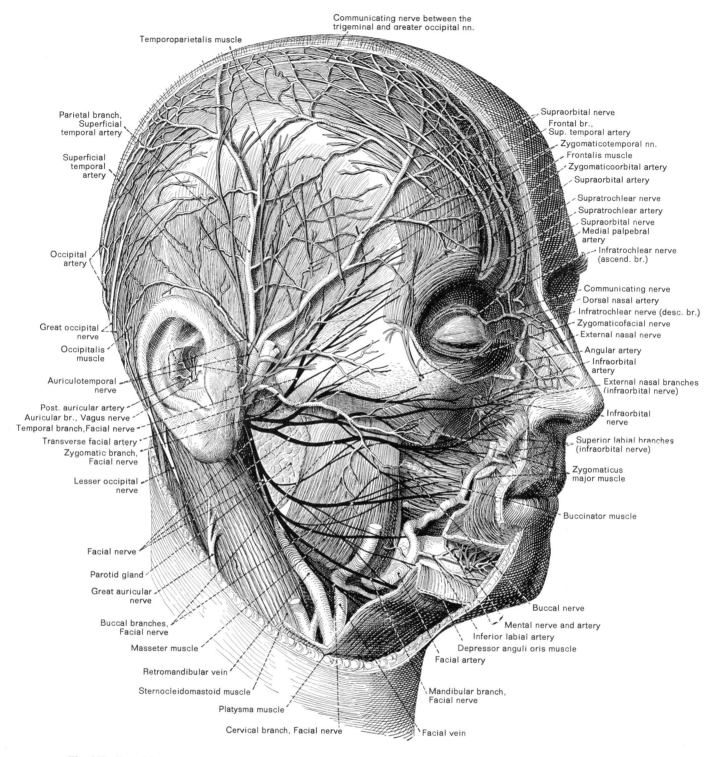

Fig. 465: Superficial Nerves and Vessels of the Face and Head

NOTE: 1) a portion of the parotid gland has been removed in order to reveal the branches of the facial nerve (black) which emerge from within the substance of the gland to supply the superficial muscles of facial expression. Identify the temporal, zygomatic, buccal, mandibular, and cervical branches. The posterior auricular branch is not shown.

2) the superficial branches of the trigeminal nerve are indicated in various colors: ophthalmic (yellow), maxillary (blue) and mandibular (green). The trigeminal nerve serves as the cutaneous nerve of the anterior and lateral face, but is also the motor nerve to the muscles of mastication. The cervical sensory nerves (white, not colored) supply the occipital region and much of the ear and neck.

3) the general distribution of the superficial temporal artery and its branches, the zygomaticoorbital and transverse facial arteries. Follow the course of the facial artery across the face to become the angular artery. Among other structures, the facial artery supplies the chin and the upper and lower lips and anastomoses with vessels emerging from the orbit.

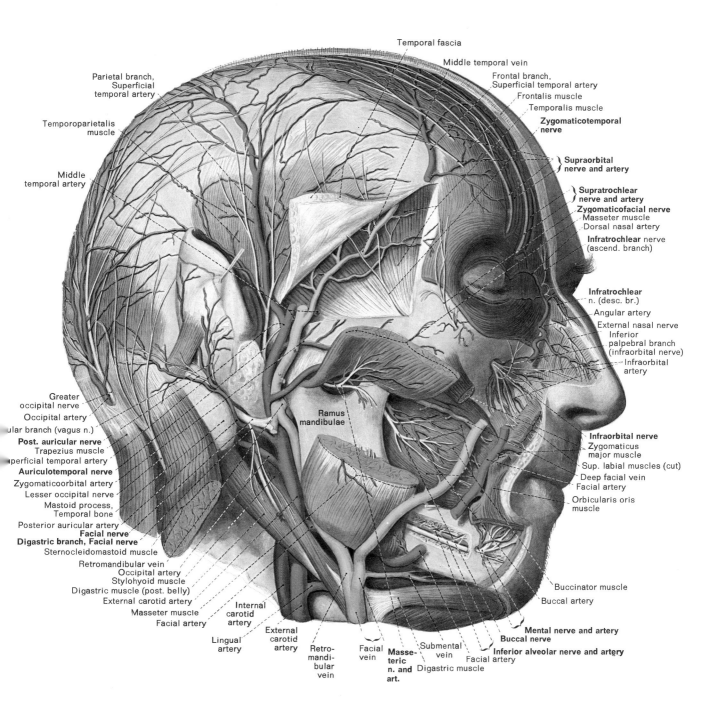

Fig. 466: Nerves and Vessels of the Superficial Head and Deeper Face

NOTE: 1) in this dissection, the temporal fascia has been cut and partially reflected. The superficial muscles on the side of the face have been removed along with the parotid gland. The main trunk of the facial nerve has been cut and its branches across the face removed. The masseter muscle has been severed and its upper half reflected upward.

2) a) the supraorbital, supratrochlear, infratrochlear and external nasal branches of the ophthalmic division of the trigeminal nerve.

b) zygomaticotemporal, zygomaticofacial and infraorbital branches of the maxillary division of the trigeminal nerve.

c) auriculotemporal, masseteric, buccal, inferior alveolar and mental branches of the mandibular division of the trigeminal nerve.

3) the posterior auricular, digastric and stylohyoid branches of the facial nerve which arise from the main nerve trunk prior to its division within the parotid gland.

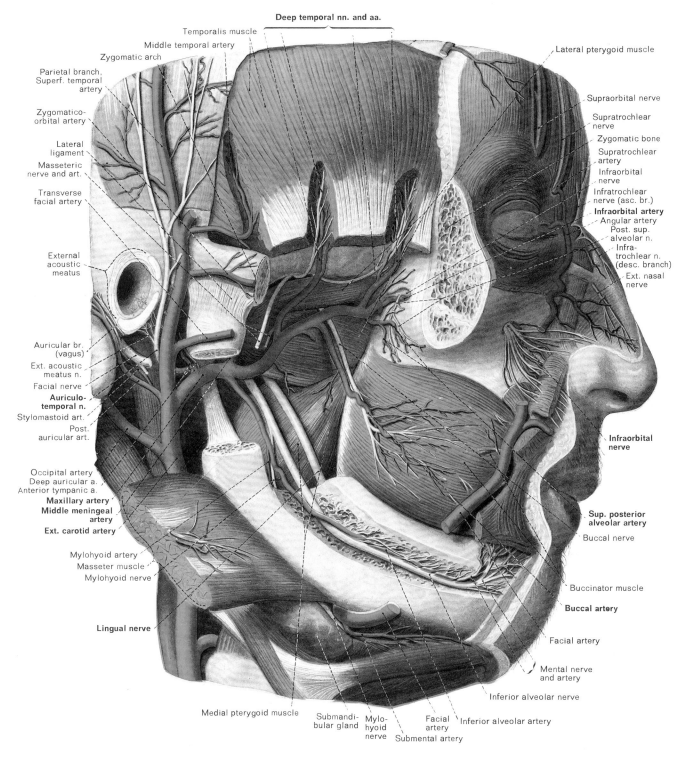

Fig. 467: The Infratemporal Region and the Maxillary Artery

NOTE: 1) the zygomatic arch and a portion of the ramus of the mandible have been removed and the temporalis and masseter muscles have been cut and partially reflected. The pterygoid venous plexus has been removed revealing the maxillary artery and its branches.

2) the infratemporal fossa lies deep to the zygomatic arch and posterior to the maxilla. It contains the medial and lateral pterygoid muscles, the inferior part of the temporalis muscle, the maxillary artery, the pterygoid plexus of veins (not shown) and the mandibular division of the trigeminal nerve.

3) the maxillary artery and a number of its branches. Seen in this dissection are the following branches of the maxillary artery: a) deep auricular, b) anterior tympanic, c) inferior alveolar, d) middle meningeal, e) masseteric (cut), f) deep temporal, g) pterygoid (not labelled), h) buccal, i) posterior superior alveolar, j) infraorbital. Branches of the maxillary artery not seen from this view are the greater palatine, the artery of the pterygoid canal, pharyngeal and the sphenopalatine.

4) the auriculotemporal, lingual, inferior alveolar, mylohyoid, masseteric and deep temporal branches of the mandibular division of the trigeminal nerve. Observe the course of the inferior alveolar nerve, accompanied by the inferior alveolar artery within the mandible.

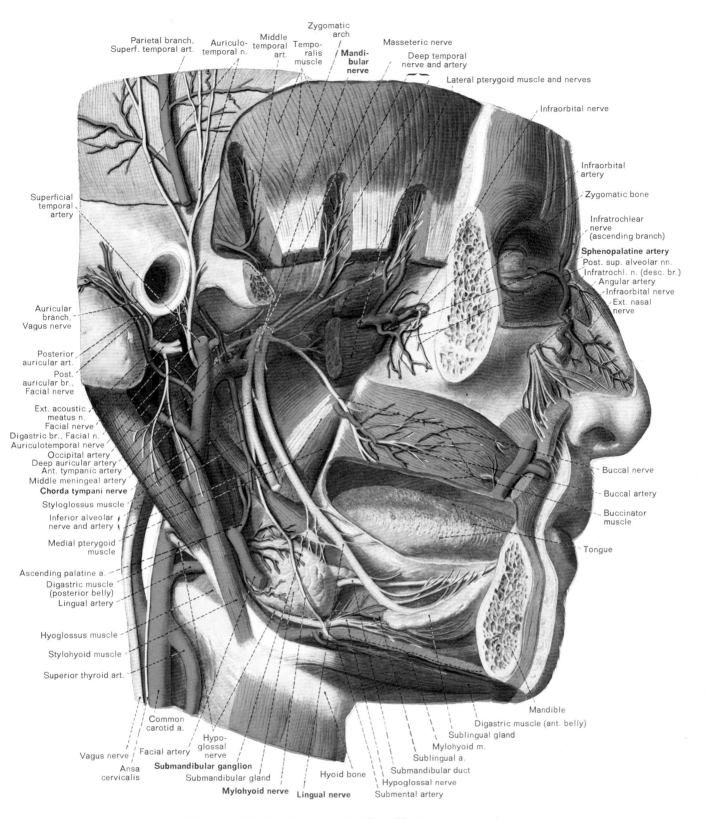

Fig. 468: The Infratemporal Region and the Branches of the Mandibular Nerve

NOTE: 1) this dissection of the deep face has removed the zygomatic arch, much of the right mandible and the lateral pterygoid muscle. A portion of the maxillary artery has been cut away along with the distal part of the inferior alveolar nerve beyond the point where the mylohyoid nerve branches.

2) the lingual nerve as it courses to the tongue. High in the infratemporal fossa, the chorda tympani nerve (which is a branch of the facial) joins the lingual. The chorda tympani not only carries special sensory fibers for taste for the anterior two-thirds of the tongue, but additionally carries the preganglionic parasympathetic fibers from the facial nerve to the submandibular ganglion.

3) the distal portion of the maxillary artery as it courses toward the sphenopalatine foramen. After giving off the infraorbital artery, the vessel passes through the foramen and enters the nasal cavity as the sphenopalatine artery, becoming the principal vessel supplying the mucosa overlying the conchae.

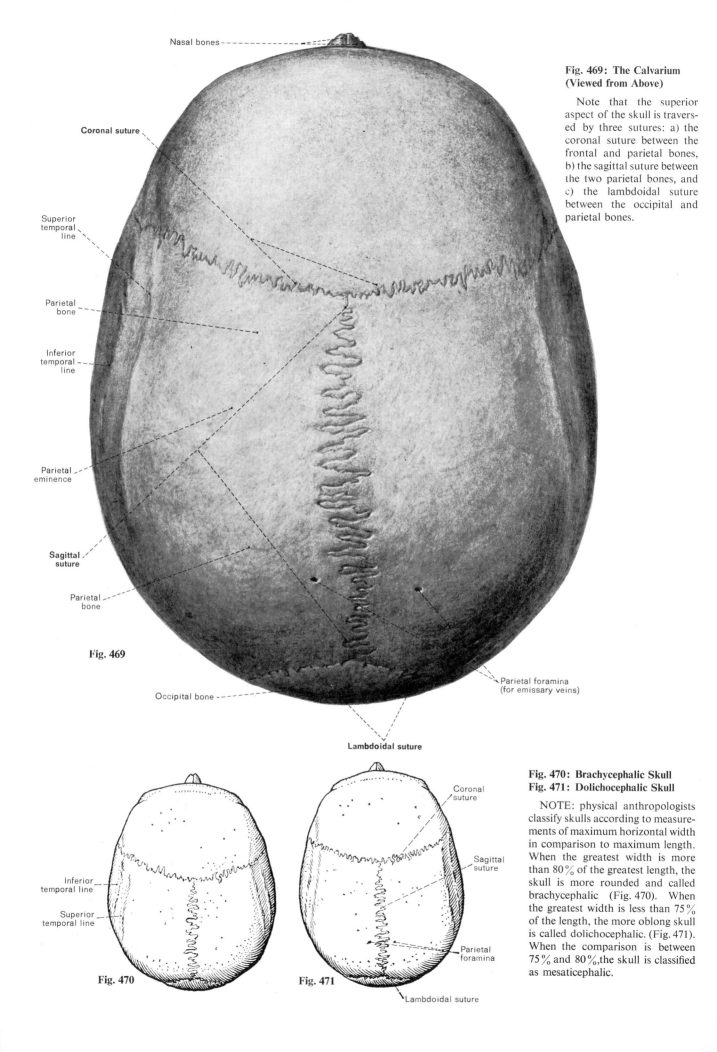

Nasal bones

Coronal suture

Superior temporal line

Parietal bone

Inferior temporal line

Parietal eminence

Sagittal suture

Parietal bone

Fig. 469

Occipital bone

Parietal foramina (for emissary veins)

Lambdoidal suture

Fig. 469: The Calvarium (Viewed from Above)

Note that the superior aspect of the skull is traversed by three sutures: a) the coronal suture between the frontal and parietal bones, b) the sagittal suture between the two parietal bones, and c) the lambdoidal suture between the occipital and parietal bones.

Coronal suture

Sagittal suture

Parietal foramina

Inferior temporal line

Superior temporal line

Fig. 470

Fig. 471

Lambdoidal suture

Fig. 470: Brachycephalic Skull
Fig. 471: Dolichocephalic Skull

NOTE: physical anthropologists classify skulls according to measurements of maximum horizontal width in comparison to maximum length. When the greatest width is more than 80% of the greatest length, the skull is more rounded and called brachycephalic (Fig. 470). When the greatest width is less than 75% of the length, the more oblong skull is called dolichocephalic. (Fig. 471). When the comparison is between 75% and 80%, the skull is classified as mesaticephalic.

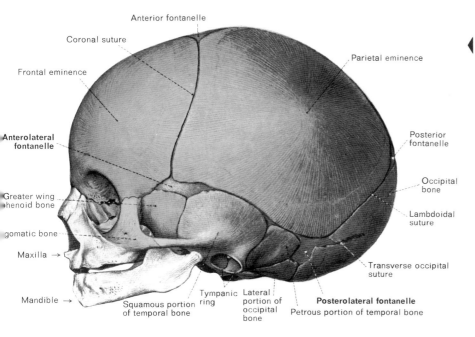

Anterior fontanelle
Coronal suture
Frontal eminence
Anterolateral fontanelle
Greater wing sphenoid bone
gomatic bone
Maxilla →
Mandible →
Squamous portion of temporal bone
Tympanic ring
Lateral portion of occipital bone
Parietal eminence
Posterior fontanelle
Occipital bone
Lambdoidal suture
Transverse occipital suture
Posterolateral fontanelle
Petrous portion of temporal bone

Fig. 472: The Skull at Birth (Lateral View)

NOTE: 1) ossification of the maturing flat bones of the skull is accomplished by the intramembranous process of bone formation. At birth this process is incomplete, thereby leaving softened membranous sites between the growing bones.

2) the nature of the skull just prior to birth is of some benefit, however, since the mobility of the bones permits some changes in its shape as might be required during the birth process.

3) the soft sites on the skull of the newborn infant are called fontanelles. From this lateral view can be seen at least two such fontanelles, the antero-lateral (or sphenoid) which is at the pterion, and the posterolateral (or mastoid) at the asterion.

Fig. 473: The Skull at Birth (Seen from Above)

NOTE: 1) the largest of the fontanelles at birth is the anterior fontanelle located at the bregma and interconnecting the frontal and parietal bones. It is approximately diamond-shaped and is situated at the junction of the coronal and sagittal sutures.

2) following the sagittal suture to its junction with the occipital bone will locate the posterior fontanelle (at the lambda). This is generally triangular in shape and is relatively small at birth.

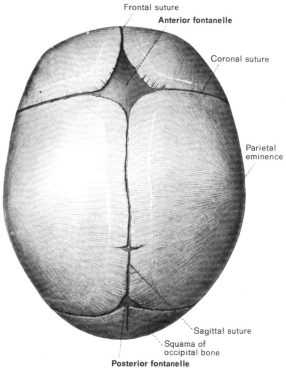

Frontal suture
Anterior fontanelle
Coronal suture
Parietal eminence
Sagittal suture
Squama of occipital bone
Posterior fontanelle

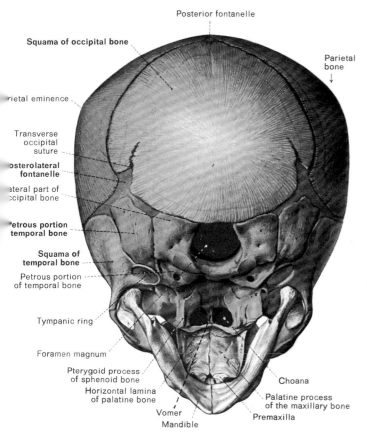

Posterior fontanelle
Squama of occipital bone
Parietal bone ↓
rietal eminence
Transverse occipital suture
osterolateral fontanelle
ateral part of ccipital bone
Petrous portion temporal bone
Squama of temporal bone
Petrous portion of temporal bone
Tympanic ring
Foramen magnum
Pterygoid process of sphenoid bone
Horizontal lamina of palatine bone
Vomer
Mandible
Choana
Palatine process of the maxillary bone
Premaxilla

Fig. 474: The Skull at Birth (Posterior-Inferior View)

NOTE: 1) the separate ossification of the petrous and squamous portions of the temporal bone as well as the basilar and squamous portions of the occipital bone. The posterolateral fontanelles are found at the articulation of the occipital, temporal and parietal bones.

2) the skull is large at birth in comparison to the size of the rest of the body, however, the facial bones (see Fig. 472) are still rudimentary and not well developed. The teeth have yet to erupt, and the sinuses and nasal cavity are small.

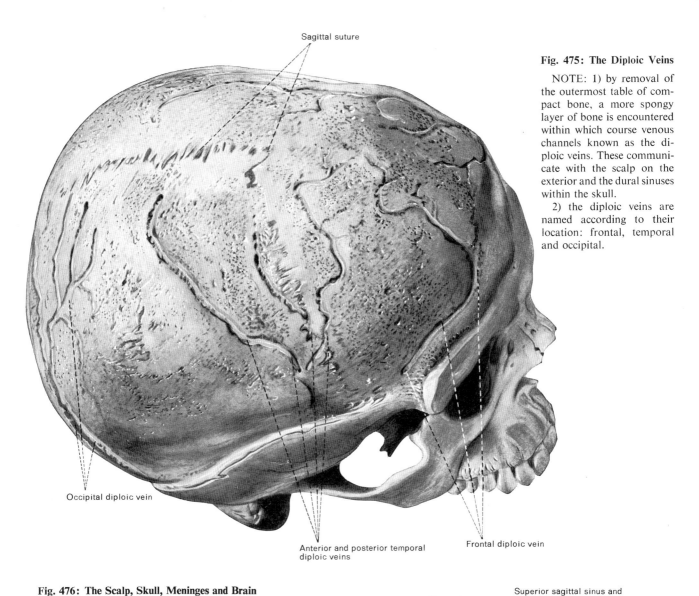

Sagittal suture

NOTE: 1) by removal of the outermost table of compact bone, a more spongy layer of bone is encountered within which course venous channels known as the diploic veins. These communicate with the scalp on the exterior and the dural sinuses within the skull.

2) the diploic veins are named according to their location: frontal, temporal and occipital.

Occipital diploic vein

Anterior and posterior temporal diploic veins

Frontal diploic vein

Fig. 476: The Scalp, Skull, Meninges and Brain

NOTE: 1) this frontal section through the cranium and upper cerebrum depicts the bony and soft coverings of the brain. The veins and dural sinuses are shown in blue. The layers of the scalp and the bony tissue of the skull lie superficial to the dura mater, arachnoid and pia mater coverings of the neural tissue of the brain.

2) the arachnoid granulations which project into the dural sinuses. These tufts of arachnoid lie next to the endothelium of the sinuses and allow the passage of cerebrospinal fluid from the subarachnoid space into the venous system.

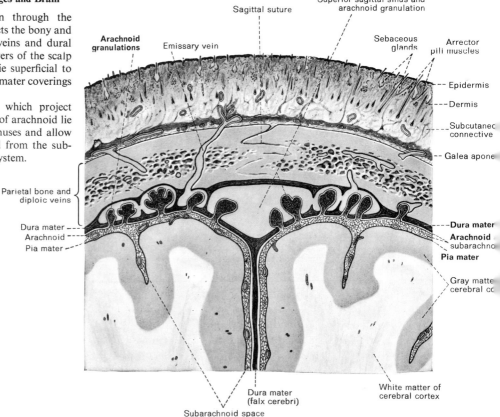

Arachnoid granulations

Emissary vein

Sagittal suture

Superior sagittal sinus and arachnoid granulation

Sebaceous glands

Arrector pili muscles

Epidermis

Dermis

Subcutaneo connective

Galea apone

Parietal bone and diploic veins

Dura mater
Arachnoid
Pia mater

Dura mater

Arachnoid subarachno

Pia mater

Gray matte cerebral co

Dura mater (falx cerebri)

Subarachnoid space

White matter of cerebral cortex

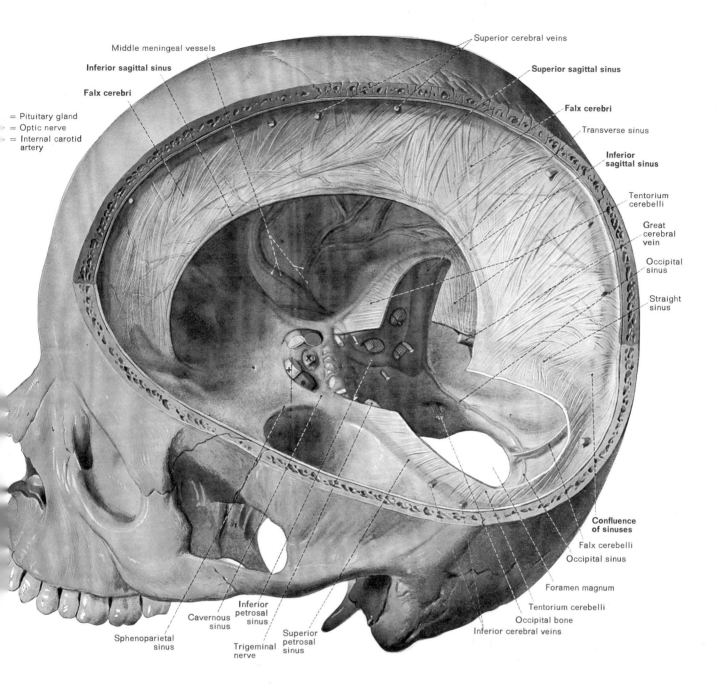

Middle meningeal vessels

Inferior sagittal sinus

Falx cerebri

= Pituitary gland
= Optic nerve
= Internal carotid
  artery

Superior cerebral veins

Superior sagittal sinus

Falx cerebri

Transverse sinus

Inferior sagittal sinus

Tentorium cerebelli

Great cerebral vein

Occipital sinus

Straight sinus

Confluence of sinuses

Falx cerebelli

Occipital sinus

Foramen magnum

Tentorium cerebelli

Occipital bone

Inferior cerebral veins

Superior petrosal sinus

Trigeminal nerve

Inferior petrosal sinus

Cavernous sinus

Sphenoparietal sinus

Fig. 477: The Intracranial Dura Mater and the Dural Sinuses

NOTE: 1) with the left skull opened and the brain removed, the reflections of the dura mater and its venous sinuses are exposed. The sinuses are colored blue while the arteries are red. Most of the left tentorium cerebelli and a portion of the right were cut away to open the posterior cranial fossa.

2) the five *unpaired* dural sinuses: the superior sagittal sinus, the inferior sagittal sinus, the straight sinus. Two other unpaired sinuses (not labelled) at the base of the skull include the intercavernous sinus and the basilar sinus. These can be seen in Figure 478.

3) the seven *paired* dural sinuses: transverse sinus, sigmoid sinus, occipital sinus, superior petrosal sinus, inferior petrosal sinus, cavernous sinus and sphenoparietal sinus. The dural sinuses consist of spaces between the two layers of dura mater which drain the cerebral blood, returning it to the internal jugular veins.

4) the sickle-shaped falx cerebri. This double layer midline reflection of dura mater extends from the crista galli anteriorly to the tentorium cerebelli posteriorly. It also extends vertically between the two cerebral hemispheres. Within the layers of the falx, observe the superior and inferior sagittal sinuses and the straight sinus which meet at the confluence of sinuses.

5) the tentorium cerebelli is a tent-like reflection of dura mater which forms a partition separating the occipital lobes of the cerebral cortex and the surface of the cerebellum. The falx cerebelli extends vertically between the two cerebellar hemispheres.

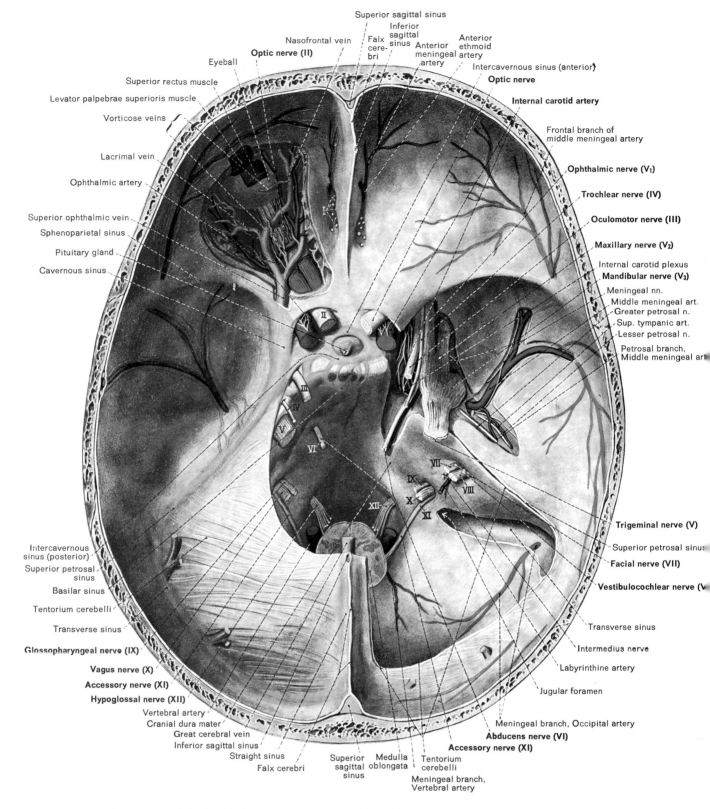

Fig. 478: The Base of the Cranial Cavity: Vessels, Nerves and Dura Mater

NOTE: 1) the base of the cranial cavity displays anterior, middle and posterior cranial fossae. The anterior fossa sustains the frontal lobes while the temporal lobes of the brain rest in the middle fossa. Posteriorly, the brain stem and the overlying cerebellum rest in the posterior fossa.

2) the dura mater and the orbital plate of the left frontal bone have been chipped away to expose the structures in the left orbit. The superior ophthalmic vein drains posteriorly and the optic nerve is seen to course from the orbit through the optic canal. Caudal to the optic foramina, observe the pituitary gland within the sella turcica.

3) the medial aspect of the middle cranial fossa shows the internal carotid artery, the 3rd, 4th, 5th and 6th cranial nerves coursing anteriorly or inferiorly toward the orbit or face and the middle meningeal artery traversing the foramen spinosum.

4) the posterior cranial fossa is marked by foramina for the last six pairs of cranial nerves. The 7th and 8th nerves pass through the internal auditory meatus while the 9th, 10th and 11th nerves emerge through the jugular foramen. The 12th nerve courses through the condyloid canal in the occipital bone.

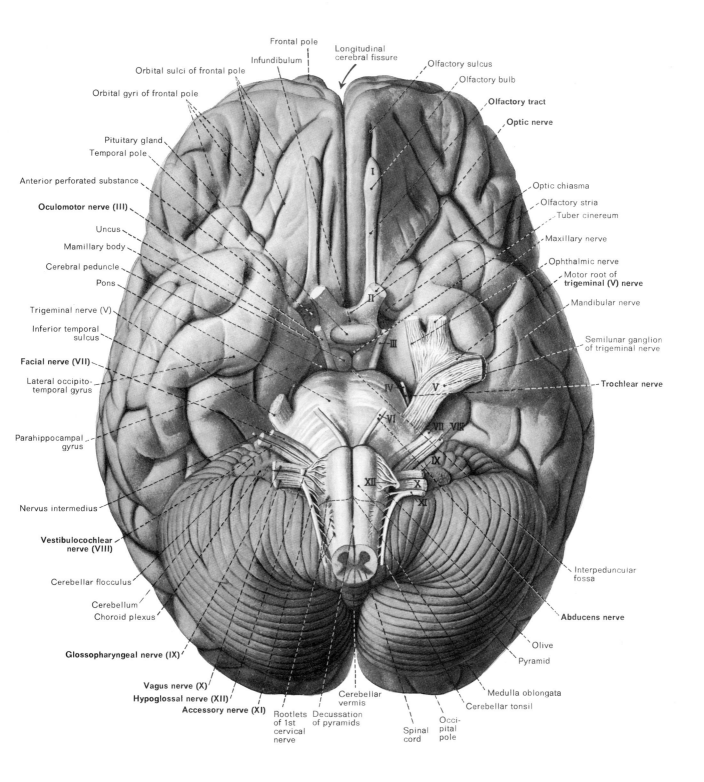

Frontal pole
Infundibulum
Longitudinal cerebral fissure
Olfactory sulcus
Olfactory bulb
Olfactory tract
Optic nerve

Orbital sulci of frontal pole
Orbital gyri of frontal pole

Pituitary gland
Temporal pole

Anterior perforated substance

Oculomotor nerve (III)

Uncus
Mamillary body
Cerebral peduncle
Pons

Trigeminal nerve (V)

Inferior temporal sulcus

Facial nerve (VII)

Lateral occipito-temporal gyrus

Parahippocampal gyrus

Nervus intermedius

Vestibulocochlear nerve (VIII)

Cerebellar flocculus

Cerebellum
Choroid plexus

Glossopharyngeal nerve (IX)

Vagus nerve (X)
Hypoglossal nerve (XII)
Accessory nerve (XI)

Optic chiasma
Olfactory stria
Tuber cinereum
Maxillary nerve
Ophthalmic nerve
Motor root of **trigeminal (V) nerve**
Mandibular nerve
Semilunar ganglion of trigeminal nerve
Trochlear nerve
Interpeduncular fossa
Abducens nerve
Olive
Pyramid
Medulla oblongata
Cerebellar tonsil

Rootlets of 1st cervical nerve
Decussation of pyramids
Cerebellar vermis
Spinal cord
Occipital pole

I II III IV V VI VII VIII IX X XI XII

Fig. 479: Ventral View of the Brain Showing the Origins of the Cranial Nerves

NOTE: 1) the cranial nerves are numbered sequentially with Roman numerals. The olfactory tracts and optic nerves (I and II) subserve receptors of special sense in the nose and eye and, as cranial nerve trunks, they attach to the base of the forebrain in contrast to all the other cranial nerves which attach at midbrain, pontine or medullary levels.

2) the oculomotor (III), trochlear (IV) and abducens (VI) nerves are motor nerves to the extraocular muscles. While the trigeminal nerve (V) is the largest of all the cranial nerves, the trochlear is the smallest. The abducens nerve emerges from the brainstem at the pontomedullary junction at about the same level, but somewhat more laterally, as the attachments of the facial (VIII) and vestibulocochlear (VIII) nerves.

3) the glossopharyngeal (IX) and vagus (X) nerves emerge from the medulla laterally in a line roughly comparable to the spinal and medullary portions of the accessory nerve (XI). In contrast, the hypoglossal (XII) nerve rootlets emerge from the ventral medulla in a line consistent with the motor ventral rootlets of the cervical segments of the spinal cord.

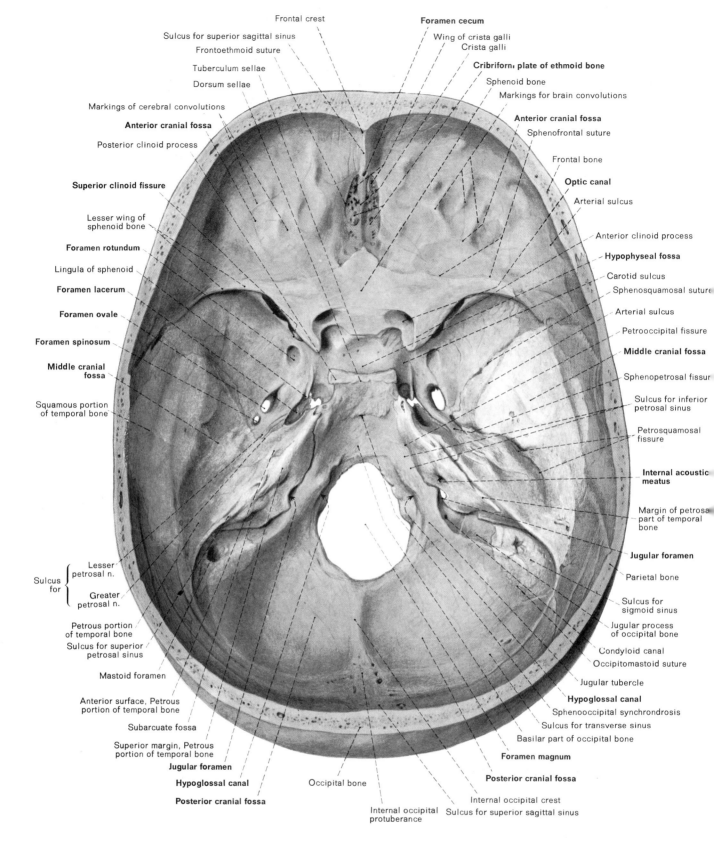

Frontal crest
Foramen cecum
Sulcus for superior sagittal sinus
Wing of crista galli
Frontoethmoid suture
Crista galli
Tuberculum sellae
Cribriform plate of ethmoid bone
Dorsum sellae
Sphenoid bone
Markings of cerebral convolutions
Markings for brain convolutions
Anterior cranial fossa
Anterior cranial fossa
Posterior clinoid process
Sphenofrontal suture
Frontal bone
Superior clinoid fissure
Optic canal
Arterial sulcus
Lesser wing of sphenoid bone
Anterior clinoid process
Foramen rotundum
Hypophyseal fossa
Lingula of sphenoid
Carotid sulcus
Foramen lacerum
Sphenosquamosal suture
Foramen ovale
Arterial sulcus
Petrooccipital fissure
Foramen spinosum
Middle cranial fossa
Middle cranial fossa
Sphenopetrosal fissure
Squamous portion of temporal bone
Sulcus for inferior petrosal sinus
Petrosquamosal fissure
Internal acoustic meatus
Margin of petrosal part of temporal bone
Lesser petrosal n.
Jugular foramen
Sulcus for
Parietal bone
Greater petrosal n.
Sulcus for sigmoid sinus
Petrous portion of temporal bone
Jugular process of occipital bone
Sulcus for superior petrosal sinus
Condyloid canal
Occipitomastoid suture
Mastoid foramen
Jugular tubercle
Anterior surface, Petrous portion of temporal bone
Hypoglossal canal
Sphenooccipital synchrondrosis
Subarcuate fossa
Sulcus for transverse sinus
Superior margin, Petrous portion of temporal bone
Basilar part of occipital bone
Jugular foramen
Foramen magnum
Hypoglossal canal
Occipital bone
Posterior cranial fossa
Posterior cranial fossa
Internal occipital crest
Internal occipital protuberance
Sulcus for superior sagittal sinus

Fig. 480: The Base of the Skull: Internal Aspect (Superior View)

NOTE: 1) the base of the cranial cavity is composed principally of the frontal (lavender) bones, the ethmoid (orange) bone, the sphenoid (green) bone, the temporal (gray) bones and the occipital (blue) bone. Additionally, the sphenoidal angle of each parietal (tan) bone is interposed between the frontal and temporal bones.

2) Important structures traverse the various foramina through the base of the skull:

Anterior Cranial Fossa: a) *foramen cecum:* a small vein. – b) *foramina of cribriform plate:* filaments of olfactory receptor neurons to olfactory bulb. – c) *anterior ethmoid foramen:* anterior ethmoidal vessels and nasociliary nerve. – d) *posterior ethmoid foramen:* posterior ethmoidal vessels and nerve.

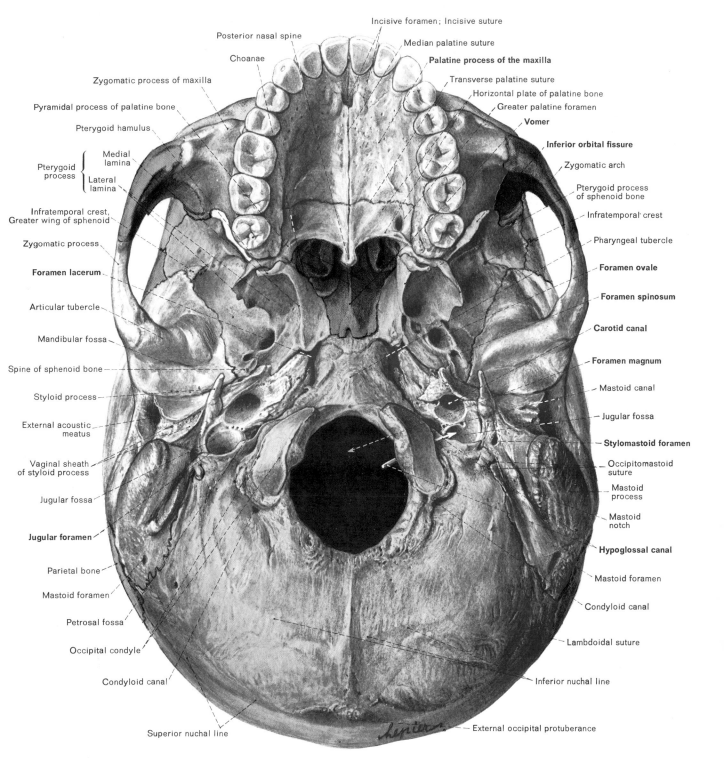

Fig. 481: The Base of the Skull: External Aspect (Inferior View)

NOTE: the base of the skull reveals a posterior region comprised of the occipital and temporal bones which are attached by muscles to the thoracic and vertebral skeleton. More anteriorly are the facial bones consisting of the maxilla, palatine, zygomatic and vomer. Interposed between these two groups of bones is the sphenoid bone.

Middle Cranial Fossa: a) *optic foramen:* optic nerve and ophthalmic artery. – b) *superior orbital fissure:* oculomotor nerve, trochlear nerve, ophthalmic nerve, abducens nerve, sympathetic fibers, superior ophthalmic vein, orbital branches of the middle meningeal artery and a dural recurrent branch from the lacrimal artery. – c) *foramen rotundum:* maxillary nerve. – d) *foramen ovale:* mandibular nerve, accessory meningeal artery. – e) *foramen spinosum:* middle meningeal artery, recurrent branch from mandibular nerve. – f) *foramen lacerum:* internal carotid artery passes across the superior part of the foramen but does not traverse it; nerve of pterygoid canal and meningeal branch of ascending pharyngeal artery traverse foramen lacerum.

Posterior Cranial Fossa: a) *internal acoustic meatus:* facial nerve, vestibulocochlear nerve, labyrinthine artery. – b) *jugular foramen:* inferior petrosal sinus and transverse sinus which together form the jugular vein; meningeal branches of occipital and ascending pharyngeal arteries; glossopharyngeal, vagus and accessory nerves. – c) *hypoglossal canal:* hypoglossal nerve. – d) *foramen magnum:* spinal cord; accessory nerve; anterior and posterior spinal arteries; vertebral arteries; tectorial membrane.

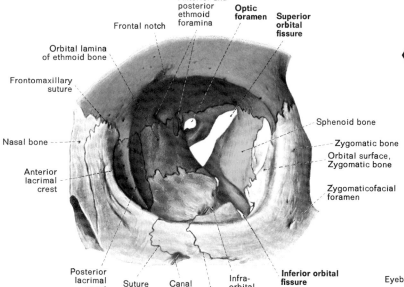

Fig. 482: The Left Bony Orbital Cavity (Anterior View)

NOTE: 1) the bony structure of the orbit is comprised of parts of seven bones: the maxilla, zygomatic, frontal, lacrimal, palatine, ethmoid and sphenoid.

2) the *roof* of the orbit is formed by the orbital plate of the frontal bone; the *floor* consists of the orbital plate of the maxilla, the palatine and zygomatic bones; the *medial wall* is thin and delicate and is formed by the frontal process of the maxilla, the orbital lamina of the ethmoid and the lacrimal bone; the strong lateral wall consists of the orbital processes of the sphenoid and zygomatic bones.

3) the optic foramen and the superior and inferior orbital fissures.

Fig. 483: The Right Eye and Eyelids

NOTE: 1) the eyeball, protected anteriorly by two thin, movable eyelids or palpebrae, is covered by a transparent mucous membrane, the conjunctiva, which is continuous along the inner surface of both eyelids as the palpebral conjunctiva.

2) at the medial angle of the eye is located a small, reddish island of skin called the caruncula lacrimalis. It contains sebaceous and sweat glands which secrete a whitish substance.

3) the pupil is the opening in the iris. Constriction and dilatation of the pupil is controlled autonomically. Parasympathetic fibers in the oculomotor nerve innervate the constrictor muscle of the pupil while sympathetic fibers from the superior cervical ganglion supply the pupillary dilator muscle.

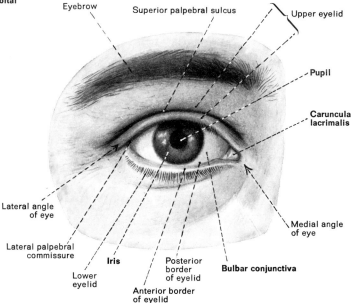

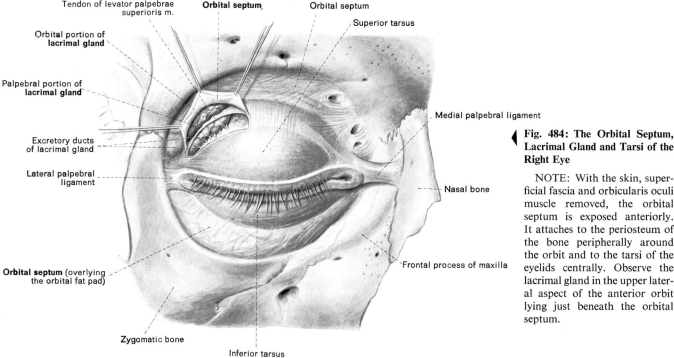

Fig. 484: The Orbital Septum, Lacrimal Gland and Tarsi of the Right Eye

NOTE: With the skin, superficial fascia and orbicularis oculi muscle removed, the orbital septum is exposed anteriorly. It attaches to the periosteum of the bone peripherally around the orbit and to the tarsi of the eyelids centrally. Observe the lacrimal gland in the upper lateral aspect of the anterior orbit lying just beneath the orbital septum.

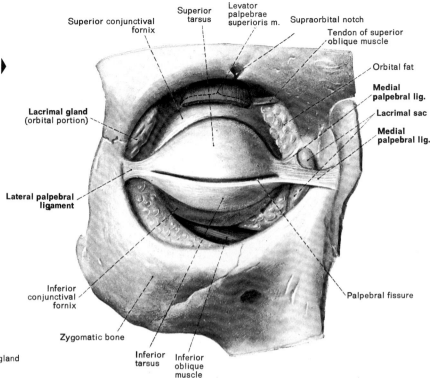

Fig. 485: The Palpebral Ligaments and Tarsal Plates

NOTE: 1) the superficial structures of the anterior orbit have been removed along with the orbital septum and the tendon of the levator palpebrae superioris muscle.

2) the lateral and medial margins of the tarsal plates are attached to the lateral and medial palpebral ligaments which in turn are attached to bone. Observe that the medial ligament is located just anterior to the lacrimal sac.

3) from this anterior view, both the tendon of the superior oblique muscle and the inferior oblique muscle can be visualized. Note also the location of the orbital portion of the lacrimal gland. Its secretions course from lateral to medial across the surface of the eye.

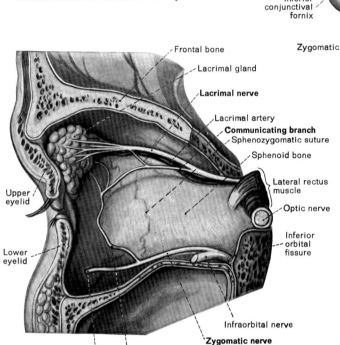

Fig. 487: The Lacrimal Canaliculi, Lacrimal Sac and Nasolacrimal Duct

NOTE: 1) at the medial edge of both the upper and lower eyelids are found single minute orifices (punkta lacrimalia) of small ducts, the lacrimal canaliculi which lead from the eyelids to the lacrimal sac. The sac forms the upper dilated end of the nasolacrimal duct which then extends a distance of about 3½ inches into the inferior meatus of the nasal cavity.

2) secretions from the lacrimal gland pass medially across the surface of the eye toward the canaliculi and then are transported to the nasal acvity by way of the nasolacrimal duct. Excessive secretions (such as during crying) cannot be handled in this manner and, thus, roll over the edge of the lower eyelid as tears.

Fig. 486: The Innervation of the Lacrimal Gland

NOTE: 1) the lacrimal gland receives postganglionic parasympathetic nerve fibers which are secretomotor in nature. The preganglionic fibers are generally said to emerge from the brain with the facial nerve (VII). The synapse between pre and postganglionic fibers occurs in the pterygopalatine ganglion.

2) the preganglionic parasympathetic fibers reach the pterygopalatine ganglion by way of the greater petrosal nerve which becomes the nerve of the pterygoid canal. The postganglionic fibers leave the ganglion and travel for a short distance with the zygomatic branch of the infraorbital nerve. From this point in the inferior aspect of the orbit, the parasympathetic fibers travel by way of a communicating branch to the lacrimal nerve by which they achieve the lacrimal gland.

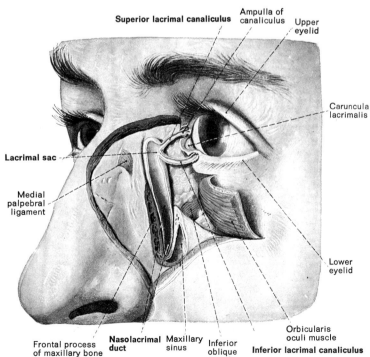

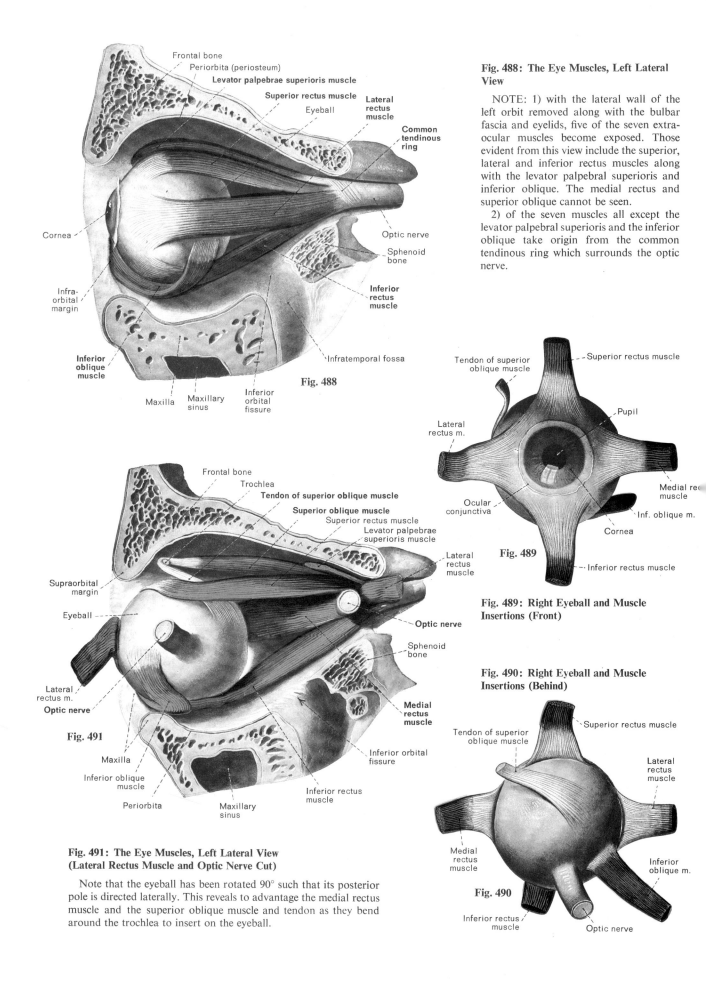

Frontal bone
Periorbita (periosteum)
Levator palpebrae superioris muscle
Superior rectus muscle
Eyeball
Lateral rectus muscle
Common tendinous ring
Cornea
Optic nerve
Sphenoid bone
Infra-orbital margin
Inferior rectus muscle
Inferior oblique muscle
Infratemporal fossa
Maxilla
Maxillary sinus
Inferior orbital fissure

Fig. 488

Fig. 488: The Eye Muscles, Left Lateral View

NOTE: 1) with the lateral wall of the left orbit removed along with the bulbar fascia and eyelids, five of the seven extra-ocular muscles become exposed. Those evident from this view include the superior, lateral and inferior rectus muscles along with the levator palpebral superioris and inferior oblique. The medial rectus and superior oblique cannot be seen.

2) of the seven muscles all except the levator palpebral superioris and the inferior oblique take origin from the common tendinous ring which surrounds the optic nerve.

Tendon of superior oblique muscle
Superior rectus muscle
Lateral rectus m.
Pupil
Ocular conjunctiva
Medial rec muscle
Inf. oblique m.
Cornea
Fig. 489
Inferior rectus muscle

Fig. 489: Right Eyeball and Muscle Insertions (Front)

Fig. 490: Right Eyeball and Muscle Insertions (Behind)

Frontal bone
Trochlea
Tendon of superior oblique muscle
Superior oblique muscle
Superior rectus muscle
Levator palpebrae superioris muscle
Lateral rectus muscle
Supraorbital margin
Eyeball
Optic nerve
Sphenoid bone
Lateral rectus m.
Optic nerve
Medial rectus muscle
Fig. 491
Inferior orbital fissure
Maxilla
Inferior oblique muscle
Periorbita
Inferior rectus muscle
Maxillary sinus

Fig. 491: The Eye Muscles, Left Lateral View (Lateral Rectus Muscle and Optic Nerve Cut)

Note that the eyeball has been rotated 90° such that its posterior pole is directed laterally. This reveals to advantage the medial rectus muscle and the superior oblique muscle and tendon as they bend around the trochlea to insert on the eyeball.

Tendon of superior oblique muscle
Superior rectus muscle
Lateral rectus muscle
Medial rectus muscle
Inferior oblique m.
Fig. 490
Inferior rectus muscle
Optic nerve

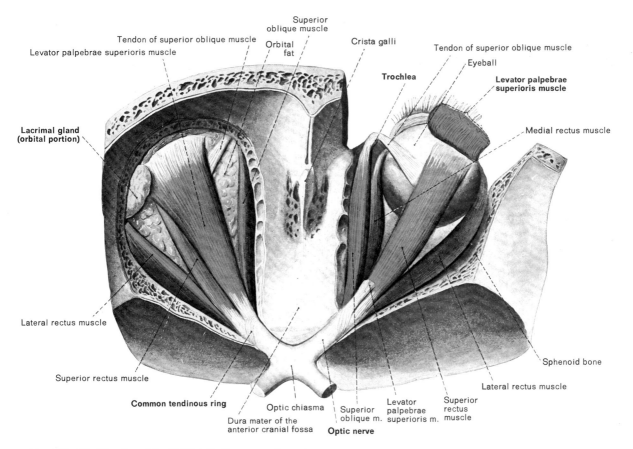

Fig. 492: The Muscles of the Orbital Cavity as seen from above

NOTE: 1) the orbital plates of the frontal bone have been removed from within the cranium. On the left side, only the bony roof of the orbit has been opened and the muscles, orbital fat and lacrimal gland have been left intact.

2) on the right side, the levator palpebrae superioris muscle has been resected and the orbital fat removed in order to expose the ocular muscles.

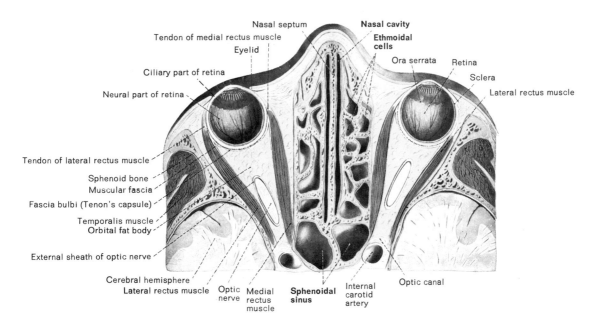

Fig. 493: A Horizontal Section Through Both Orbits at the Level of the Sphenoid Sinus

NOTE: 1) between the orbital cavities is situated the ethmoid bone containing the ethmoidal air sinuses (air cells). The vertically oriented perpendicular plate of the ethmoid serves as the nasal septum which subdivides the nasal cavity into two symmetrical chambers.

2) the posterior portion of the orbits are separated by the sphenoidal sinuses, located within the body of the sphenoid bone. These sinuses usually are not symmetrical.

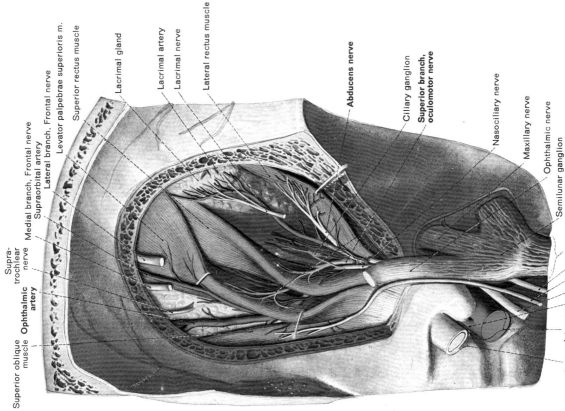

Medial branch, Frontal nerve

Supra-
trochlear
nerve

Superior oblique muscle **Ophthalmic artery**

Lacrimal gland

Lacrimal artery

Lacrimal nerve

Lateral rectus muscle

Medial branch, Frontal nerve

Supraorbital artery

Lateral branch, Frontal nerve

Levator palpebrae superioris m.

Superior rectus muscle

Abducens nerve

Ciliary ganglion

Superior branch, oculomotor nerve

Nasociliary nerve

Maxillary nerve

Ophthalmic nerve

Semilunar ganglion

Trigeminal nerve

Abducens nerve

Trochlear nerve

Oculomotor nerve

Optic nerve

Internal carotid art.

Ophthalmic artery

Fig. 495: Nerves and Arteries of the Orbit (Stage 2)
Superior View: the Trochlear and Abducens Nerves

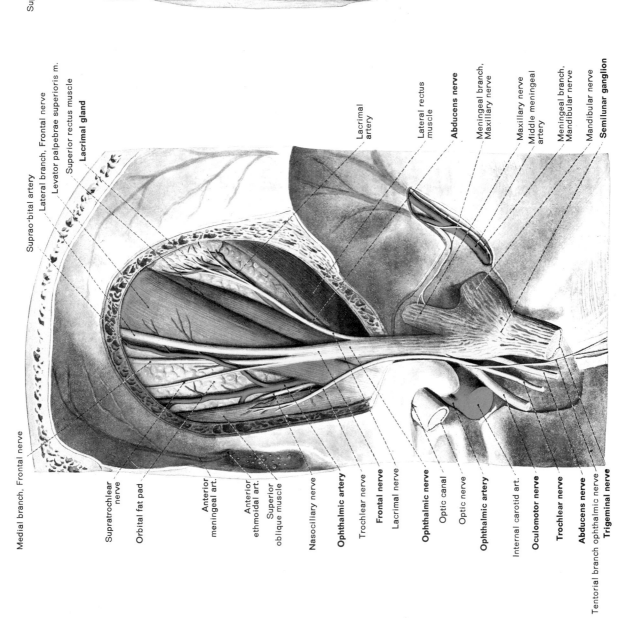

Medial branch, Frontal nerve

Suprao-bital artery

Lateral branch, Frontal nerve

Levator palpebrae superioris m.

Superior rectus muscle

Lacrimal gland

Supratrochlear
nerve

Orbital fat pad

Anterior
meningeal art.

Anterior
ethmoidal art.

Superior
oblique muscle

Nasociliary nerve

Ophthalmic artery

Trochlear nerve

Frontal nerve

Lacrimal nerve

Ophthalmic nerve

Optic canal

Optic nerve

Ophthalmic artery

Internal carotid art.

Oculomotor nerve

Trochlear nerve

Abducens nerve

Tentorial branch ophthalmic nerve

Trigeminal nerve

Lacrimal
artery

Lateral rectus
muscle

Abducens nerve

Meningeal branch,
Maxillary nerve

Maxillary nerve

Middle meningeal
artery

Meningeal branch,
Mandibular nerve

Mandibular nerve

Semilunar ganglion

Fig. 494: Nerves and Arteries of the Orbit (Stage 1)
Superior View: Ophthalmic Nerve and Artery

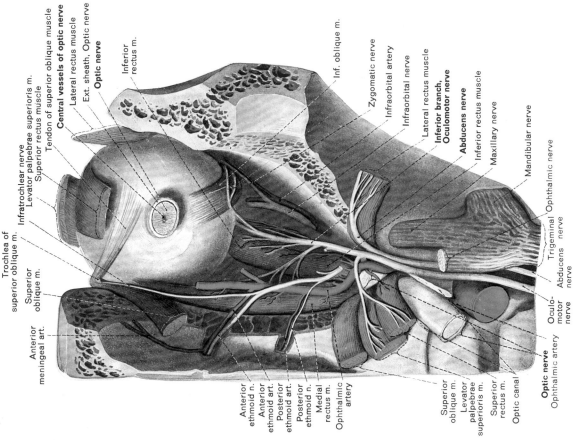

**Fig. 497: Nerves and Arteries of the Orbit (Stage 4)
Superior View: the Oculomotor Nerve (Inferior Branch)**

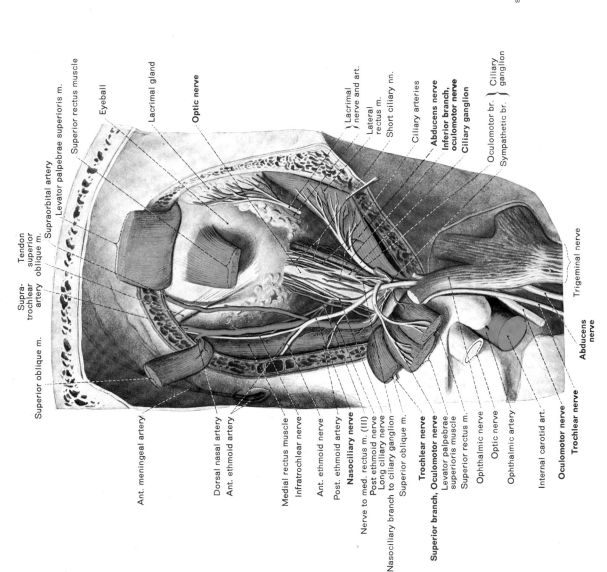

**Fig. 496: Nerves and Arteries of the Orbit (Stage 3)
Superior View: the Optic Nerve and Ciliary Ganglion**

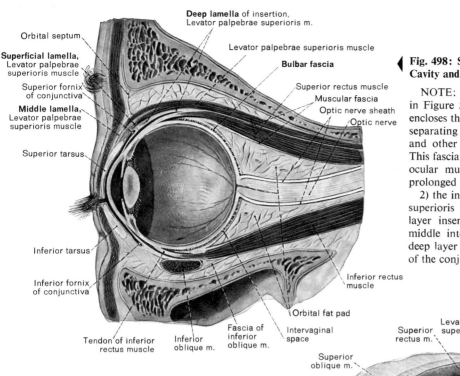

Fig. 498 labels: Orbital septum, Superficial lamella, Levator palpebrae superioris muscle, Superior fornix of conjunctiva, Middle lamella, Levator palpebrae superioris muscle, Superior tarsus, Inferior tarsus, Inferior fornix of conjunctiva, Tendon of inferior rectus muscle, Inferior oblique m., Fascia of inferior oblique m., Intervaginal space, Deep lamella of insertion, Levator palpebrae superioris m., Levator palpebrae superioris muscle, Bulbar fascia, Superior rectus muscle, Muscular fascia, Optic nerve sheath, Optic nerve, Inferior rectus muscle, Orbital fat pad

Fig. 498: Sagittal View of the Orbital Cavity and Eyeball

NOTE: 1) the bulbar fascia (also seen in Figure 500) is a thin membrane which encloses the posterior 3/4ths of the eyeball, separating the eyeball from the orbital fat and other contents of the orbital cavity. This fascia is pierced by the tendons of the ocular muscles over which the fascia is prolonged like a tubular sheath.

2) the insertion of the levator palpebrae superioris is trilaminar. The superficial layer inserts into the upper eyelid, the middle into the superior tarsus and the deep layer inserts into the superior fornix of the conjunctiva.

Fig. 499: Origins of the Ocular Muscles, Apex of Left Orbit

NOTE: 1) this anterior view of the apex of the left orbit shows the stumps of the ocular muscles which have been cut close to their origins.

2) the four rectus muscles arise from a common tendinous ring surrounding the optic canal. The levator palpebrae superioris and superior oblique muscles arise from the sphenoid bone close to the tendinous ring while the inferior oblique (not shown) arises from the orbital surface of the maxilla.

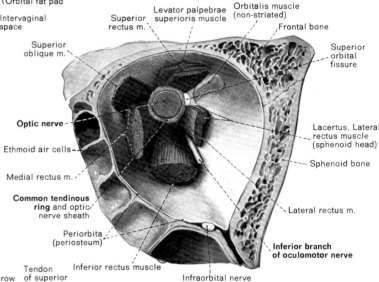

Fig. 499 labels: Superior oblique m., Superior rectus m., Levator palpebrae superioris muscle, Orbitalis muscle (non-striated), Frontal bone, Superior orbital fissure, Optic nerve, Ethmoid air cells, Medial rectus m., Common tendinous ring and optic nerve sheath, Periorbita (periosteum), Inferior rectus muscle, Infraorbital nerve, Lacertus, Lateral rectus muscle (sphenoid head), Sphenoid bone, Lateral rectus m., Inferior branch of oculomotor nerve

Fig. 500 labels: Tarsal glands, Superior rectus muscle, Eyebrow, Tendon of superior oblique m., Anterior palpebral border, Eyelashes, Posterior palpebral border, Medial rectus m., Sup. lacrimal papilla, Medial palpebral commissure, Lacrimal caruncle, Inf. lacrimal papilla, Anterior margin of bulbar fascia, Lateral rectus m., Lateral palpebral commissure, Orbital fat pad, Inferior oblique m., Optic nerve, Inferior rectus m., Inferior tarsus, Openings of tarsal glands, Bulbar fascia

Fig. 500: The Bulbar Fascia (Capsule of Tenon), Right Eye

NOTE: 1) longitudinal incisions have been made down the middle of each eyelid and the flaps have been reflected to expose the orbital cavity anteriorly.

2) the optic nerve has been severed at the optic disc and the eyeball, along with the insertions of the ocular muscles, has been removed from the orbital cavity.

3) the bulbar fascia which envelopes the posterior aspect of the eyeball (from the sclerocorneal junction to the optic nerve) has been left within the orbit. Observe how the bulbar fascia is perforated by the tendons of the ocular muscles. It is also pierced from behind by the ciliary vessels and nerves.

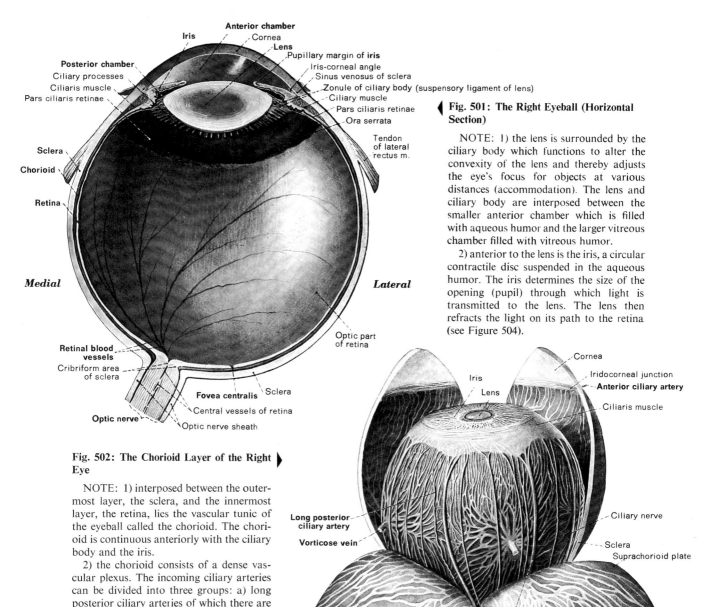

Fig. 501: The Right Eyeball (Horizontal Section)

Labels for upper left figure:
- Iris
- Anterior chamber
- Cornea
- Lens
- Pupillary margin of **iris**
- Iris-corneal angle
- Sinus venosus of sclera
- Zonule of ciliary body (suspensory ligament of lens)
- Ciliary muscle
- Pars ciliaris retinae
- Ora serrata
- Posterior chamber
- Ciliary processes
- Ciliaris muscle
- Pars ciliaris retinae
- Sclera
- Chorioid
- Retina
- Medial
- Lateral
- Tendon of lateral rectus m.
- Optic part of retina
- Retinal blood vessels
- Cribriform area of sclera
- Fovea centralis
- Sclera
- Central vessels of retina
- Optic nerve
- Optic nerve sheath

NOTE: 1) the lens is surrounded by the ciliary body which functions to alter the convexity of the lens and thereby adjusts the eye's focus for objects at various distances (accommodation). The lens and ciliary body are interposed between the smaller anterior chamber which is filled with aqueous humor and the larger vitreous chamber filled with vitreous humor.

2) anterior to the lens is the iris, a circular contractile disc suspended in the aqueous humor. The iris determines the size of the opening (pupil) through which light is transmitted to the lens. The lens then refracts the light on its path to the retina (see Figure 504).

Fig. 502: The Chorioid Layer of the Right Eye

NOTE: 1) interposed between the outermost layer, the sclera, and the innermost layer, the retina, lies the vascular tunic of the eyeball called the chorioid. The chorioid is continuous anteriorly with the ciliary body and the iris.

2) the chorioid consists of a dense vascular plexus. The incoming ciliary arteries can be divided into three groups: a) long posterior ciliary arteries of which there are generally two, b) five to seven short posterior ciliary arteries and c) the anterior ciliary arteries. These vessels are derived from the ophthalmic or its lacrimal branch and they drain into the vorticose veins which pass through the sclera to flow into ophthalmic veins.

Labels for right figure:
- Cornea
- Iridocorneal junction
- **Anterior ciliary artery**
- Iris
- Lens
- Ciliaris muscle
- **Long posterior ciliary artery**
- **Vorticose vein**
- Ciliary nerve
- Sclera
- Suprachorioid plate
- Ciliary nerves
- Posterior ciliary artery
- Optic nerve

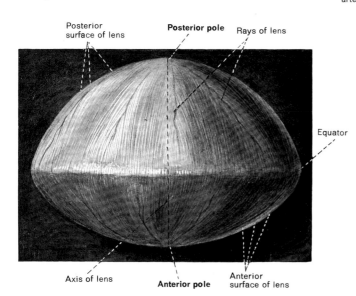

Labels for lower left figure:
- Posterior surface of lens
- **Posterior pole**
- Rays of lens
- Equator
- Axis of lens
- **Anterior pole**
- Anterior surface of lens

Fig. 503: The Lens (Equatorial View)

NOTE: 1) the lens is a biconvex structure situated between the iris and the vitreous body. Its shape is less convex anteriorly than posteriorly and the lens is composed of a series of concentrically arranged laminae surrounded by a transparent membrane.

2) the adult lens is colorless and contains no blood vessels. With increasing age, it becomes more flattened and less capable of altering its shape to accommodate for short distances.

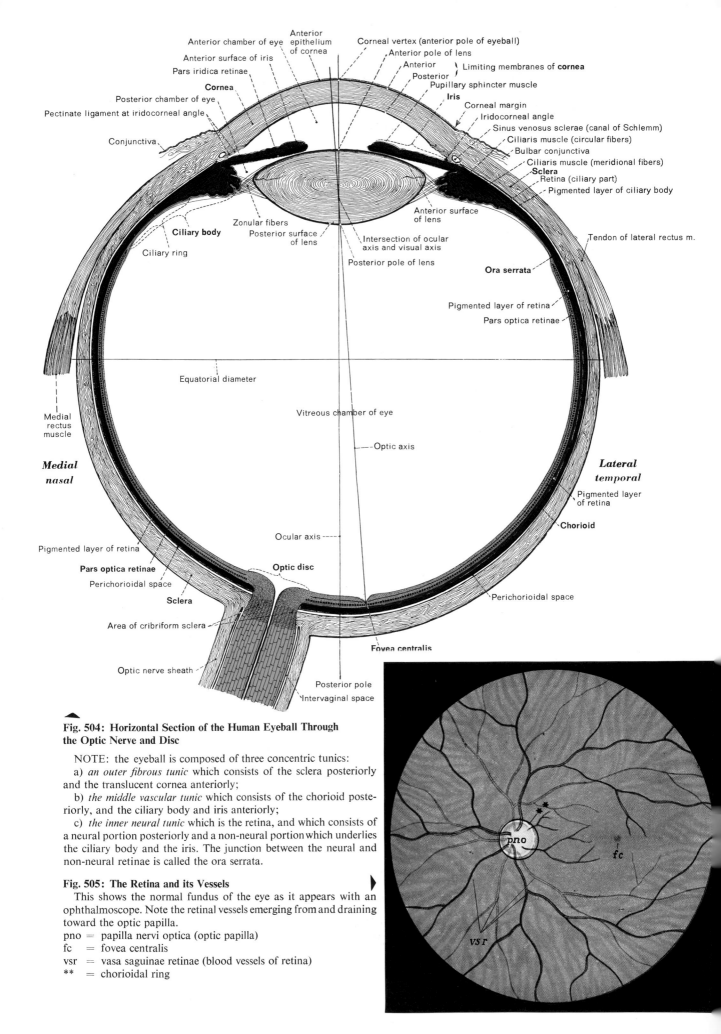

Anterior
Anterior chamber of eye   epithelium   Corneal vertex (anterior pole of eyeball)
of cornea
Anterior surface of iris   Anterior pole of lens
Pars iridica retinae   Anterior   Limiting membranes of **cornea**
Posterior
Cornea   Pupillary sphincter muscle
Posterior chamber of eye   **Iris**
Pectinate ligament at iridocorneal angle   Corneal margin
Iridocorneal angle
Conjunctiva   Sinus venosus sclerae (canal of Schlemm)
Ciliaris muscle (circular fibers)
Bulbar conjunctiva
Ciliaris muscle (meridional fibers)
Sclera
Retina (ciliary part)
Pigmented layer of ciliary body
Ciliary body   Anterior surface
Zonular fibers   of lens
Posterior surface
of lens
Ciliary ring   Tendon of lateral rectus m.
Intersection of ocular
axis and visual axis
Posterior pole of lens   **Ora serrata**

Pigmented layer of retina
Pars optica retinae

Equatorial diameter

Vitreous chamber of eye

Medial
rectus   Optic axis
muscle

Medial   *Lateral*
nasal   *temporal*

Pigmented layer
of retina

Ocular axis   **Chorioid**

Pigmented layer of retina
Pars optica retinae
Perichorioidal space   **Optic disc**
Sclera   Perichorioidal space
Area of cribriform sclera

Fovea centralis

Optic nerve sheath   Posterior pole
Intervaginal space

Fig. 504: **Horizontal Section of the Human Eyeball Through
the Optic Nerve and Disc**

NOTE: the eyeball is composed of three concentric tunics:
a) *an outer fibrous tunic* which consists of the sclera posteriorly
and the translucent cornea anteriorly;
b) *the middle vascular tunic* which consists of the chorioid posteriorly, and the ciliary body and iris anteriorly;
c) *the inner neural tunic* which is the retina, and which consists of
a neural portion posteriorly and a non-neural portion which underlies
the ciliary body and the iris. The junction between the neural and
non-neural retinae is called the ora serrata.

Fig. 505: **The Retina and its Vessels**
This shows the normal fundus of the eye as it appears with an
ophthalmoscope. Note the retinal vessels emerging from and draining
toward the optic papilla.
pno = papilla nervi optica (optic papilla)
fc = fovea centralis
vsr = vasa saguinae retinae (blood vessels of retina)
** = chorioidal ring

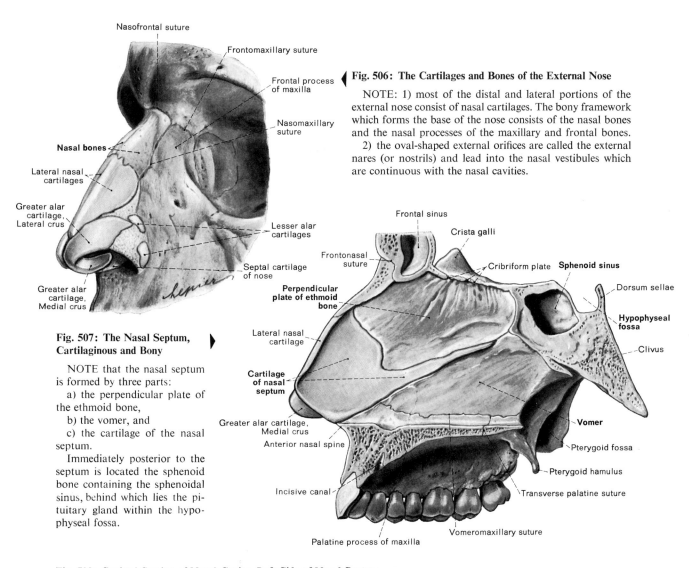

Fig. 506 labels: Nasofrontal suture, Frontomaxillary suture, Frontal process of maxilla, Nasomaxillary suture, **Nasal bones**, Lateral nasal cartilages, Greater alar cartilage, Lateral crus, Lesser alar cartilages, Septal cartilage of nose, Greater alar cartilage, Medial crus

Fig. 506: The Cartilages and Bones of the External Nose

NOTE: 1) most of the distal and lateral portions of the external nose consist of nasal cartilages. The bony framework which forms the base of the nose consists of the nasal bones and the nasal processes of the maxillary and frontal bones.

2) the oval-shaped external orifices are called the external nares (or nostrils) and lead into the nasal vestibules which are continuous with the nasal cavities.

Fig. 507: The Nasal Septum, Cartilaginous and Bony

NOTE that the nasal septum is formed by three parts:

a) the perpendicular plate of the ethmoid bone,

b) the vomer, and

c) the cartilage of the nasal septum.

Immediately posterior to the septum is located the sphenoid bone containing the sphenoidal sinus, behind which lies the pituitary gland within the hypophyseal fossa.

Fig. 507 labels: Frontal sinus, Crista galli, Cribriform plate, **Sphenoid sinus**, Dorsum sellae, **Hypophyseal fossa**, Clivus, Frontonasal suture, **Perpendicular plate of ethmoid bone**, Lateral nasal cartilage, **Cartilage of nasal septum**, Greater alar cartilage, Medial crus, Anterior nasal spine, **Vomer**, Pterygoid fossa, Pterygoid hamulus, Transverse palatine suture, Incisive canal, Vomeromaxillary suture, Palatine process of maxilla

Fig. 508: Sagittal Section of Nasal Cavity, Left Side of Nasal Septum

NOTE that the mucosa in the upper aspect of the nasal cavity and nasal septum contains the filaments of the olfactory nerves which subserve the special sense of smell. These filaments of olfactory receptors penetrate the cribriform plate of the ethmoid bone and enter the olfactory bulb.

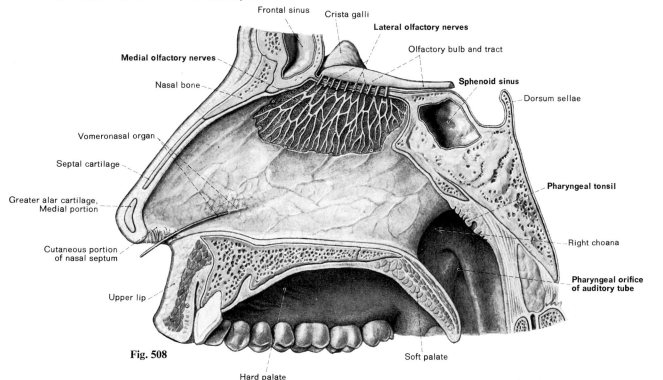

Fig. 508 labels: Frontal sinus, Crista galli, **Lateral olfactory nerves**, Olfactory bulb and tract, **Medial olfactory nerves**, **Sphenoid sinus**, Dorsum sellae, Nasal bone, Vomeronasal organ, Septal cartilage, **Pharyngeal tonsil**, Greater alar cartilage, Medial portion, Right choana, Cutaneous portion of nasal septum, **Pharyngeal orifice of auditory tube**, Upper lip, Fig. 508, Hard palate, Soft palate

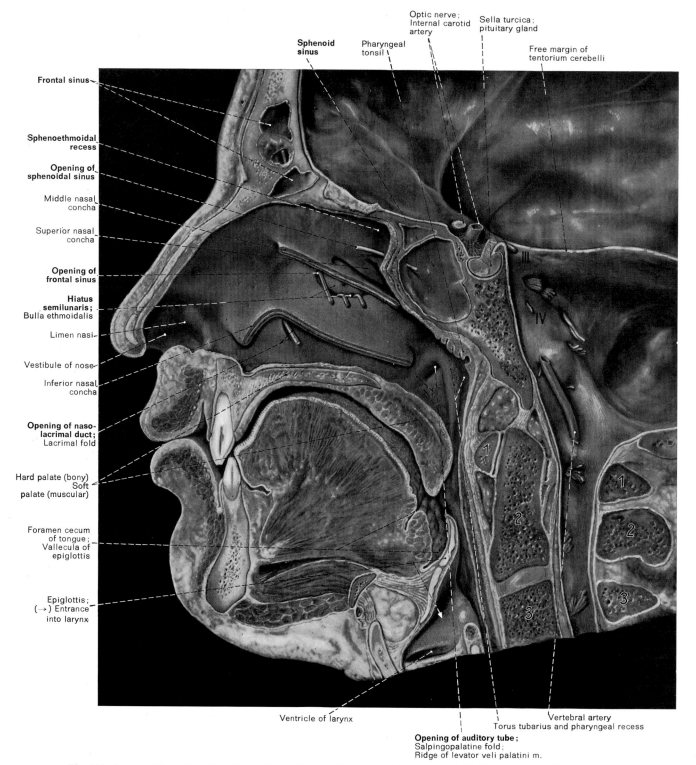

Frontal sinus

Sphenoethmoidal recess

Opening of sphenoidal sinus

Middle nasal concha

Superior nasal concha

Opening of frontal sinus

Hiatus semilunaris; Bulla ethmoidalis

Limen nasi

Vestibule of nose

Inferior nasal concha

Opening of naso- lacrimal duct; Lacrimal fold

Hard palate (bony) Soft palate (muscular)

Foramen cecum of tongue; Vallecula of epiglottis

Epiglottis; (→) Entrance into larynx

Sphenoid sinus

Pharyngeal tonsil

Optic nerve; Internal carotid artery

Sella turcica; pituitary gland

Free margin of tentorium cerebelli

Ventricle of larynx

Torus tubarius and pharyngeal recess

Vertebral artery

Opening of auditory tube; Salpingopalatine fold; Ridge of levator veli palatini m.

Fig. 509: Lateral Wall of the Right Nasal Cavity Showing Openings of the Paranasal Air Sinuses and the Nasopharynx

NOTE: 1) this median sagittal section of the adult head displays the right nasal cavity with the middle and inferior nasal conchae removed. The nasal cavity communicates anteriorly with the environment through the vestibule and nostril and posteriorly with the pharynx (nasopharynx).

2) openings of the various paranasal sinuses and other structures. These include:

a) the *sphenoid sinus* which opens into the sphenoethmoidal recess above the superior concha.

b) the *frontal sinus* and *maxillary sinus* both of which open into a groove called the hiatus semilunaris in the middle meatus below the middle concha.

c) the *nasolacrimal duct* which opens into the inferior meatus below the inferior concha.

d) the *auditory tube* which opens into the nasopharynx just behind the inferior concha. This tube stretches between the cavity of the middle ear (tympanic cavity) and the nasopharynx, thereby allowing the cavity of the middle ear to alter its air pressure consistent with the environment. This mechanism equalizes the air pressure on both sides of the tympanic membrane.

3) the nasal cavity, oral cavity and laryngeal cavity all communicate with the pharynx, forming, in turn, the nasopharynx, oral pharynx and laryngeal pharynx.

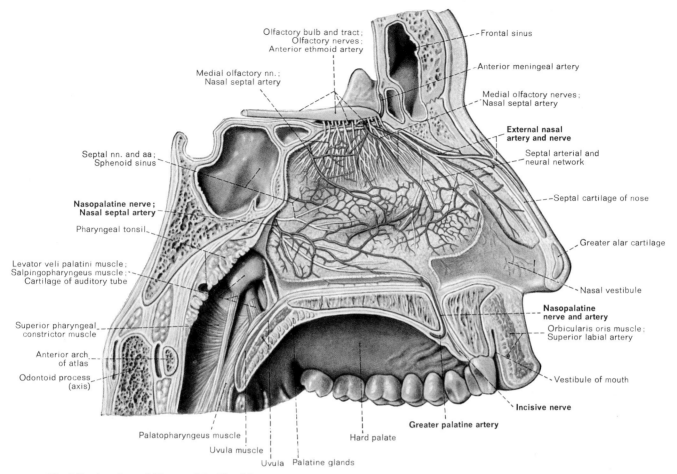

Fig. 510: Arteries and Nerves of the Nasal Septum

Note that the mucous membrane has been removed from the nasal septum and nasopharynx revealing the septal vessels and nerves and the nasopharyngeal muscles.

Fig. 511: The Lateral Wall of the Left Nasal Cavity

NOTE: the mucous membrane overlying the lateral olfactory nerves has been removed. The lateral wall of the nasal cavity is marked by the superior, middle and inferior nasal conchae. Beneath each concha courses its corresponding nasal passage or meatus.

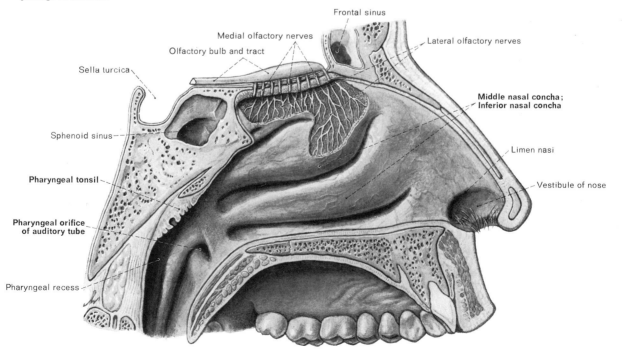

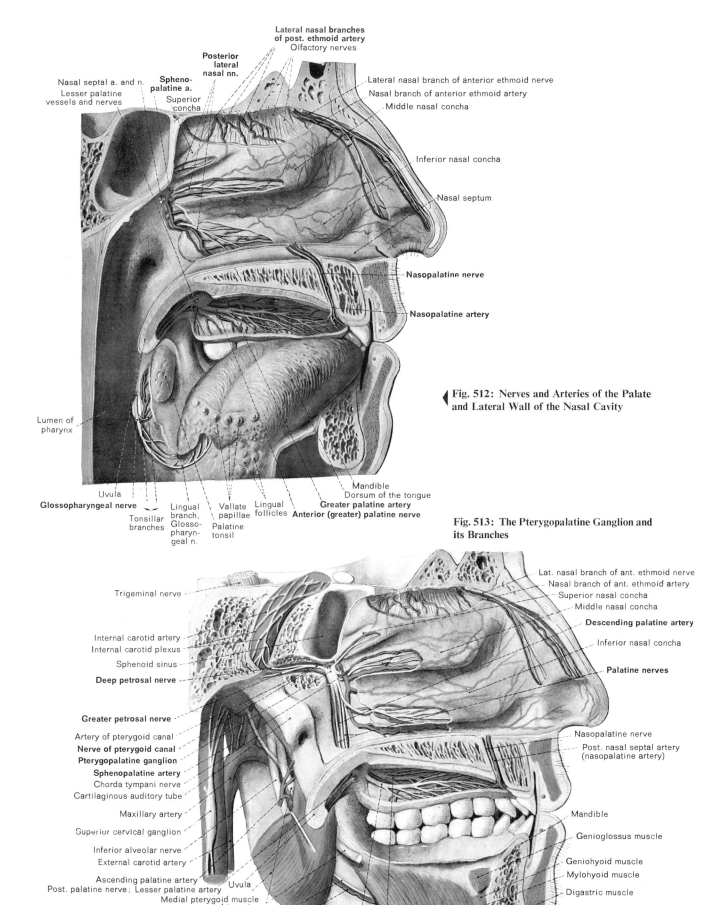

Lateral nasal branches
of post. ethmoid artery
Olfactory nerves

Posterior
lateral
nasal nn.

Nasal septal a. and n.
Lesser palatine
vessels and nerves

Spheno-
palatine a.

Sphenopalatine a.

Superior
concha

Lateral nasal branch of anterior ethmoid nerve
Nasal branch of anterior ethmoid artery
Middle nasal concha

Inferior nasal concha

Nasal septum

Nasopalatine nerve

Nasopalatine artery

Lumen of
pharynx

◀ **Fig. 512: Nerves and Arteries of the Palate
and Lateral Wall of the Nasal Cavity**

Uvula

Glossopharyngeal nerve

Tonsillar
branches

Lingual
branch,
Glosso-
pharyn-
geal n.

Vallate
papillae

Palatine
tonsil

Lingual
follicles

Mandible
Dorsum of the tongue
Greater palatine artery
Anterior (greater) palatine nerve

**Fig. 513: The Pterygopalatine Ganglion and
its Branches**

Trigeminal nerve

Internal carotid artery
Internal carotid plexus
Sphenoid sinus
Deep petrosal nerve

Greater petrosal nerve
Artery of pterygoid canal
Nerve of pterygoid canal
Pterygopalatine ganglion
Sphenopalatine artery
Chorda tympani nerve
Cartilaginous auditory tube

Maxillary artery
Superior cervical ganglion
Inferior alveolar nerve
External carotid artery
Ascending palatine artery
Post. palatine nerve; Lesser palatine artery
Medial pterygoid muscle
Mylohyoid
nerve and artery

Uvula

Lingual nerve

**Anterior (greater)
palatine nerve**

Greater palatine artery

Lat. nasal branch of ant. ethmoid nerve
Nasal branch of ant. ethmoid artery
Superior nasal concha
Middle nasal concha
Descending palatine artery

Inferior nasal concha

Palatine nerves

Nasopalatine nerve
Post. nasal septal artery
(nasopalatine artery)

Mandible
Genioglossus muscle
Geniohyoid muscle
Mylohyoid muscle
Digastric muscle

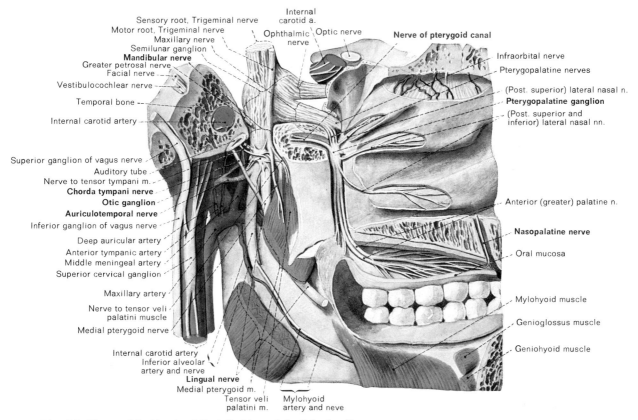

Fig. 514: Nerves of the Nasal and Oral Cavities and the Otic Ganglion

Note the junction of the chorda tympani nerve with the lingual nerve and the position of the otic ganglion in relation to the mandibular branch of the trigeminal. This ganglion receives preganglionic parasympathetic fibers by way of the tympanic branch of the glossopharyngeal nerve. Its postganglionic fibers supply the parotid gland.

Fig. 515: The Maxillary Nerve, the Petrosal Nerves and the Facial Nerve

Note that the nerve of the pterygoid canal is formed by the union of the deep petrosal and greater petrosal nerves. The deep petrosal nerve transmits postganglionic sympathetic fibers while the greater petrosal nerve contains sensory fibers from the geniculate ganglion of the facial nerve and preganglionic parasympathetic fibers from the nervus intermedius portion of the facial nerve. The lesser petrosal nerve carries preganglionic fibers of the glossopharyngeal nerve to the otic ganglion (see Figure 514).

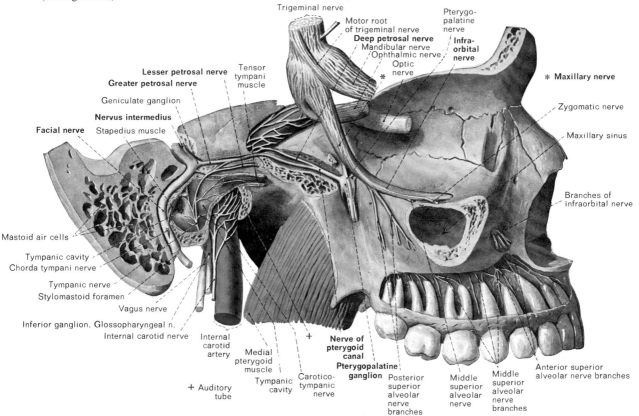

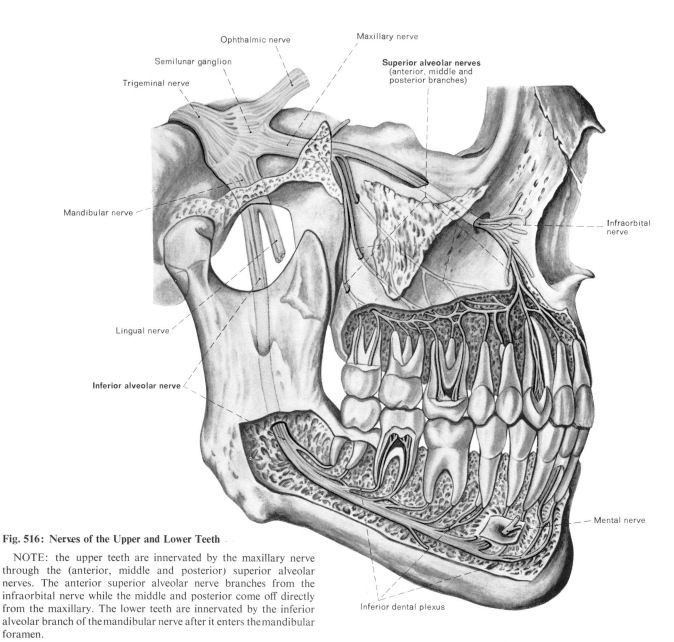

Ophthalmic nerve

Maxillary nerve

Semilunar ganglion

Superior alveolar nerves
(anterior, middle and
posterior branches)

Trigeminal nerve

Mandibular nerve

Infraorbital
nerve

Lingual nerve

Inferior alveolar nerve

Mental nerve

Inferior dental plexus

Fig. 516: Nerves of the Upper and Lower Teeth

NOTE: the upper teeth are innervated by the maxillary nerve through the (anterior, middle and posterior) superior alveolar nerves. The anterior superior alveolar nerve branches from the infraorbital nerve while the middle and posterior come off directly from the maxillary. The lower teeth are innervated by the inferior alveolar branch of the mandibular nerve after it enters the mandibular foramen.

Condylar process

Coronoid process

Ramus of mandible

Alveolar part
(sockets for teeth)

Ramus
of mandible

Oblique line

Mandibular
angle

Mental foramen

Mental tubercle   Mental protuberance

Fig. 517: The Mandible as seen from the Front

NOTE: 1) the anterior aspect of the mandible forms the bony substructure of the mentum or chin. The two vertical rami of the mandible are continuous with the body of the mandible at the mandibular angle.

2) the mental foramen transmits the mental branch of the inferior alveolar nerve to the skin of the chin and lower lip on each side. The mental branch of the inferior alveolar artery accompanies the mental nerve and participates in the vascular supply of the lower lip.

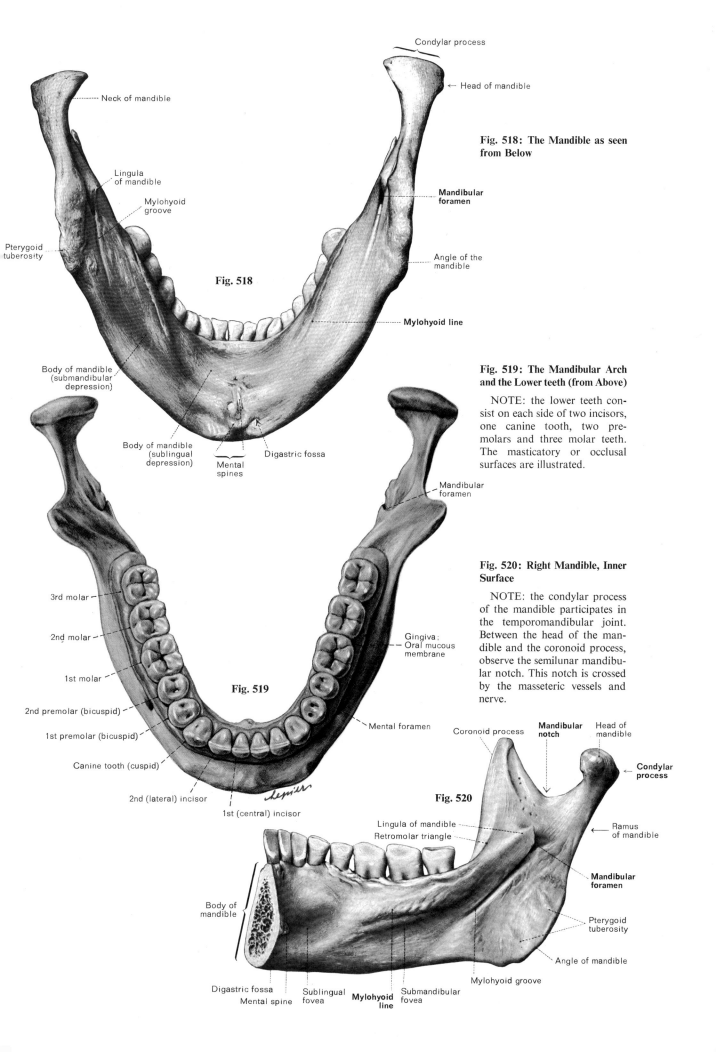

Neck of mandible

Condylar process

← Head of mandible

Fig. 518: The Mandible as seen from Below

Lingula of mandible

Mylohyoid groove

Mandibular foramen

Pterygoid tuberosity

Angle of the mandible

Fig. 518

Mylohyoid line

Fig. 519: The Mandibular Arch and the Lower teeth (from Above)

NOTE: the lower teeth consist on each side of two incisors, one canine tooth, two premolars and three molar teeth. The masticatory or occlusal surfaces are illustrated.

Body of mandible (submandibular depression)

Body of mandible (sublingual depression)

Digastric fossa

Mental spines

Mandibular foramen

Fig. 520: Right Mandible, Inner Surface

NOTE: the condylar process of the mandible participates in the temporomandibular joint. Between the head of the mandible and the coronoid process, observe the semilunar mandibular notch. This notch is crossed by the masseteric vessels and nerve.

3rd molar

2nd molar

1st molar

2nd premolar (bicuspid)

1st premolar (bicuspid)

Canine tooth (cuspid)

2nd (lateral) incisor

1st (central) incisor

Gingiva; Oral mucous membrane

Fig. 519

Mental foramen

Coronoid process

Mandibular notch

Head of mandible

Condylar process

Fig. 520

Ramus of mandible

Lingula of mandible

Retromolar triangle

Mandibular foramen

Body of mandible

Pterygoid tuberosity

Angle of mandible

Digastric fossa

Mental spine

Sublingual fovea

Mylohyoid line

Submandibular fovea

Mylohyoid groove

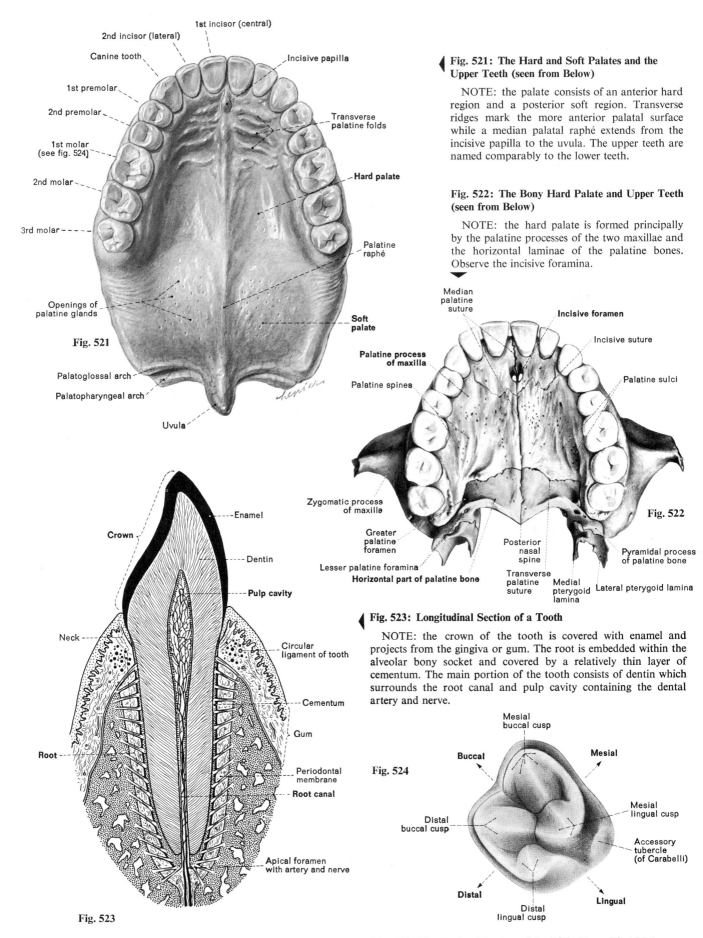

1st incisor (central)

2nd incisor (lateral)

Canine tooth

1st premolar

2nd premolar

1st molar
(see fig. 524)

2nd molar

3rd molar

Openings of
palatine glands

Incisive papilla

Transverse
palatine folds

Hard palate

Palatine
raphé

Soft palate

Fig. 521

Palatoglossal arch

Palatopharyngeal arch

Uvula

Fig. 521: The Hard and Soft Palates and the Upper Teeth (seen from Below)

NOTE: the palate consists of an anterior hard region and a posterior soft region. Transverse ridges mark the more anterior palatal surface while a median palatal raphé extends from the incisive papilla to the uvula. The upper teeth are named comparably to the lower teeth.

Fig. 522: The Bony Hard Palate and Upper Teeth (seen from Below)

NOTE: the hard palate is formed principally by the palatine processes of the two maxillae and the horizontal laminae of the palatine bones. Observe the incisive foramina.

Median palatine suture

Incisive foramen

Incisive suture

Palatine process of maxilla

Palatine spines

Palatine sulci

Zygomatic process of maxilla

Greater palatine foramen

Lesser palatine foramina

Horizontal part of palatine bone

Posterior nasal spine

Transverse palatine suture

Medial pterygoid lamina

Lateral pterygoid lamina

Pyramidal process of palatine bone

Fig. 522

Fig. 523: Longitudinal Section of a Tooth

NOTE: the crown of the tooth is covered with enamel and projects from the gingiva or gum. The root is embedded within the alveolar bony socket and covered by a relatively thin layer of cementum. The main portion of the tooth consists of dentin which surrounds the root canal and pulp cavity containing the dental artery and nerve.

Crown

Enamel

Dentin

Pulp cavity

Neck

Circular ligament of tooth

Cementum

Gum

Root

Periodontal membrane

Root canal

Apical foramen with artery and nerve

Fig. 523

Fig. 524

Mesial buccal cusp

Buccal

Mesial

Distal buccal cusp

Mesial lingual cusp

Accessory tubercle (of Carabelli)

Distal

Distal lingual cusp

Lingual

Fig. 524: The Occlusal Surface of the Right Upper First Molar

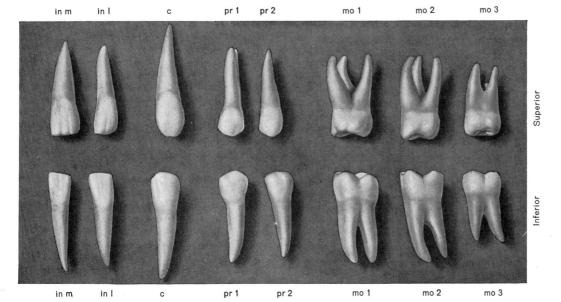

| in m | in l | c | pr 1 | pr 2 | mo 1 | mo 2 | mo 3 |

in m = Medial incisor
in l = Lateral incisor
c = Canine
pr 1 = 1st premolar
pr 2 = 2nd premolar
mo 1 = 1st molar
mo 2 = 2nd molar
mo 3 = 3rd molar

Superior

Inferior

Fig. 525

| in m | in l | c | pr 1 | pr 2 | mo 1 | mo 2 | mo 3 |

Fig. 525: The Maxillary and Mandibular Permanent Teeth (Buccal Surfaces)

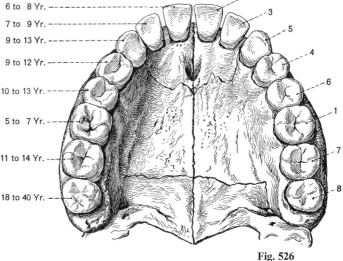

6 to 9 M.
8 to 12 M.
16 to 20 M.
12 to 16 M.
20 to 30 M.

Fig. 527

Fig. 527: Diagram Showing Eruption Times of Deciduous Upper Teeth

NOTE: on the left side of the illustration the times of eruption are shown in *months* for each tooth while the sequential order of appearance of the erupted *deciduous* teeth is indicated on the right side by numbers.

Fig. 526: Diagram Showing Eruption Times of Permanent Upper Teeth

NOTE: on the left side of the illustration the times of eruption are shown in *years* for each tooth while the sequential order of appearance of the erupted *permanent* teeth is indicated on the right side by numbers.

6 to 8 Yr.
7 to 9 Yr.
9 to 13 Yr.
9 to 12 Yr.
10 to 13 Yr.
5 to 7 Yr.
11 to 14 Yr.
18 to 40 Yr.

Fig. 526

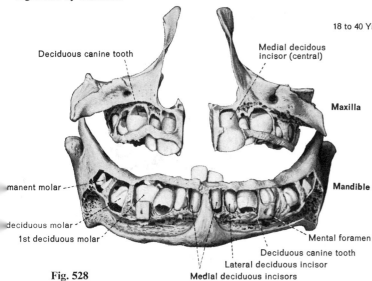

Deciduous canine tooth
Medial decidous incisor (central)
Maxilla
-manent molar
-deciduous molar
1st deciduous molar
Mandible
Mental foramen
Deciduous canine tooth
Lateral deciduous incisor
Medial deciduous incisors

Fig. 528

Fig. 528: Dentition of a Child of Nearly One Year of Age

NOTE: 1) the deciduous or "milk teeth" number 20 in all, including two incisors, one canine and two molars in each jaw quadrant. The earliest of these teeth to erupt are the incisors which generally penetrate through the gum line before the end of the first year.

2) generally speaking:
a 1 year old child has 6 teeth,
a 1½ year old child has 12 teeth,
a 2 year old child has 16 teeth, and
a 2½ year old child has 20 teeth.

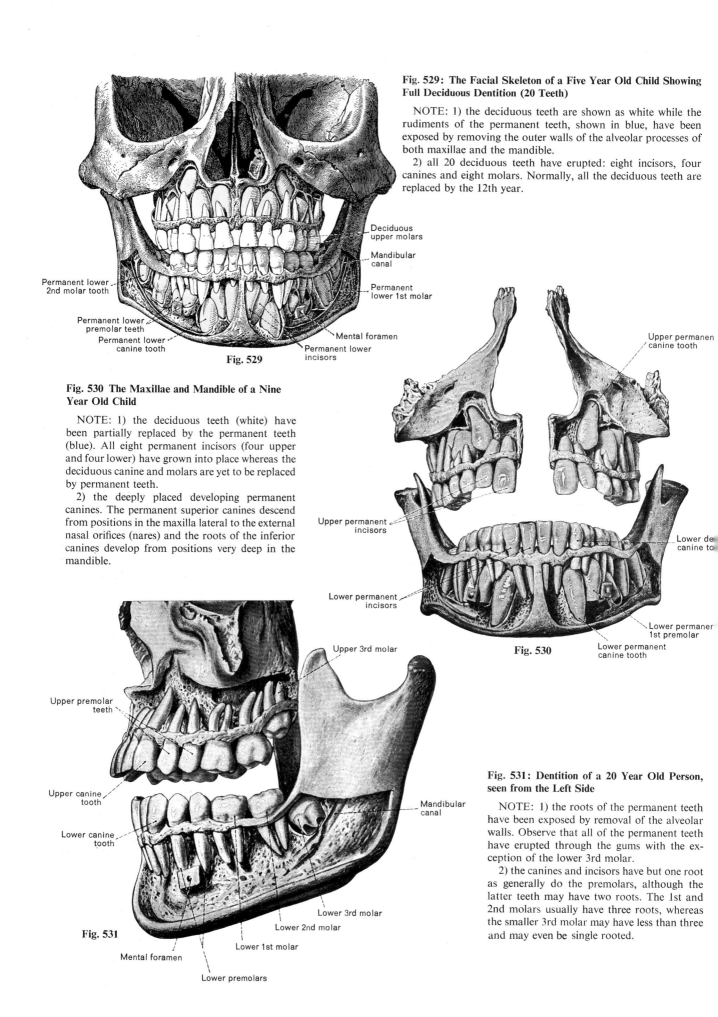

Fig. 529: The Facial Skeleton of a Five Year Old Child Showing Full Deciduous Dentition (20 Teeth)

NOTE: 1) the deciduous teeth are shown as white while the rudiments of the permanent teeth, shown in blue, have been exposed by removing the outer walls of the alveolar processes of both maxillae and the mandible.

2) all 20 deciduous teeth have erupted: eight incisors, four canines and eight molars. Normally, all the deciduous teeth are replaced by the 12th year.

Deciduous upper molars

Mandibular canal

Permanent lower 2nd molar tooth

Permanent lower 1st molar

Permanent lower premolar teeth

Permanent lower canine tooth

Mental foramen

Permanent lower incisors

Fig. 529

Fig. 530 The Maxillae and Mandible of a Nine Year Old Child

NOTE: 1) the deciduous teeth (white) have been partially replaced by the permanent teeth (blue). All eight permanent incisors (four upper and four lower) have grown into place whereas the deciduous canine and molars are yet to be replaced by permanent teeth.

2) the deeply placed developing permanent canines. The permanent superior canines descend from positions in the maxilla lateral to the external nasal orifices (nares) and the roots of the inferior canines develop from positions very deep in the mandible.

Upper permanent canine tooth

Upper permanent incisors

Lower deciduous canine tooth

Lower permanent incisors

Lower permanent 1st premolar

Lower permanent canine tooth

Fig. 530

Upper premolar teeth

Upper 3rd molar

Upper canine tooth

Lower canine tooth

Mandibular canal

Lower 3rd molar

Lower 2nd molar

Lower 1st molar

Mental foramen

Lower premolars

Fig. 531

Fig. 531: Dentition of a 20 Year Old Person, seen from the Left Side

NOTE: 1) the roots of the permanent teeth have been exposed by removal of the alveolar walls. Observe that all of the permanent teeth have erupted through the gums with the exception of the lower 3rd molar.

2) the canines and incisors have but one root as generally do the premolars, although the latter teeth may have two roots. The 1st and 2nd molars usually have three roots, whereas the smaller 3rd molar may have less than three and may even be single rooted.

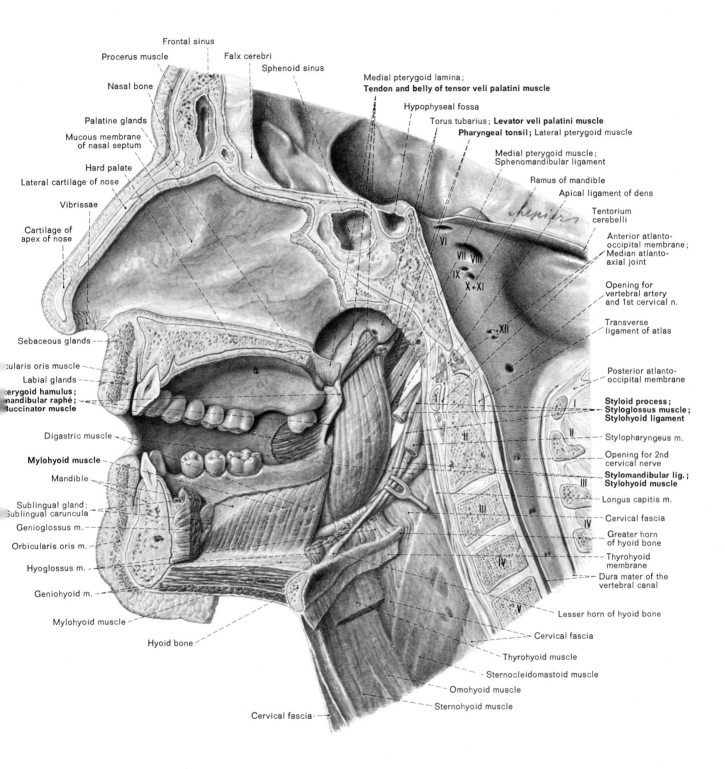

Fig. 532: Paramedian Sagittal View of the Face and Neck

NOTE: 1) this dissection has exposed the right half of the oral cavity and the nasal septum. The mucous membrane has been removed from the floor of the mouth exposing the mylohyoid muscle; the pharyngeal constrictors have also been removed. Observe the pterygomandibular raphé and the buccinator muscle.

2) the tendon of the tensor veli palatini muscle as it turns medially around the pterygoid hamulus. The tendon has been severed at its insertion into the palatine aponeurosis. This muscle tightens the soft palate and, being derived from the first or mandibular branchial arch, it is innervated by the trigeminal nerve.

3) the stylohyoid ligament and the styloglossus and stylopharyngeus muscles which have been cut. These three structures all attach to the styloid process, as do the stylomandibular ligament and the stylohyoid muscles which have not been cut.

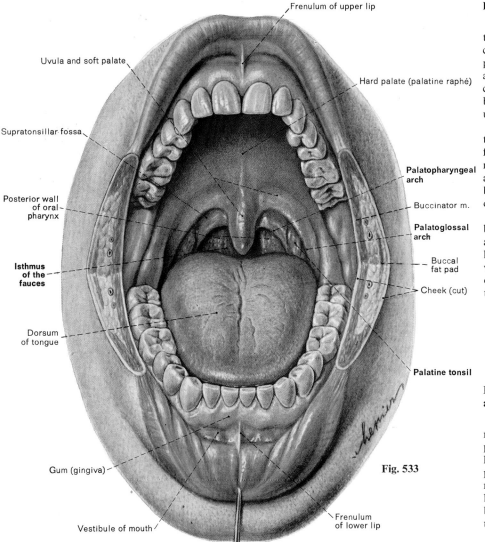

Frenulum of upper lip

Uvula and soft palate

Hard palate (palatine raphé)

Supratonsillar fossa

Palatopharyngeal arch

Posterior wall of oral pharynx

Buccinator m.

Palatoglossal arch

Isthmus of the fauces

Buccal fat pad

Cheek (cut)

Dorsum of tongue

Palatine tonsil

Gum (gingiva)

Fig. 533

Vestibule of mouth

Frenulum of lower lip

Fig. 533: The Oral Cavity

NOTE: 1) the position of the palatine tonsils located on each side of the oral cavity within fossae between the palatoglossal and palatopharyngeal arches. These soft folds are formed by correspondingly named muscles covered by oral mucous membrane (see Figure 535).

2) the passage between the oral cavity and the oral pharynx is called the fauces. This aperture or isthmus commences anteriorly at the palatoglossal arches on each side and is also bounded by the soft palate superiorly and the dorsum of the tongue inferiorly.

3) that portion of the oral cavity between the teeth and the lips anteriorly and between the teeth and cheeks laterally is called the vestibule. The vestibule communicates with the larger oral cavity proper behind the 3rd molar teeth.

Fig. 535: The Palate: Muscular Folds and Glands ▶

NOTE: the oral mucosa has been removed from both the hard and soft palate revealing the palatal musculature, vessels and glands. Observe the palatoglossus and palatopharyngeus muscles along with the greater and lesser palatine nerves and vessels. A branch of lesser palatine artery contributes to the tonsillar blood supply.

Fig. 534: The Lips Viewed from Within the Oral Cavity

NOTE: 1) this dissection demonstrates the muscles of the mouth from within the oral cavity after the oral mucous membrane has been removed. Observe the numerous small labial glands.

2) the contour of the lips as they surround the oral orifice depends on the arrangement of the muscular bundles which interlace at the labial margins. These include the elevators and depressors of the lips and their angles along with the orbicularis oris and buccinator muscles.

3) the fibers of the buccinator muscle converging at the angle of the mouth. Many of these fibers decussate, becoming continuous with the fibers of the orbicularis oris muscle of both the upper and lower lips.

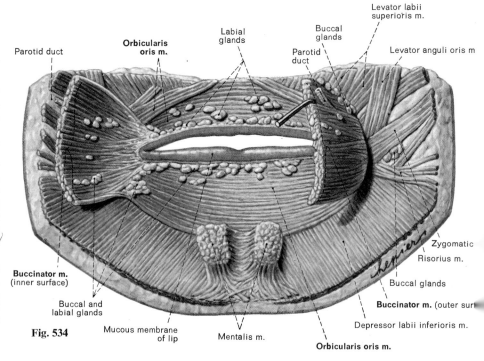

Parotid duct

Orbicularis oris m.

Labial glands

Buccal glands

Parotid duct

Levator labii superioris m.

Levator anguli oris m

Zygomatic

Risorius m.

Buccal glands

Buccinator m. (outer sur

Depressor labii inferioris m.

Buccinator m. (inner surface)

Buccal and labial glands

Mucous membrane of lip

Mentalis m.

Orbicularis oris m.

Fig. 534

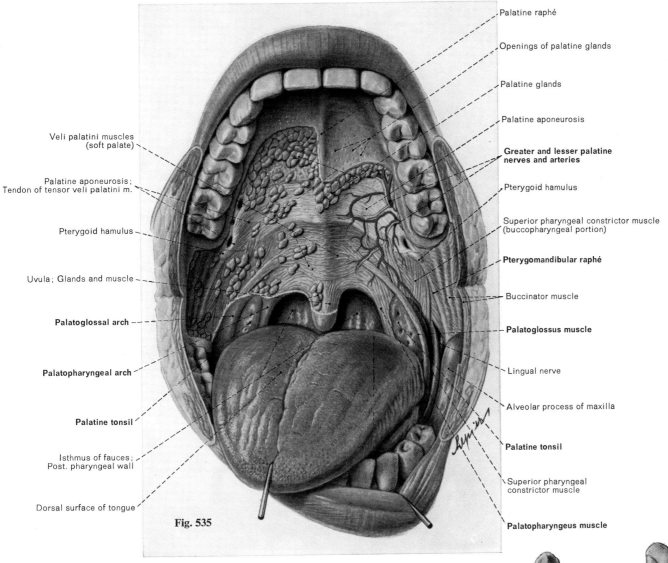

Palatine raphé

Openings of palatine glands

Palatine glands

Palatine aponeurosis

Greater and lesser palatine nerves and arteries

Pterygoid hamulus

Superior pharyngeal constrictor muscle (buccopharyngeal portion)

Pterygomandibular raphé

Buccinator muscle

Palatoglossus muscle

Lingual nerve

Alveolar process of maxilla

Palatine tonsil

Superior pharyngeal constrictor muscle

Palatopharyngeus muscle

Veli palatini muscles (soft palate)

Palatine aponeurosis; Tendon of tensor veli palatini m.

Pterygoid hamulus

Uvula; Glands and muscle

Palatoglossal arch

Palatopharyngeal arch

Palatine tonsil

Isthmus of fauces; Post. pharyngeal wall

Dorsal surface of tongue

Fig. 535

Fig. 536: The Submandibular and Sublingual Glands

NOTE: 1) with the tongue removed, and the genioglossus and geniohyoid muscles cut anteriorly, the submandibular and sublingual glands have been exposed and their relationship to the inner aspect of the right mandible demonstrated.

2) the submandibular duct which measures about 2 inches in length and which courses anteriorly between the sublingual gland and the genioglossus muscle (which is cut). This duct opens into the floor of the mouth on each side of the frenulum of the tongue (sublingual caruncle).

3) the sublingual gland lies along the lingual surface of the body of the mandible and its 10 to 20 small ducts open along the sublingual fold. The most anterior duct frequently joins the submandibular duct at its orifice.

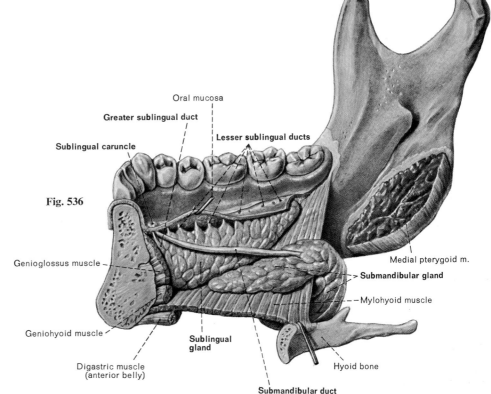

Oral mucosa

Greater sublingual duct

Lesser sublingual ducts

Sublingual caruncle

Fig. 536

Genioglossus muscle

Medial pterygoid m.

Submandibular gland

Mylohyoid muscle

Geniohyoid muscle

Sublingual gland

Digastric muscle (anterior belly)

Hyoid bone

Submandibular duct

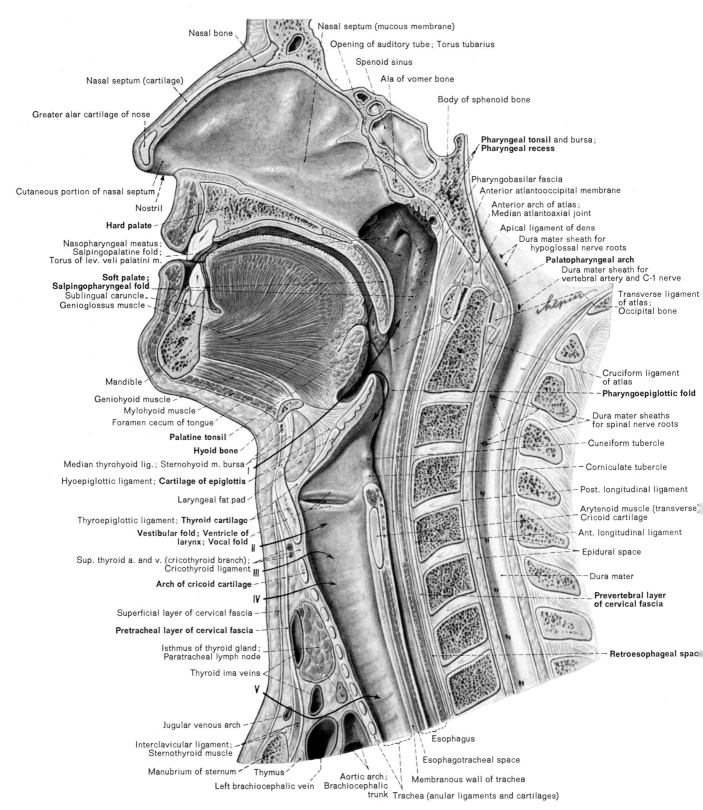

Nasal bone

Nasal septum (mucous membrane)

Opening of auditory tube; Torus tubarius

Spenoid sinus

Ala of vomer bone

Body of sphenoid bone

Nasal septum (cartilage)

Greater alar cartilage of nose

Pharyngeal tonsil and bursa;
Pharyngeal recess

Pharyngobasilar fascia
Anterior atlantooccipital membrane

Anterior arch of atlas;
Median atlantoaxial joint

Apical ligament of dens
Dura mater sheath for
hypoglossal nerve roots

Palatopharyngeal arch
Dura mater sheath for
vertebral artery and C-1 nerve

Transverse ligament
of atlas;
Occipital bone

Cutaneous portion of nasal septum

Nostril

Hard palate

Nasopharyngeal meatus;
Salpingopalatine fold;
Torus of lev. veli palatini m.

**Soft palate;
Salpingopharyngeal fold**
Sublingual caruncle
Genioglossus muscle

Mandible

Geniohyoid muscle
Mylohyoid muscle
Foramen cecum of tongue

Palatine tonsil

Hyoid bone

Median thyrohyoid lig.; Sternohyoid m. bursa

Hyoepiglottic ligament; **Cartilage of epiglottis**

Laryngeal fat pad

Thyroepiglottic ligament; **Thyroid cartilage**

**Vestibular fold; Ventricle of
larynx; Vocal fold** II

Sup. thyroid a. and v. (cricothyroid branch);
Cricothyroid ligament III

Arch of cricoid cartilage

IV

Superficial layer of cervical fascia

Pretracheal layer of cervical fascia

Isthmus of thyroid gland;
Paratracheal lymph node

Thyroid ima veins

V

Jugular venous arch

Interclavicular ligament;
Sternothyroid muscle

Manubrium of sternum — Thymus
Left brachiocephalic vein
Aortic arch;
Brachiocephalic
trunk
Esophagus
Esophagotracheal space
Membranous wall of trachea
Trachea (anular ligaments and cartilages)

Cruciform ligament
of atlas
Pharyngoepiglottic fold

Dura mater sheaths
for spinal nerve roots

Cuneiform tubercle

Corniculate tubercle

Post. longitudinal ligament

Arytenoid muscle (transverse)
Cricoid cartilage

Ant. longitudinal ligament

Epidural space

Dura mater

**Prevertebral layer
of cervical fascia**

Retroesophageal spac

Fig. 537: The Viscera of the Head and Neck: Mid-sagittal Section

NOTE: 1) the closed oral cavity is occupied principally by the tongue. Observe that the posterior aspect of the oral cavity opens into the oropharanyx. Superiorly, the posterior nasal cavities are continuous with the nasopharynx, whereas inferiorly the laryngeal portion of the pharynx (between the levels of the epiglottis and cricoid cartilages) opens into the larynx.

2) the pharynx continues inferiorly as the esophagus while the larynx becomes the trachea below the level of the cricoid cartilage.

3) during the act of swallowing (deglutition), as food is directed toward the posterior part of the oral cavity, the soft palate is both elevated and tensed (by the levator and tensor veli palatini muscles) and directed toward the posterior wall of the pharynx, thereby closing off the nasopharynx. Simultaneously the larynx is drawn superiorly toward the epiglottis to the level of the hyoid bone and the pharynx also ascends. This action closes the laryngeal orifice, thereby preventing food from entering the larynx.

4) arrows I to V: surgical approaches to pharynx, larynx and trachea.

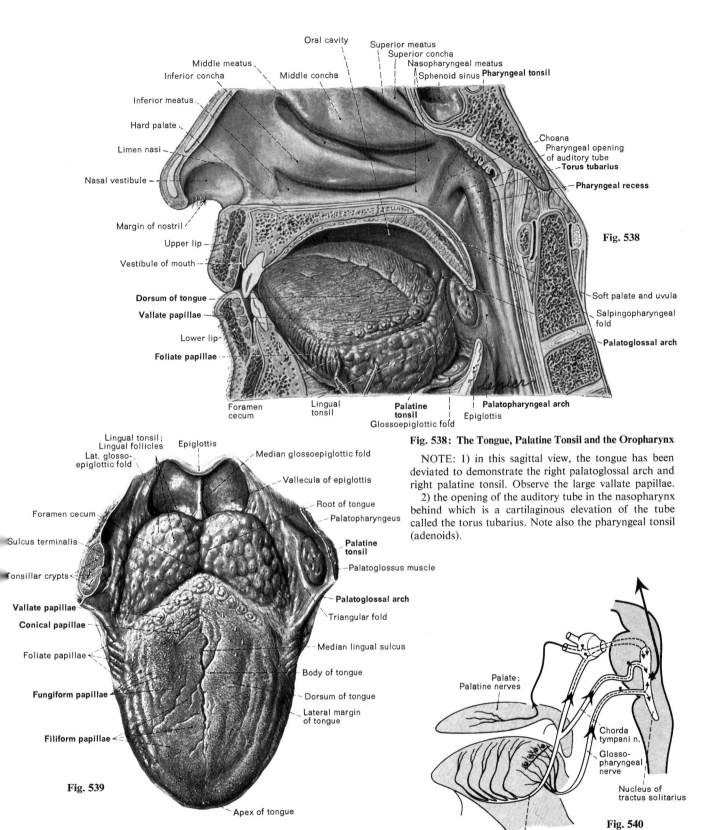

Fig. 538: The Tongue, Palatine Tonsil and the Oropharynx

NOTE: 1) in this sagittal view, the tongue has been deviated to demonstrate the right palatoglossal arch and right palatine tonsil. Observe the large vallate papillae.

2) the opening of the auditory tube in the nasopharynx behind which is a cartilaginous elevation of the tube called the torus tubarius. Note also the pharyngeal tonsil (adenoids).

Fig. 539: Dorsal Surface of the Tongue

NOTE: 1) the dorsum of the tongue is marked by numerous elevations called papillae. These serve as receptor sites for the special sense of taste. Observe the inverted V-shaped group of large vallate papillae.

2) the fungiform papillae which are found principally at the sides and apex of the tongue. These are relatively large and round and have a deep red color.

3) the filiform (conical) papillae. These are very small and generally arranged in rows which course parallel to the vallate papillae.

Fig. 540: The Taste Pathways: Peripheral Nerves

Note that the sense of taste is transmitted to the brain along several peripheral nerves: a) chorda tympani nerve: anterior part of tongue; b) glossopharyngeal nerve: vallate papillae and posterior or pharyngeal part of tongue; c) middle and posterior palatine nerves: palatal region; d) vagus nerve (not shown): epiglottis and the most posterior part of the tongue.

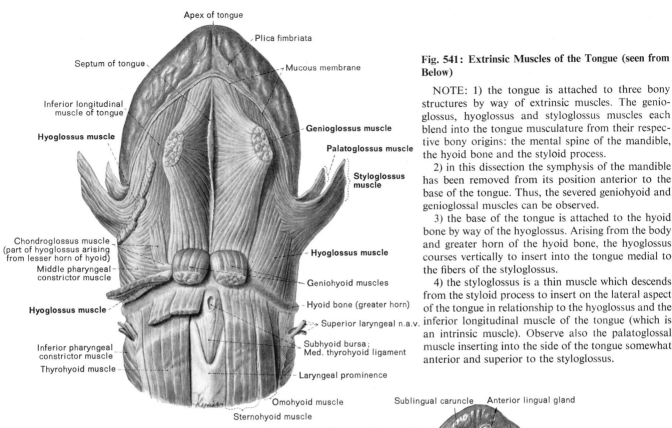

Apex of tongue

Plica fimbriata

Septum of tongue

Mucous membrane

Inferior longitudinal muscle of tongue

Hyoglossus muscle

Genioglossus muscle

Palatoglossus muscle

Styloglossus muscle

Chondroglossus muscle (part of hyoglossus arising from lesser horn of hyoid)

Middle pharyngeal constrictor muscle

Hyoglossus muscle

Hyoglossus muscle

Geniohyoid muscles

Hyoid bone (greater horn)

Superior laryngeal n.a.v.

Subhyoid bursa; Med. thyrohyoid ligament

Laryngeal prominence

Inferior pharyngeal constrictor muscle

Thyrohyoid muscle

Omohyoid muscle

Sternohyoid muscle

Fig. 541: Extrinsic Muscles of the Tongue (seen from Below)

NOTE: 1) the tongue is attached to three bony structures by way of extrinsic muscles. The genioglossus, hyoglossus and styloglossus muscles each blend into the tongue musculature from their respective bony origins: the mental spine of the mandible, the hyoid bone and the styloid process.

2) in this dissection the symphysis of the mandible has been removed from its position anterior to the base of the tongue. Thus, the severed geniohyoid and genioglossal muscles can be observed.

3) the base of the tongue is attached to the hyoid bone by way of the hyoglossus. Arising from the body and greater horn of the hyoid bone, the hyoglossus courses vertically to insert into the tongue medial to the fibers of the styloglossus.

4) the styloglossus is a thin muscle which descends from the styloid process to insert on the lateral aspect of the tongue in relationship to the hyoglossus and the inferior longitudinal muscle of the tongue (which is an intrinsic muscle). Observe also the palatoglossal muscle inserting into the side of the tongue somewhat anterior and superior to the styloglossus.

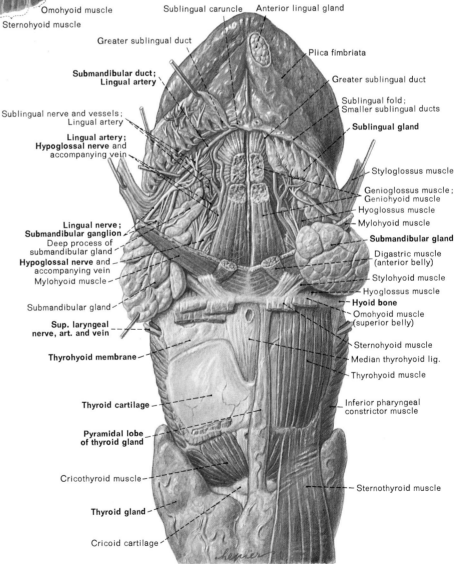

Sublingual caruncle

Anterior lingual gland

Greater sublingual duct

Plica fimbriata

Submandibular duct; Lingual artery

Greater sublingual duct

Sublingual fold; Smaller sublingual ducts

Sublingual nerve and vessels; Lingual artery

Sublingual gland

Lingual artery; Hypoglossal nerve and accompanying vein

Styloglossus muscle

Genioglossus muscle; Geniohyoid muscle

Hyoglossus muscle

Mylohyoid muscle

Lingual nerve; Submandibular ganglion

Submandibular gland

Deep process of submandibular gland

Digastric muscle (anterior belly)

Hypoglossal nerve and accompanying vein

Stylohyoid muscle

Mylohyoid muscle

Hyoglossus muscle

Submandibular gland

Hyoid bone

Omohyoid muscle (superior belly)

Sup. laryngeal nerve, art. and vein

Sternohyoid muscle

Median thyrohyoid lig.

Thyrohyoid muscle

Thyrohyoid membrane

Inferior pharyngeal constrictor muscle

Thyroid cartilage

Pyramidal lobe of thyroid gland

Cricothyroid muscle

Sternothyroid muscle

Thyroid gland

Cricoid cartilage

Fig. 542: The Inferior Aspect of the Tongue and Other Oral and Cervical Viscera

NOTE: 1) with the extrinsic muscles of the tongue severed and the mandible removed, the sublingual and submandibular glands are observed in their suprahyoid location. On the left side of the figure (right side of the tongue), these glands have been pulled aside to expose the lingual nerve and submandibular duct, the hypoglossal nerve and vein, and the lingual artery and its sublingual branch.

2) the thyroid cartilage, the thyrohyoid membrane and the pyramidal lobe of the larger thyroid gland (seen below). Observe the internal branch of the superior laryngeal nerve, artery and vein as they pierce the thyrohyoid membrane to enter the larynx.

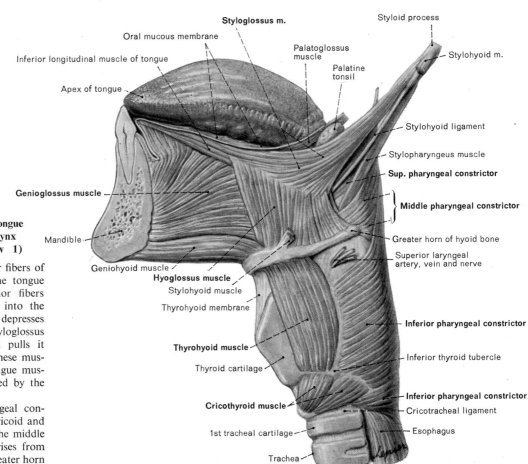

Fig. 543: The Extrinsic Tongue Muscles: the External Larynx and Pharynx (Lateral View 1)

NOTE: 1) the posterior fibers of the genioglossus draw the tongue forward while its anterior fibers retract the tongue back into the mouth. The hyoglossus depresses the tongue while the styloglossus elevates the tongue and pulls it backward. All three of these muscles and the intrinsic tongue muscles as well are innervated by the hypoglossal nerve.

2) the inferior pharyngeal constrictor arises from the cricoid and thyroid cartilages while the middle pharyngeal constrictor arises from the entire length of the greater horn of the hyoid bone, from the stylohyoid ligament and from the lesser horn (seen in Fig. 544).

3) the thyrohyoid muscle covering the lateral surface of the thyroid cartilage and the two parts of the cricothyroid muscle.

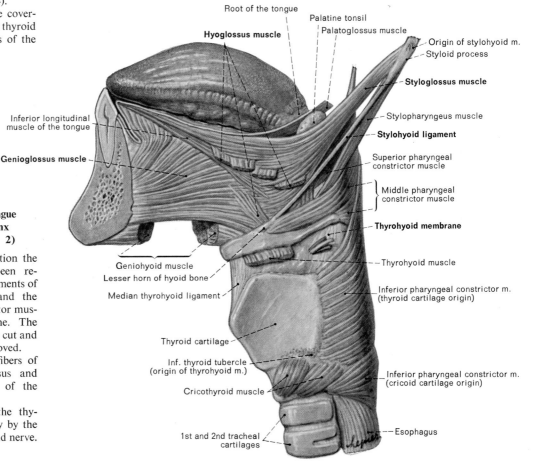

Fig. 544: The Extrinsic Tongue Muscles: the External Larynx and Pharynx (Lateral View 2)

NOTE: 1) in this dissection the hyoglossus muscle has been removed, revealing the attachments of the stylohyoid ligament and the middle pharyngeal constrictor muscle along the hyoid bone. The geniohyoid muscle has been cut and the thyrohyoid muscle removed.

2) the blending of the fibers of the styloglossus, hyoglossus and genioglossus at the base of the tongue.

3) the penetration of the thyrohyoid membrane laterally by the internal laryngeal vessels and nerve.

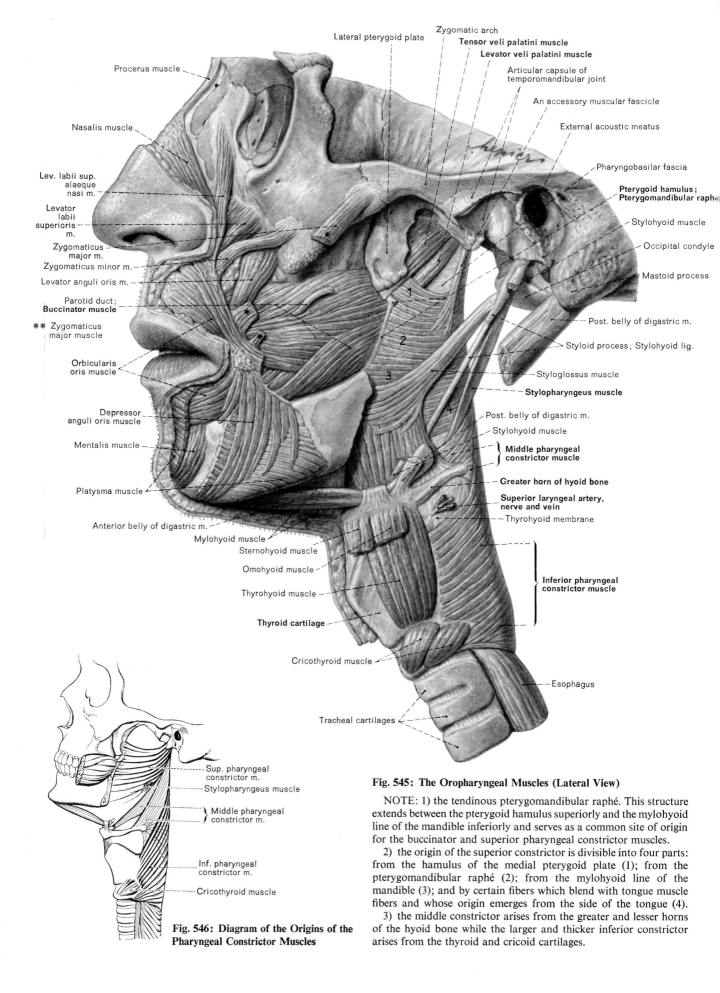

Procerus muscle

Nasalis muscle

Lev. labii sup. alaeque nasi m.

Levator labii superioris m.

Zygomaticus major m.

Zygomaticus minor m.

Levator anguli oris m.

Parotid duct;
Buccinator muscle

✳✳ Zygomaticus major muscle

Orbicularis oris muscle

Depressor anguli oris muscle

Mentalis muscle

Platysma muscle

Anterior belly of digastric m.

Mylohyoid muscle

Sternohyoid muscle

Omohyoid muscle

Thyrohyoid muscle

Thyroid cartilage

Cricothyroid muscle

Tracheal cartilages

Lateral pterygoid plate

Zygomatic arch

Tensor veli palatini muscle

Levator veli palatini muscle

Articular capsule of temporomandibular joint

An accessory muscular fascicle

External acoustic meatus

Pharyngobasilar fascia

Pterygoid hamulus; Pterygomandibular raphe

Stylohyoid muscle

Occipital condyle

Mastoid process

Post. belly of digastric m.

Styloid process; Stylohyoid lig.

Styloglossus muscle

Stylopharyngeus muscle

Post. belly of digastric m.

Stylohyoid muscle

Middle pharyngeal constrictor muscle

Greater horn of hyoid bone

Superior laryngeal artery, nerve and vein

Thyrohyoid membrane

Inferior pharyngeal constrictor muscle

Esophagus

Fig. 545: The Oropharyngeal Muscles (Lateral View)

NOTE: 1) the tendinous pterygomandibular raphé. This structure extends between the pterygoid hamulus superiorly and the mylohyoid line of the mandible inferiorly and serves as a common site of origin for the buccinator and superior pharyngeal constrictor muscles.

2) the origin of the superior constrictor is divisible into four parts: from the hamulus of the medial pterygoid plate (1); from the pterygomandibular raphé (2); from the mylohyoid line of the mandible (3); and by certain fibers which blend with tongue muscle fibers and whose origin emerges from the side of the tongue (4).

3) the middle constrictor arises from the greater and lesser horns of the hyoid bone while the larger and thicker inferior constrictor arises from the thyroid and cricoid cartilages.

Sup. pharyngeal constrictor m.

Stylopharyngeus muscle

Middle pharyngeal constrictor m.

Inf. pharyngeal constrictor m.

Cricothyroid muscle

Fig. 546: Diagram of the Origins of the Pharyngeal Constrictor Muscles

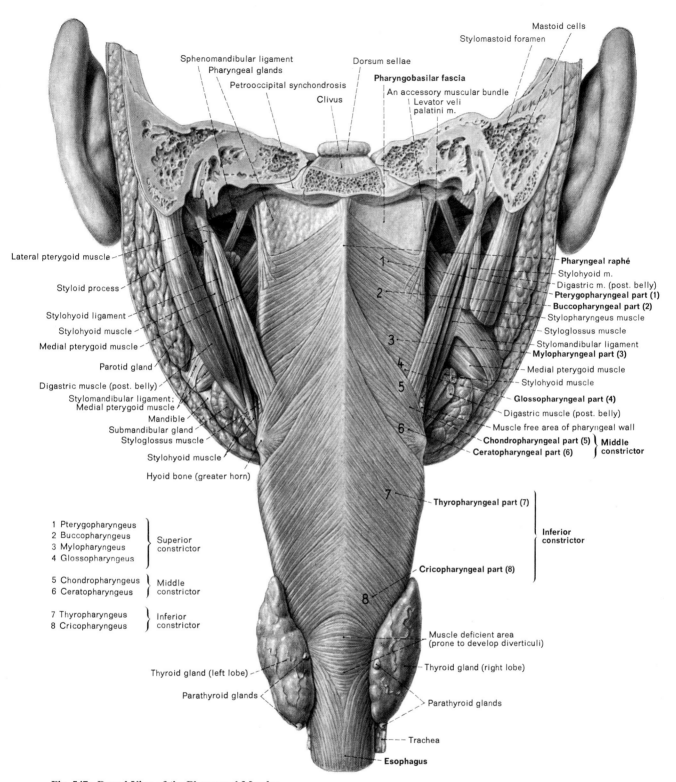

Mastoid cells
Stylomastoid foramen
Sphenomandibular ligament
Pharyngeal glands
Dorsum sellae
Petrooccipital synchondrosis
Pharyngobasilar fascia
Clivus
An accessory muscular bundle
Levator veli palatini m.

Lateral pterygoid muscle
Styloid process
Stylohyoid ligament
Stylohyoid muscle
Medial pterygoid muscle
Parotid gland
Digastric muscle (post. belly)
Stylomandibular ligament;
Medial pterygoid muscle
Mandible
Submandibular gland
Styloglossus muscle
Stylohyoid muscle
Hyoid bone (greater horn)

Pharyngeal raphé
Stylohyoid m.
Digastric m. (post. belly)
Pterygopharyngeal part (1)
Buccopharyngeal part (2)
Stylopharyngeus muscle
Styloglossus muscle
Stylomandibular ligament
Mylopharyngeal part (3)
Medial pterygoid muscle
Stylohyoid muscle
Glossopharyngeal part (4)
Digastric muscle (post. belly)
Muscle free area of pharyngeal wall
Chondropharyngeal part (5) } **Middle**
Ceratopharyngeal part (6) } **constrictor**

Thyropharyngeal part (7) } **Inferior constrictor**

Cricopharyngeal part (8)

1 Pterygopharyngeus
2 Buccopharyngeus   } Superior
3 Mylopharyngeus   constrictor
4 Glossopharyngeus

5 Chondropharyngeus } Middle
6 Ceratopharyngeus   constrictor

7 Thyropharyngeus   } Inferior
8 Cricopharyngeus   constrictor

Muscle deficient area
(prone to develop diverticuli)

Thyroid gland (left lobe)
Parathyroid glands

Thyroid gland (right lobe)
Parathyroid glands

Trachea

Esophagus

Fig. 547: Dorsal View of the Pharyngeal Muscles

NOTE: 1) this posterior view of the pharynx was achieved by making a frontal transection through the petrous and mastoid portions of the temporal bones and through the body of the occipital bone. The styloid processes and their muscular attachments have been left intact.

2) the arrangement of the divisions of the pharyngeal constrictors. Their muscle fibers arise laterally to insert in a posterior median pharyngeal raphé. The superior constrictor is divisible into four parts while the middle and inferior constrictor are each divisible into two. Above the superior constrictor, observe the fibrous pharyngobasilar fascia which attaches to the basal portion of the occipital bone and to the temporal bones. Below the inferior constrictor, the pharynx is continuous with the muscular esophagus.

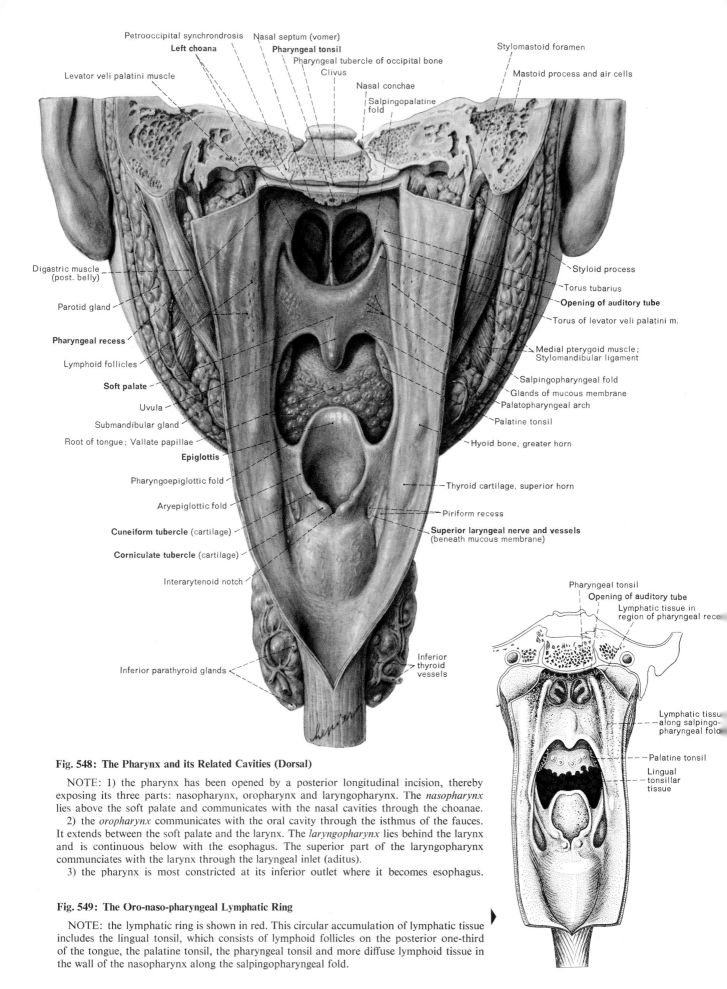

Petrooccipital synchrondrosis
Nasal septum (vomer)
Left choana
Pharyngeal tonsil
Pharyngeal tubercle of occipital bone
Clivus
Nasal conchae
Salpingopalatine fold
Levator veli palatini muscle
Stylomastoid foramen
Mastoid process and air cells

Digastric muscle (post. belly)
Parotid gland
Pharyngeal recess
Lymphoid follicles
Soft palate
Uvula
Submandibular gland
Root of tongue; Vallate papillae
Epiglottis
Pharyngoepiglottic fold
Aryepiglottic fold
Cuneiform tubercle (cartilage)
Corniculate tubercle (cartilage)
Interarytenoid notch
Inferior parathyroid glands

Styloid process
Torus tubarius
Opening of auditory tube
Torus of levator veli palatini m.
Medial pterygoid muscle; Stylomandibular ligament
Salpingopharyngeal fold
Glands of mucous membrane
Palatopharyngeal arch
Palatine tonsil
Hyoid bone, greater horn
Thyroid cartilage, superior horn
Piriform recess
Superior laryngeal nerve and vessels (beneath mucous membrane)
Inferior thyroid vessels

Pharyngeal tonsil
Opening of auditory tube
Lymphatic tissue in region of pharyngeal rece
Lymphatic tissu along salpingo-pharyngeal fol
Palatine tonsil
Lingual tonsillar tissue

Fig. 548: The Pharynx and its Related Cavities (Dorsal)

NOTE: 1) the pharynx has been opened by a posterior longitudinal incision, thereby exposing its three parts: nasopharynx, oropharynx and laryngopharynx. The *nasopharynx* lies above the soft palate and communicates with the nasal cavities through the choanae.

2) the *oropharynx* communicates with the oral cavity through the isthmus of the fauces. It extends between the soft palate and the larynx. The *laryngopharynx* lies behind the larynx and is continuous below with the esophagus. The superior part of the laryngopharynx communicates with the larynx through the laryngeal inlet (aditus).

3) the pharynx is most constricted at its inferior outlet where it becomes esophagus.

Fig. 549: The Oro-naso-pharyngeal Lymphatic Ring

NOTE: the lymphatic ring is shown in red. This circular accumulation of lymphatic tissue includes the lingual tonsil, which consists of lymphoid follicles on the posterior one-third of the tongue, the palatine tonsil, the pharyngeal tonsil and more diffuse lymphoid tissue in the wall of the nasopharynx along the salpingopharyngeal fold.

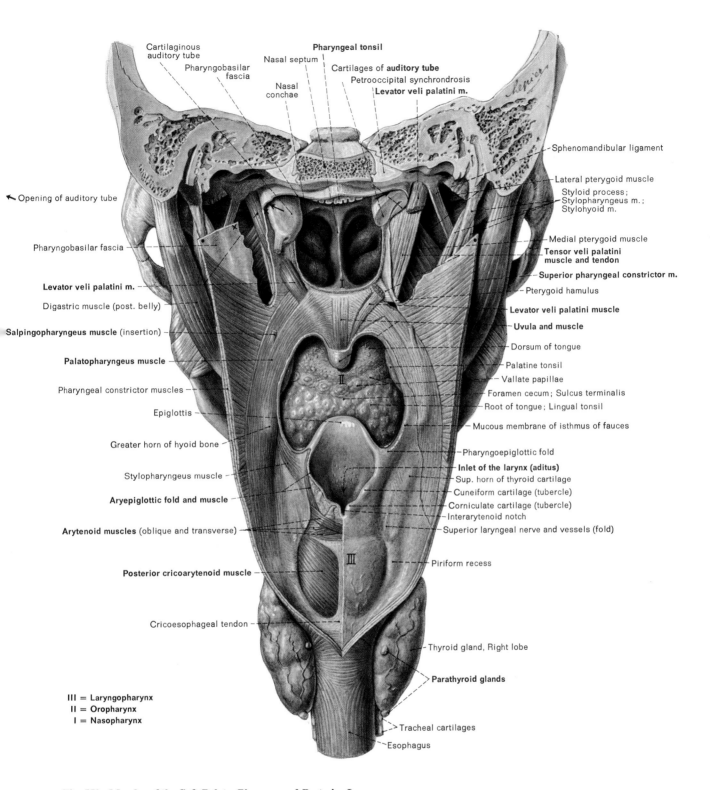

Fig. 550: Muscles of the Soft Palate, Pharynx, and Posterior Larynx

NOTE: 1) the dissection in this figure is similar to that in Figure 548. The pharynx has been opened dorsally by a midline incision and the mucous membrane has been removed from the soft palate, pharynx and the left posterior larynx. On the right side, a portion of the levator veli palatini muscle has been removed in order to expose the adjacent belly and tendon of the tensor veli palatini muscle.

2) the muscles of the soft palate. Both the muscle of the uvula and the levator veli palatini muscle are innervated by the vagus and accessory nerve contributions to the pharyngeal plexus, whereas the tensor veli palatini muscle is innervated by the mandibular division of the trigeminal nerve.

3) the palatopharyngeus muscle arising by two fascicles from the soft palate. The muscle fibers of these two fascicles arise posterior and anterior to the insertion of the levator veli palatini muscle. The fascicles descend and merge and then insert into the posterior border of the thyroid cartilage and onto the adjacent pharyngeal wall.

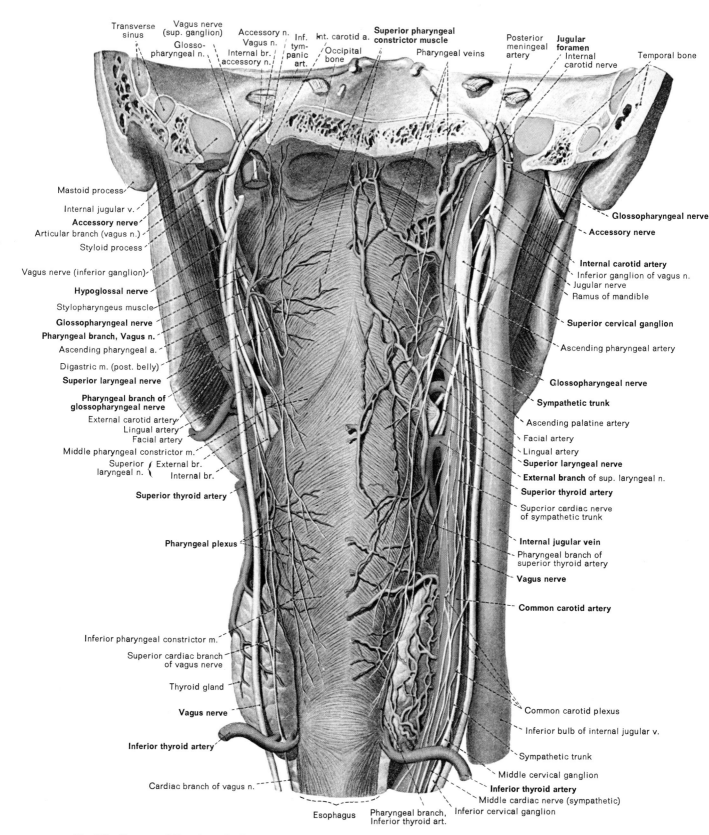

Fig. 551: Nerves and Vessels on the Dorsal and Lateral Walls of the Pharynx

NOTE: 1) the head has been split longitudinally. The pharynx, larynx and facial structures were separated from the vertebral column and its associated muscles. This posterior view of the pharynx also shows the large nerves and blood vessels which course through the neck. On the right side, observe the carotid artery, internal jugular vein, vagus nerve and sympathetic trunk.

2) on the left side, the glossopharyngeal and hypoglossal nerves were exposed by the removal of the carotid arteries and internal jugular vein. Along with the jugular vein, the jugular foramen transmits the 9th, 10th and 11th cranial nerves.

3) the thyroid gland and its superior and inferior thyroid arteries. The superior and middle thyroid veins drain into the internal jugular vein while the inferior thyroid veins (not shown) usually drain into the left brachiocephalic vein.

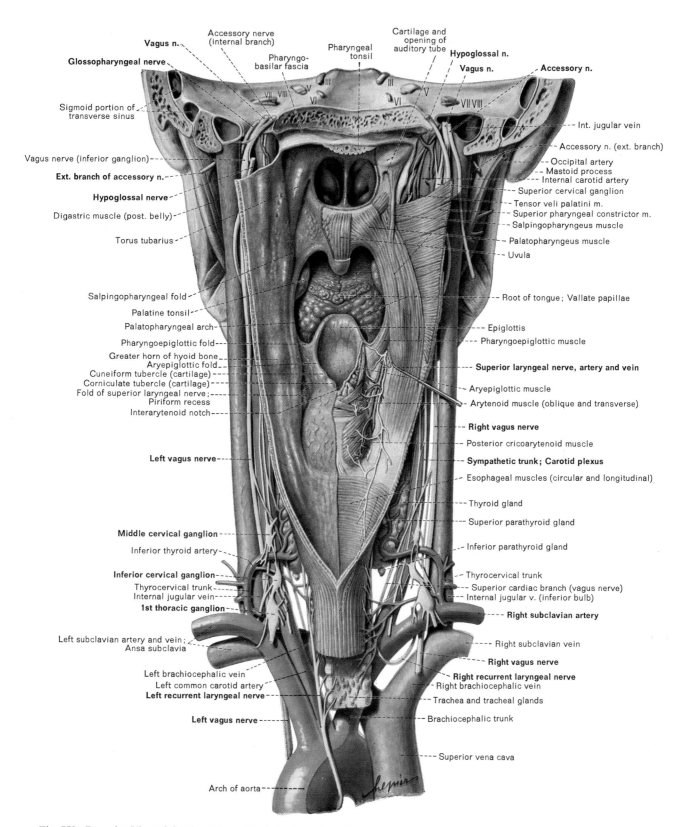

Vagus n.
Accessory nerve (internal branch)
Pharyngo-basilar fascia
Pharyngeal tonsil
Cartilage and opening of auditory tube
Hypoglossal n.
Vagus n.
Accessory n.

Glossopharyngeal nerve

Sigmoid portion of transverse sinus

Vagus nerve (inferior ganglion)

Ext. branch of accessory n.

Hypoglossal nerve

Digastric muscle (post. belly)

Torus tubarius

Salpingopharyngeal fold

Palatine tonsil

Palatopharyngeal arch

Pharyngoepiglottic fold

Greater horn of hyoid bone
Aryepiglottic fold
Cuneiform tubercle (cartilage)
Corniculate tubercle (cartilage)
Fold of superior laryngeal nerve;
Piriform recess
Interarytenoid notch

Left vagus nerve

Middle cervical ganglion

Inferior thyroid artery

Inferior cervical ganglion
Thyrocervical trunk
Internal jugular vein
1st thoracic ganglion

Left subclavian artery and vein;
Ansa subclavia

Left brachiocephalic vein
Left common carotid artery
Left recurrent laryngeal nerve

Left vagus nerve

Arch of aorta

Int. jugular vein

Accessory n. (ext. branch)

Occipital artery
Mastoid process
Internal carotid artery
Superior cervical ganglion

Tensor veli palatini m.
Superior pharyngeal constrictor m.
Salpingopharyngeus muscle
Palatopharyngeus muscle
Uvula

Root of tongue; Vallate papillae

Epiglottis

Pharyngoepiglottic muscle

Superior laryngeal nerve, artery and vein

Aryepiglottic muscle
Arytenoid muscle (oblique and transverse)

Right vagus nerve

Posterior cricoarytenoid muscle

Sympathetic trunk; Carotid plexus

Esophageal muscles (circular and longitudinal)

Thyroid gland

Superior parathyroid gland

Inferior parathyroid gland

Thyrocervical trunk
Superior cardiac branch (vagus nerve)
Internal jugular v. (inferior bulb)

Right subclavian artery

Right subclavian vein

Right vagus nerve
Right recurrent laryngeal nerve
Right brachiocephalic vein
Trachea and tracheal glands

Brachiocephalic trunk

Superior vena cava

Fig. 552: Posterior View of Cervical Viscera: Muscles, Vessels and Nerves

NOTE: 1) in this posterior view of the vessels and nerves of the neck, the dorsal wall of the pharynx has been opened longitudinally, revealing the nasal, oral and laryngeal orifices which communicate with the pharynx. Observe the superior laryngeal artery, vein and nerve entering the larynx from above.

2) the recurrent laryngeal nerves ascending from the thorax to the larynx in the tracheoesophageal groove. On the left side, the recurrent laryngeal nerve courses around the arch of the aorta to reach this groove while on the right side the recurrent laryngeal nerve curves around the subclavian artery.

3) the inferior cervical ganglion (at the level of 7th cervical vertebra). This ganglion is fused with the 1st thoracic sympathetic ganglion in about 80% of cases. The fused 1st thoracic and inferior cervical ganglion is called the stellate ganglion.

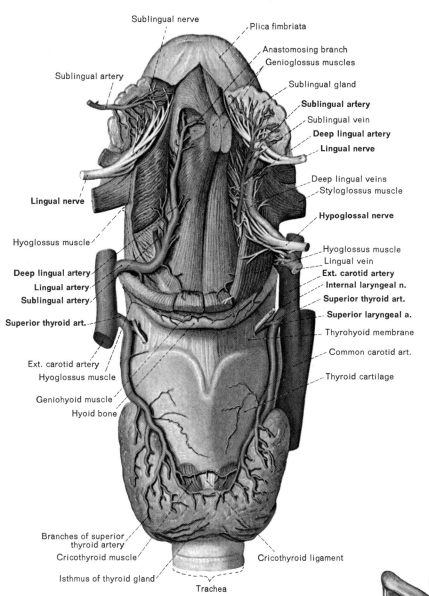

Sublingual nerve
Plica fimbriata
Anastomosing branch
Genioglossus muscles
Sublingual artery
Sublingual gland
Sublingual artery
Sublingual vein
Deep lingual artery
Lingual nerve
Deep lingual veins
Styloglossus muscle
Hypoglossal nerve
Hyoglossus muscle
Lingual vein
Ext. carotid artery
Internal laryngeal n.
Superior thyroid art.
Superior laryngeal a.
Thyrohyoid membrane
Common carotid art.
Thyroid cartilage

Sublingual artery
Lingual nerve
Hyoglossus muscle
Deep lingual artery
Lingual artery
Sublingual artery
Superior thyroid art.
Ext. carotid artery
Hyoglossus muscle
Geniohyoid muscle
Hyoid bone

Branches of superior thyroid artery
Cricothyroid muscle
Isthmus of thyroid gland
Cricothyroid ligament
Trachea

Fig. 553: Ventral View of Larynx, Tongue and Thyroid Gland: Vessels and Nerves

NOTE: 1) the superior thyroid arteries descending to the thyroid gland. In their course they give off the superior laryngeal arteries which penetrate the thyrohyoid membrane to gain entrance to the interior of the larynx, accompanied by the internal laryngeal branch of the superior laryngeal nerve. Observe also the cranial and medial course of the lingual artery deep to the hyoglossus muscle and its suprahyoid, sublingual and deep lingual branches.

2) the lingual nerves as they enter the tongue to supply its anterior two-thirds with general sensation. The motor nerve to the tongue is the hypoglossal and it is seen coursing along with accompanying veins (venae comitantes). The hypoglossal nerve enters the base of the tongue just above the hyoid bone passing anteriorly across the external carotid and lingual arteries.

Fig. 554: The Cartilages and Ligaments of the Larynx (Ventral View)

NOTE: 1) the laryngeal cartilages comprise the skeletal framework of the larynx and they are interconnected by ligaments and membranes. There are *three larger unpaired* cartilages, the cricoid, thyroid and epiglottis and *three sets of paired* cartilages, the arytenoid, cuneiform and corniculate. In this anterior view the unpaired cricoid, thyroid and epiglottis cartilages are all visible.

2) the thyrohyoid membrane and the centrally located thyrohyoid ligament. Attached at the cranial border of the thyroid cartilage, this membrane stretches across the posterior surfaces of the greater horns of the hyoid bone. The medial thyrohyoid ligament extends from the thyroid notch to the body of the hyoid bone. The membrane is pierced by the superior laryngeal vessels and the internal laryngeal nerve.

3) the cricothyroid ligament attaching the contiguous margins of the cricoid and thyroid cartilages. This is a strong ligament and its lateral portions underlie the cricothyroid muscles. Below, the cricotracheal ligament connects the inferior margin of the cricoid cartilage with the first tracheal ring.

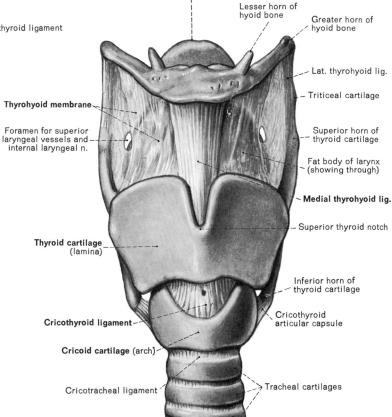

Epiglottis
Lesser horn of hyoid bone
Greater horn of hyoid bone
Thyrohyoid membrane
Lat. thyrohyoid lig.
Triticeal cartilage
Foramen for superior laryngeal vessels and internal laryngeal n.
Superior horn of thyroid cartilage
Fat body of larynx (showing through)
Medial thyrohyoid lig.
Superior thyroid notch
Thyroid cartilage (lamina)
Inferior horn of thyroid cartilage
Cricothyroid articular capsule
Cricothyroid ligament
Cricoid cartilage (arch)
Cricotracheal ligament
Tracheal cartilages

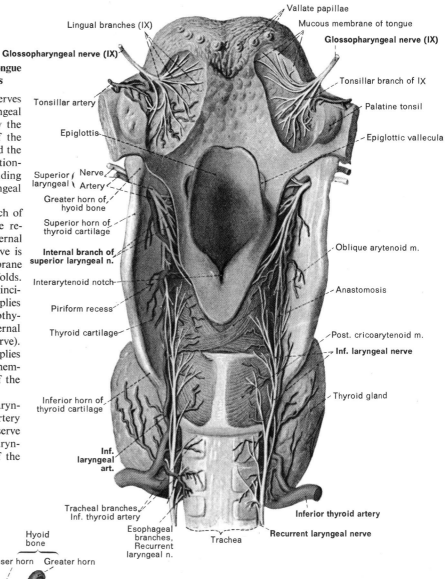

Fig. 555: Dorsal View of Larynx, Tongue and Thyroid Gland: Vessels and Nerves

NOTE: 1) the glossopharyngeal nerves (IX) as they enter the root or pharyngeal part of the tongue in order to supply the posterior one-third of the surface of the tongue with both general sensation and the special sense of taste. Observe the relationship of the tonsillar branch of the ascending palatine artery with the glossopharyngeal nerve.

2) the courses of the internal branch of the superior laryngeal nerve and the recurrent laryngeal nerve. The internal branch of the superior laryngeal nerve is sensory to the laryngeal mucous membrane as far down as the level of the vocal folds. The recurrent laryngeal nerve is the principal motor nerve of the larynx and supplies all laryngeal muscles except the cricothyroid (which is supplied by the external branch of the superior laryngeal nerve). Additionally, the recurrent nerve supplies sensory innervation to the mucous membrane of the larynx below the level of the vocal folds.

3) the relationships of recurrent laryngeal nerves to the inferior thyroid artery and its inferior laryngeal branches. Observe also the proximity of the recurrent laryngeal nerves to the posterior aspect of the thyroid glands.

Labels for Fig. 555 (left to right, top to bottom): Lingual branches (IX); Glossopharyngeal nerve (IX); Vallate papillae; Mucous membrane of tongue; Glossopharyngeal nerve (IX); Tonsillar artery; Tonsillar branch of IX; Palatine tonsil; Epiglottis; Epiglottic vallecula; Superior laryngeal Nerve, Artery; Greater horn of hyoid bone; Superior horn of thyroid cartilage; Internal branch of superior laryngeal n.; Oblique arytenoid m.; Interarytenoid notch; Anastomosis; Piriform recess; Post. cricoarytenoid m.; Thyroid cartilage; Inf. laryngeal nerve; Inferior horn of thyroid cartilage; Thyroid gland; Inf. laryngeal art.; Tracheal branches, Inf. thyroid artery; Esophageal branches, Recurrent laryngeal n.; Trachea; Inferior thyroid artery; Recurrent laryngeal nerve

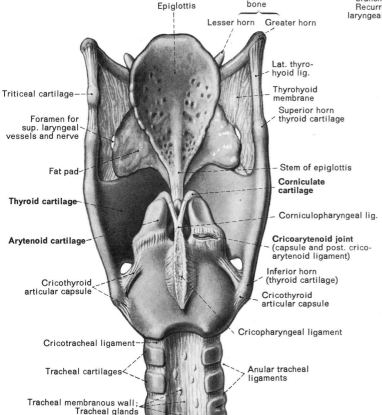

Labels for Fig. 556: Epiglottis; Hyoid bone; Lesser horn; Greater horn; Lat. thyrohyoid lig.; Thyrohyoid membrane; Superior horn thyroid cartilage; Triticeal cartilage; Foramen for sup. laryngeal vessels and nerve; Fat pad; Stem of epiglottis; Corniculate cartilage; Thyroid cartilage; Corniculopharyngeal lig.; Arytenoid cartilage; Cricoarytenoid joint (capsule and post. cricoarytenoid ligament); Inferior horn (thyroid cartilage); Cricothyroid articular capsule; Cricothyroid articular capsule; Cricotracheal ligament; Cricopharyngeal ligament; Tracheal cartilages; Anular tracheal ligaments; Tracheal membranous wall; Tracheal glands

Fig. 556: The Cartilages and Ligaments of the Larynx

NOTE: 1) the articulation of the paired arytenoid cartilages with the cricoid cartilage below. These synovial cricoarytenoid joints are surrounded by articular capsules and strengthened by the posterior cricoarytenoid ligaments.

2) the cricoarytenoid joints allow for a) *rotation of the arytenoid cartilage* on an axis which is nearly vertical and b) *the horizontal gliding movement* of the arytenoid cartilages.

3) rotation of the arytenoid cartilages results in medial or lateral displacement of the vocal folds, thereby increasing or decreasing the size of the opening between the folds, the rima glottidis. The horizontal gliding action of the arytenoid cartilages permits the bases of these cartilages to be approximated or moved apart. Medial rotation and medial gliding of the arytenoid cartilages occur simultaneously as do the two lateral movements.

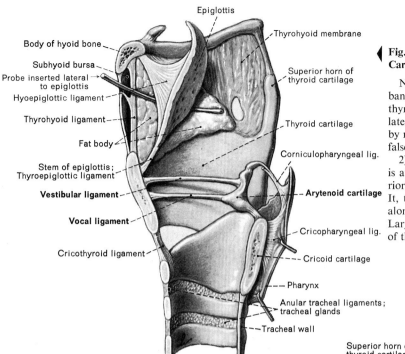

Epiglottis

Thyrohyoid membrane

Body of hyoid bone

Superior horn of thyroid cartilage

Subhyoid bursa

Probe inserted lateral to epiglottis

Hyoepiglottic ligament

Thyrohyoid ligament

Thyroid cartilage

Fat body

Corniculopharyngeal lig.

Stem of epiglottis; Thyroepiglottic ligament

Vestibular ligament

Arytenoid cartilage

Vocal ligament

Cricopharyngeal lig.

Cricothyroid ligament

Cricoid cartilage

Pharynx

Anular tracheal ligaments; tracheal glands

Tracheal wall

Fig. 557: The Right Half of the Larynx Showing the Cartilages and the Vestibular and Vocal Ligaments

NOTE: 1) the vestibular ligament is a compact band of fibrous tissue attached anteriorly to the thyroid cartilage and posteriorly to the anterior and lateral surface of the arytenoid cartilage. It is enclosed by mucous membrane to form the vestibular fold (or false vocal fold).

2) the vocal ligament consists of elastic tissue which is attached anteriorly to thyroid cartilage and posteriorly to the vocal process of the arytenoid cartilage. It, too, is surrounded by mucous membrane which, along with the vocalis muscle, forms the vocal fold. Laryngeal sound waves are produced by oscillations of the vocal folds initiated by puffs of air.

Fig. 558: The Vocal Ligaments and Conus Elasticus from Above ▶

Note that the conus elasticus is a membrane consisting principally of yellow elastic fibers which interconnects the thyroid, cricoid and arytenoid cartilages. It underlies the mucous membrane below the vocal folds and is overlain to some extent by the cricothyroid muscle on the exterior of the larynx. Observe the symmetry of the arytenoid cartilages and their related vocal ligaments.

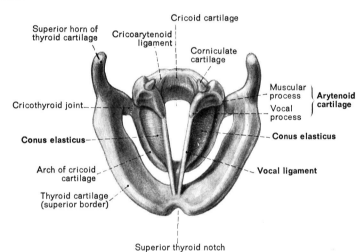

Cricoid cartilage

Superior horn of thyroid cartilage

Cricoarytenoid ligament

Corniculate cartilage

Muscular process

Vocal process

Arytenoid cartilage

Cricothyroid joint

Conus elasticus

Conus elasticus

Arch of cricoid cartilage

Vocal ligament

Thyroid cartilage (superior border)

Superior thyroid notch

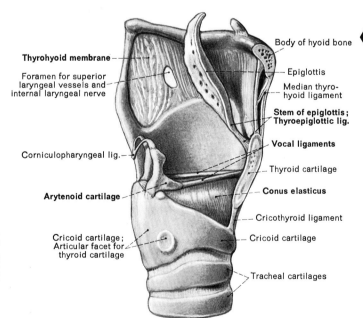

Thyrohyoid membrane

Foramen for superior laryngeal vessels and internal laryngeal nerve

Body of hyoid bone

Epiglottis

Median thyrohyoid ligament

Stem of epiglottis; Thyroepiglottic lig.

Vocal ligaments

Corniculopharyngeal lig.

Thyroid cartilage

Arytenoid cartilage

Conus elasticus

Cricothyroid ligament

Cricoid cartilage; Articular facet for thyroid cartilage

Cricoid cartilage

Tracheal cartilages

Fig. 559: The Upper Left Part of the Larynx

NOTE: 1) the right halves of the hyoid bone, epiglottis and thyroid cartilage have been removed to reveal the interior of the upper left portion of the larynx. The two vocal ligaments, the arytenoid cartilages and the conus elasticus are also displayed.

2) the broad thyrohyoid membrane and its foramen. Observe the attachment of the stem of the epiglottis to the thyroid cartilage by means of the thyroepiglottic ligament.

3) the conus elasticus as it attaches to the vocal fold and the arytenoid, thyroid and cricoid cartilages.

4) although laryngeal sounds are initiated at the vocal folds, the pitch, quality, volume, range, tone and overtone characteristics of the human voice incorporate not only the vocal folds but also the structures in the mouth (tongue, teeth, and palate), the nasal cavities (sinuses), the pharynx, the rest of the larynx, the lungs, diaphragm and abdominal musculature.

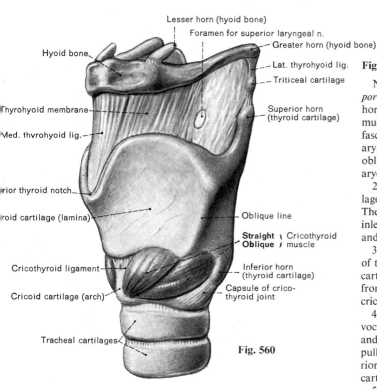

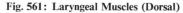

Fig. 560: Labels reading (top to bottom, clockwise): Lesser horn (hyoid bone), Foramen for superior laryngeal n., Greater horn (hyoid bone), Lat. thyrohyoid lig., Triticeal cartilage, Superior horn (thyroid cartilage), Oblique line, Straight \ Oblique / Cricothyroid muscle, Inferior horn (thyroid cartilage), Capsule of cricothyroid joint, Tracheal cartilages, Cricoid cartilage (arch), Cricothyroid ligament, roid cartilage (lamina), rior thyroid notch, Med. thyrohyoid lig., Thyrohyoid membrane, Hyoid bone

Fig. 560: Ventrolateral View of the Exterior Larynx and the Cricothyroid Muscle

NOTE: 1) the cricothyroid muscle consists of straight and oblique heads. The *straight head* is more vertical and inserts into the lower border of the lamina of the thyroid cartilage while the *oblique head* is more horizontal and inserts onto the inferior horn of the thyroid cartilage.

2) the cricothyroid muscle tilts the anterior part of the cricoid cartilage superiorly. In so doing, the arytenoid cartilages which are attached to the cricoid are pulled dorsally. In addition, the thyroid cartilage is pulled forward and downward. These actions increase the distance between the arytenoid and thyroid cartilages, thereby increasing the tension of and elongating the vocal folds.

Fig. 561: Laryngeal Muscles (Dorsal)

NOTE: 1) the *arytenoid muscle* consisting of a *transverse portion* which spans the zone between the two arytenoid cartilages horizontally, and an *oblique portion* which consists of two muscular fascicles that cross one another. Thus, each of the two fascicles of the oblique portion extends from the base of one arytenoid cartilage to the apex of the other cartilage. Some oblique arytenoid fibers continue to the epiglottis along the aryepiglottic fold. These constitute the *aryepiglottis muscle*.

2) the *transverse arytenoid* approximates the arytenoid cartilages and, therefore, closes the posterior part of the rima glottis. The *oblique arytenoid and aryepiglottic muscles* tend to close the inlet into the larynx by pulling the aryepiglottic folds together and approximating the arytenoid cartilages and the epiglottis.

3) the *posterior cricoarytenoid* muscle extends from the lamina of the cricoid cartilage to the muscular process of the arytenoid cartilage while the *lateral cricoarytenoid* muscle arises laterally from the arch of the cricoid cartilage to insert with the posterior cricoarytenoid muscle onto the arytenoid cartilage.

4) the *posterior cricoarytenoids* are the only abductors of the vocal folds while the *lateral cricoarytenoids* act as antagonists, and adduct the vocal folds. The posterior muscle abducts by pulling the base of the arytenoid cartilages medially and posteriorly, while the lateral muscle adducts by pulling these same cartilages anteriorly and laterally.

5) the *thyroarytenoid muscle* is a thin sheet of muscle radiating from the thyroid cartilage principally backward toward the arytenoid cartilage. Its upper fibers continue to the epiglottis and, joining the aryepiglottic fibers, become the *thyroepiglottic muscle*. Its deepest (and most medial) fibers form the *vocalis muscle* which is attached to the lateral aspect of the vocal fold.

6) the thyroarytenoid muscles draw the arytenoid cartilages toward the thyroid cartilage and thus shorten (relax) the vocal folds.

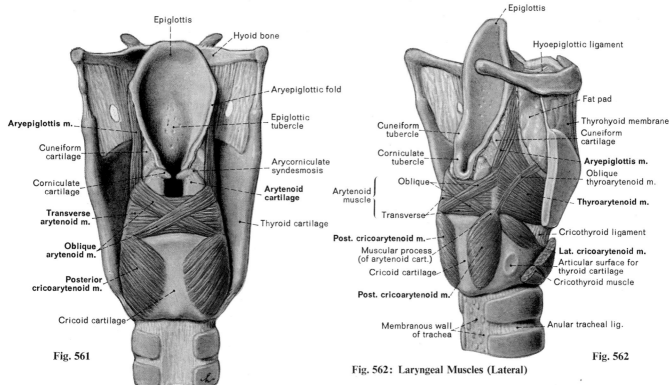

Fig. 561

Labels: Epiglottis, Hyoid bone, Aryepiglottic fold, Epiglottic tubercle, Arycorniculate syndesmosis, **Arytenoid cartilage**, Thyroid cartilage, Cricoid cartilage, Cricoid cartilage, **Posterior cricoarytenoid m.**, **Oblique arytenoid m.**, **Transverse arytenoid m.**, Corniculate cartilage, Cuneiform cartilage, **Aryepiglottis m.**

Fig. 562: Laryngeal Muscles (Lateral)

Labels: Epiglottis, Hyoepiglottic ligament, Fat pad, Thyrohyoid membrane, Cuneiform cartilage, **Aryepiglottis m.**, Oblique thyroarytenoid m., **Thyroarytenoid m.**, Cricothyroid ligament, **Lat. cricoarytenoid m.**, Articular surface for thyroid cartilage, Cricothyroid muscle, Anular tracheal lig., Membranous wall of trachea, **Post. cricoarytenoid m.**, Cricoid cartilage, Muscular process (of arytenoid cart.), **Post. cricoarytenoid m.**, Arytenoid muscle { Oblique, Transverse }, Corniculate tubercle, Cuneiform tubercle

Fig. 562

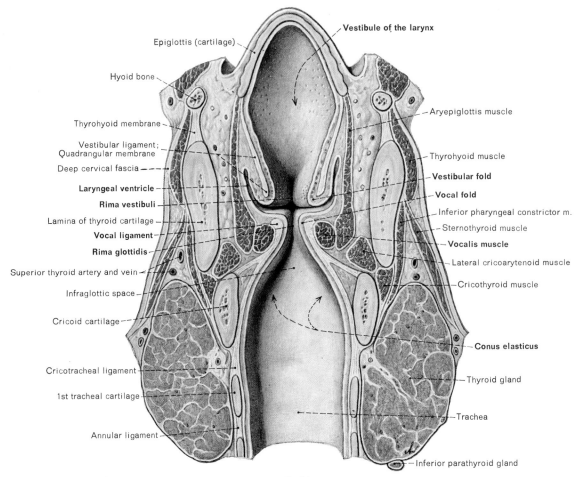

Fig. 563: Frontal Section of Larynx Showing Laryngeal Folds and Cavities

NOTE: 1) the paired vocal folds consisting of mucous membrane overlying the vocal ligaments and vocalis muscles. Just superior to the vocal folds observe the vestibular folds. On each side, the vestibular fold is separated from the vocal folds by a recess called the laryngeal ventricle (or sinus).

2) that above the vestibular folds is the vestibule of the larynx which lies just below the laryngeal inlet. Below the vocal folds observe the infraglottic space. This space communicates with the trachea below and is limited by the rima glottidis between the vocal folds above.

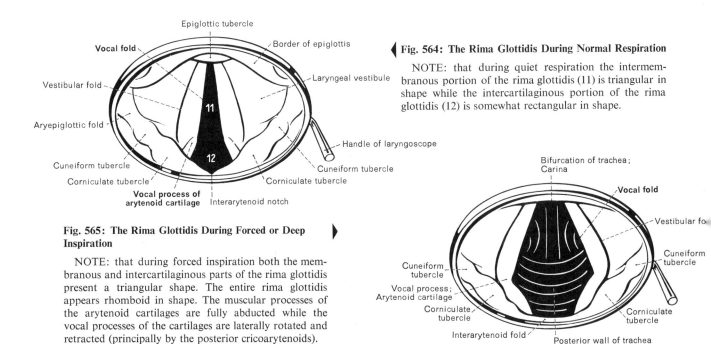

Fig. 564: The Rima Glottidis During Normal Respiration

NOTE: that during quiet respiration the intermembranous portion of the rima glottidis (11) is triangular in shape while the intercartilaginous portion of the rima glottidis (12) is somewhat rectangular in shape.

Fig. 565: The Rima Glottidis During Forced or Deep Inspiration

NOTE: that during forced inspiration both the membranous and intercartilaginous parts of the rima glottidis present a triangular shape. The entire rima glottidis appears rhomboid in shape. The muscular processes of the arytenoid cartilages are fully abducted while the vocal processes of the cartilages are laterally rotated and retracted (principally by the posterior cricoarytenoids).

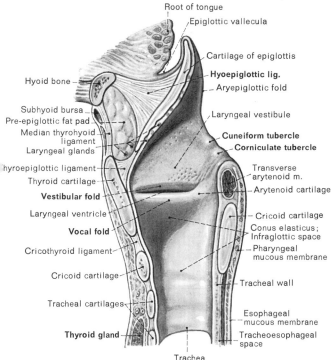

Fig. 566: Midsagittal Section of Larynx

NOTE: 1) the laryngeal inlet through which the larynx communicates with the pharynx. This aperture leads to the laryngeal vestibule, the anterior border of which is the epiglottis. On each side the aryepiglottic folds define the borders of the inlet, which are marked by oval elevations, the cuneiform and corniculate cartilages.

2) the space between the vestibular folds and the vocal folds is known as the ventricle or laryngeal sinus. Below the vocal fold observe how the conus elasticus bounds the infraglottic space laterally, and the communication of this space with the trachea.

3) the attachments of the epiglottis. Superiorly its hyoepiglottic ligament stretches to the hyoid bone; inferiorly the thyroepiglottic ligament connects the stem of the epiglottis to the thyroid cartilage; laterally the aryepiglottic folds extend between the epiglottis and the arytenoid cartilages.

Fig. 567: Cross Section of Larynx at the Vocal Folds

I = intermembranous portion of rima glottidis

II = intercartilaginous portion of rima glottidis

NOTE: the orientation of the arytenoid cartilages and their articulations with the cricoid cartilage. The vocal folds consist of mucous membrane overlying the vocal ligaments lateral to which extend the deeper vocalis portions of the thyroarytenoid muscle. By drawing the arytenoid cartilages forward, the thyroarytenoids shorten and relax the vocal folds. Simultaneously they medially rotate the arytenoid cartilages and, thus, approximate the vocal folds.

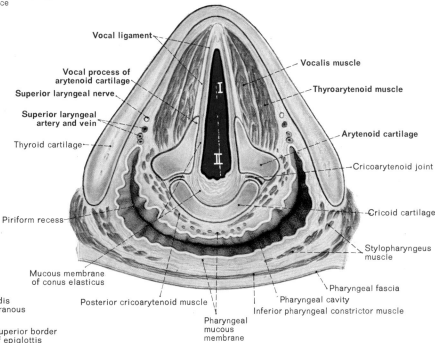

Fig. 568: The Rima Glottidis During Phonation (Shrill Tones)

NOTE: that during the emission of shrill tones, the vocal folds are approximated and the vocal ligaments tensed resulting in a narrowing of the rima glottidis to a thin slit.

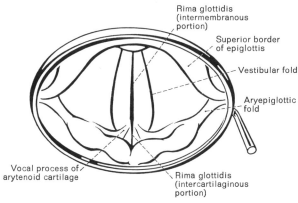

Fig. 569: The Rima Glottidis During Whispering

NOTE: that during the production of whispering sounds the intermembranous portion of the vocal folds are approximated while the intercartilaginous portion of the folds are kept separated. The anterior part of the rima glottidis is narrow and slit-like and the posterior, intercartilaginous portion remains open.

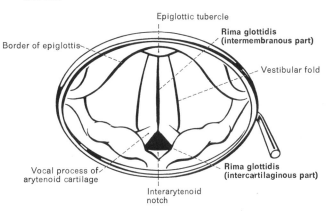

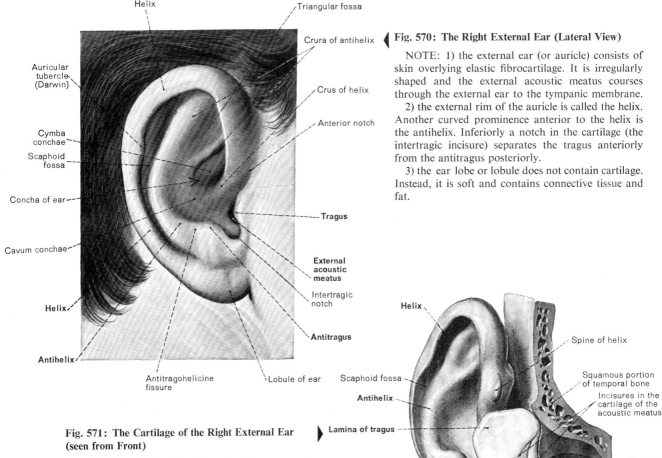

Helix

Triangular fossa

Crura of antihelix

Auricular tubercle (Darwin)

Crus of helix

Anterior notch

Cymba conchae

Scaphoid fossa

Concha of ear

Tragus

Cavum conchae

External acoustic meatus

Helix

Intertragic notch

Antihelix

Antitragus

Antitragohelicine fissure

Lobule of ear

Fig. 570: The Right External Ear (Lateral View)

NOTE: 1) the external ear (or auricle) consists of skin overlying elastic fibrocartilage. It is irregularly shaped and the external acoustic meatus courses through the external ear to the tympanic membrane.

2) the external rim of the auricle is called the helix. Another curved prominence anterior to the helix is the antihelix. Inferiorly a notch in the cartilage (the intertragic incisure) separates the tragus anteriorly from the antitragus posteriorly.

3) the ear lobe or lobule does not contain cartilage. Instead, it is soft and contains connective tissue and fat.

Fig. 571: The Cartilage of the Right External Ear (seen from Front)

NOTE: 1) with the skin of the external ear removed, the contours of the single cartilage conform generally with those of the intact auricle. The cartilage is seen to be absent inferiorly at the site of the ear lobe.

2) the attachment of the auricular cartilage to the temporal bone. This attachment is strengthened by the anterior and posterior ligaments (not shown in this figure) which articulate the tragus and spine of the helix to the temporal bone anteriorly and the concha to the mastoid process posteriorly. The continuous overlying skin completes the attachment.

Helix

Spine of helix

Squamous portion of temporal bone

Incisures in the cartilage of the acoustic meatus

Scaphoid fossa

Antihelix

Lamina of tragus

Tympanic part of temporal bone

Antitragohelicine fissure

Tail of helix

Styloid process

Cartilage of acoustic meatus

Mastoid process

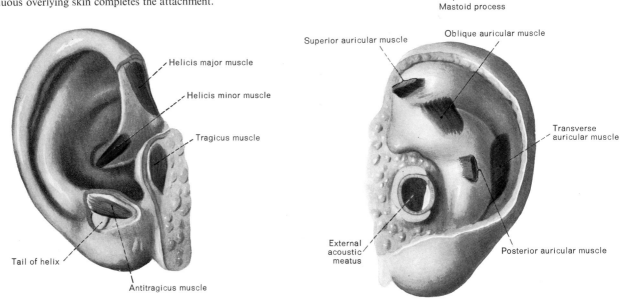

Helicis major muscle

Helicis minor muscle

Tragicus muscle

Tail of helix

Antitragicus muscle

Fig. 572: Intrinsic Muscles of External Ear (Lateral Surface)

Superior auricular muscle

Oblique auricular muscle

Transverse auricular muscle

External acoustic meatus

Posterior auricular muscle

Fig. 573: Muscles Attaching to the Medial Surface of External Ear

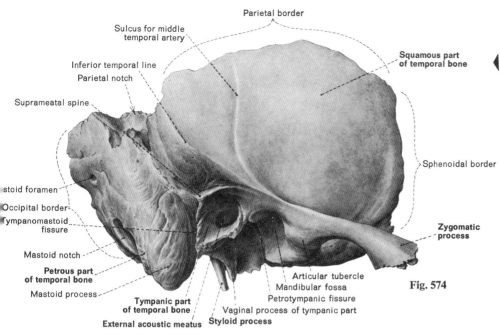

Parietal border

Sulcus for middle temporal artery

Inferior temporal line
Parietal notch

Suprameatal spine

Mastoid foramen

Occipital border

Tympanomastoid fissure

Mastoid notch

Petrous part of temporal bone

Mastoid process

Tympanic part of temporal bone

External acoustic meatus

Styloid process

Vaginal process of tympanic part

Petrotympanic fissure

Mandibular fossa

Articular tubercle

Squamous part of temporal bone

Sphenoidal border

Zygomatic process

Fig. 574

◀ Fig. 574: The Right Temporal Bone (Lateral View)

NOTE: 1) the temporal bone which forms the osseous encasement for the middle and internal ear, consists of three parts: *squamous*, *tympanic* and *petrous*.

2) the *squamous part* is broad in shape, thin and flat. From it extends the zygomatic process. The *tympanic part* is interposed below the squamous and anterior to the petrous parts. The external acoustic meatus which leads to the tympanic membrane is surrounded by the tympanic part of the temporal bone.

3) the hard *petrous part* contains the organ of hearing and the vestibular canals. Its mastoid process is not solid but contains many air cells and its external surface affords attachment to several muscles.

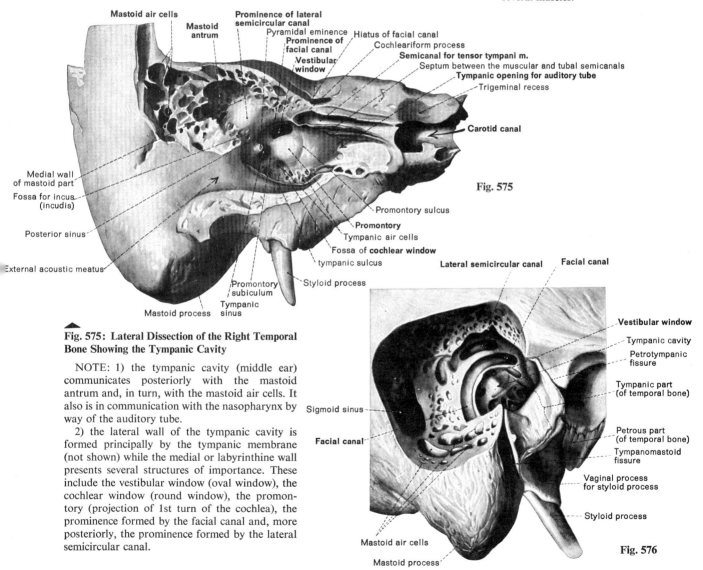

Mastoid air cells

Mastoid antrum

Prominence of lateral semicircular canal

Pyramidal eminence

Prominence of facial canal

Hiatus of facial canal

Cochleariform process

Vestibular window

Semicanal for tensor tympani m.

Septum between the muscular and tubal semicanals

Tympanic opening for auditory tube

Trigeminal recess

Carotid canal

Fig. 575

Medial wall of mastoid part

Fossa for incus (incudis)

Posterior sinus

External acoustic meatus

Mastoid process

Promontory subiculum

Tympanic sinus

Styloid process

Promontory sulcus

Promontory

Tympanic air cells

Fossa of **cochlear window**

tympanic sulcus

Fig. 575: Lateral Dissection of the Right Temporal Bone Showing the Tympanic Cavity

NOTE: 1) the tympanic cavity (middle ear) communicates posteriorly with the mastoid antrum and, in turn, with the mastoid air cells. It also is in communication with the nasopharynx by way of the auditory tube.

2) the lateral wall of the tympanic cavity is formed principally by the tympanic membrane (not shown) while the medial or labyrinthine wall presents several structures of importance. These include the vestibular window (oval window), the cochlear window (round window), the promontory (projection of 1st turn of the cochlea), the prominence formed by the facial canal and, more posteriorly, the prominence formed by the lateral semicircular canal.

Lateral semicircular canal

Facial canal

Vestibular window

Tympanic cavity

Petrotympanic fissure

Tympanic part (of temporal bone)

Petrous part (of temporal bone)

Tympanomastoid fissure

Vaginal process for styloid process

Styloid process

Sigmoid sinus

Facial canal

Mastoid air cells

Mastoid process

Fig. 576

Fig. 576: The Facial and Lateral Semicircular Canals Exposed by a Lateral Approach (right)

NOTE: bone has been removed from the medial wall of the tympanic cavity in order to expose the facial nerve canal and the lateral semicircular canal. Observe the anatomical relationship of the facial canal (and nerve) to the vestibular window.

Fig. 577: Frontal Section Through Left External, Middle and Internal Ear

NOTE: 1) the external auditory meatus commences at the auricle and leads to the external surface of the tympanic membrane. Through the meatus course the sound waves which cause vibration of the tympanum.

2) the middle ear (or tympanic cavity) contains three ossicles (malleus, incus and stapes) and two muscles (tensor tympani and stapedius [not shown]). The cavity of the middle ear communicates with the mastoid antrum and mastoid air cells posteriorly and the nasopharynx by way of the auditory tube. From the middle ear this tube courses downward, forward and medially. The ossicles interconnect the tympanic membrane with the inner ear.

3) the inner ear contains the coiled cochlea (or organ of hearing) and the three semicircular canals (the vestibular organ) and their associated structures and nerves.

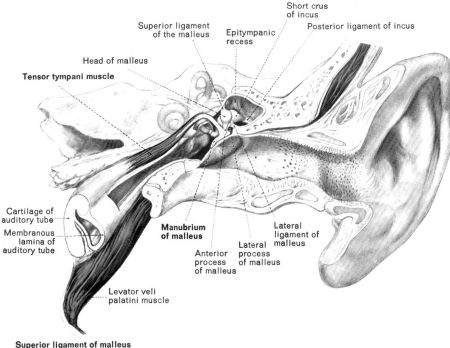

Short crus of incus — Posterior ligament of incus — Superior ligament of the malleus — Epitympanic recess — Head of malleus — Tensor tympani muscle — Cartilage of auditory tube — Membranous lamina of auditory tube — Manubrium of malleus — Anterior process of malleus — Lateral process of malleus — Lateral ligament of malleus — Levator veli palatini muscle

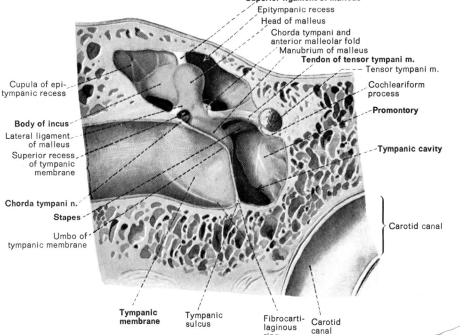

Superior ligament of malleus — Epitympanic recess — Head of malleus — Chorda tympani and anterior malleolar fold — Manubrium of malleus — Tendon of tensor tympani m. — Tensor tympani m. — Cochleariform process — Promontory — Tympanic cavity — Carotid canal — Cupula of epi-tympanic recess — Body of incus — Lateral ligament of malleus — Superior recess of tympanic membrane — Chorda tympani n. — Stapes — Umbo of tympanic membrane — Tympanic membrane — Tympanic sulcus — Fibrocartilaginous ring — Carotid canal

Fig. 578: Frontal Section Through Right External and Middle Ear

NOTE: 1) the slender tendon of the tensor tympani muscle as it turns sharply upon reaching the tympanic cavity to terminate on the manubrium of the malleus.

2) the tympanic cavity is extended superiorly by the epitympanic recess and inferiorly by the hypotympanic recess. On the medial wall of the middle ear observe the promontory which protrudes into the tympanic cavity and which contains the spiral chochlea.

3) the lateral and superior ligaments attaching to the head of the malleus.

Fig. 579: Frontal Section of Left Ear Through the Middle Ear Bones

NOTE: 1) when sound waves are received at the tympanic membrane, they cause medial displacements of the manubrium of the malleus. The head of the malleus is tilted laterally, pulling with it the body of the incus. At the same time the long process of the incus is displaced medially as is the articulation between the incus and the stapes.

2) the base of the stapes rocks as though it were on a fulcrum at the vestibular window thereby establishing waves in the perilymph. These waves stimulate the auditory receptors and become dissipated at the secondary tympanic membrane covering the cochlear window.

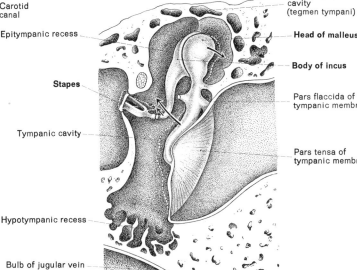

Roof of tympanic cavity (tegmen tympani) — Head of malleus — Body of incus — Pars flaccida of tympanic membrane — Pars tensa of tympanic membrane — Epitympanic recess — Stapes — Tympanic cavity — Hypotympanic recess — Bulb of jugular vein

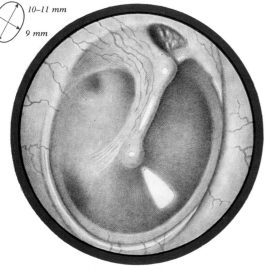

10–11 mm

9 mm

Fig. 581: Labeled Diagram of Fig. 580

NOTE: 1) the tympanic membrane has been divided into quadrants. The most depressed point is the umbo and is found at the rounded extremity of the handle of the malleus.

2) the anterior and posterior malleolar folds. The more lax part (pars flaccida) of the tympanic membrane lies above and between these folds while the rest is more tightly stretched (pars tensa).

Fig. 580: Right Tympanic Membrane as seen with an Otoscope in a Living Person

NOTE: that the tympanic membrane is oval in shape and measures about 9 mm. across and from 10 to 11 mm vertically (upper inset, actual size). Its blood supply is derived from the deep auricular and anterior tympanic branches of the maxillary artery and the stylomastoid branch of the posterior auricular artery.

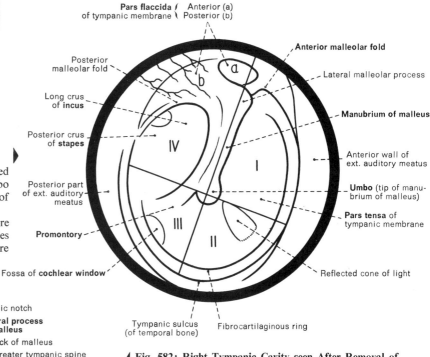

Pars flaccida / Anterior (a)
of tympanic membrane \ Posterior (b)

Posterior
malleolar fold

Long crus
of incus

Posterior crus
of stapes

Posterior part
of ext. auditory
meatus

Promontory

Fossa of cochlear window

Anterior malleolar fold

Lateral malleolar process

Manubrium of malleus

Anterior wall of
ext. auditory meatus

Umbo (tip of manu-
brium of malleus)

Pars tensa of
tympanic membrane

Reflected cone of light

Tympanic sulcus
(of temporal bone)

Fibrocartilaginous ring

Fig. 582: Right Tympanic Cavity seen After Removal of Tympanic Membrane

NOTE: that from this lateral view the lateral process and manubrium of the malleus, the lenticular process and long crus of the incus as well as the stapes can be observed upon the removal of the tympanic membrane. Note also the chorda tympani nerve and the tendons of the stapedius and tensor tympani muscles.

Lesser tympanic spine

Tympanic notch

Lateral process
of malleus

Neck of malleus

Greater tympanic spine

Ant. malleolar fold;
Chorda tympani nerve

Tendon of tensor
tympani muscle

Manubrium of malleus

Septum covering
tensor tympani muscle
(septum canalis
musculotubarii)

acoustic meatus

a tympani
and fold

us of incus

ramidal
minence

endon of
s muscle

artilaginous ring

Fossa of
cochlear window

Lenticular process
of incus

Stapes

Promontory

Fig. 583: Lateral Wall of the Right Middle Ear (Tympanic Membrane Viewed from within the Tympanic Cavity)

NOTE: 1) the manubrium of the malleus has been severed from the remainder of the ossicle and left attached to the tympanic membrane. The fibrocartilaginous tympanic ring is deficient superiorly forming the tympanic notch (of Rivinus). The looser portion of the tympanic membrane (pars flaccida) covers this zone.

2) the tympanic membrane below the malleolar folds is the pars tensa. This portion is made taut by the tensor tympani muscle which attaches to the manubrium of the malleus.

3) the innervation of external surface of the tympanic membrane comes from the auriculotemporal branch of the mandibular nerve (V) and the auricular branch of the vagus (X). The inner surface of the membrane receives innervation from the tympanic branch of the glossopharyngeal nerve (IX).

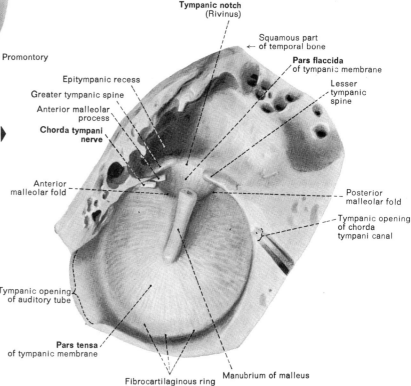

Tympanic notch
(Rivinus)

Squamous part
← of temporal bone

Pars flaccida
of tympanic membrane

Lesser
tympanic
spine

Epitympanic recess

Greater tympanic spine

Anterior malleolar
process

Chorda tympani
nerve

Anterior
malleolar fold

Posterior
malleolar fold

Tympanic opening
of chorda
tympani canal

Tympanic opening
of auditory tube

Pars tensa
of tympanic membrane

Fibrocartilaginous ring

Manubrium of malleus

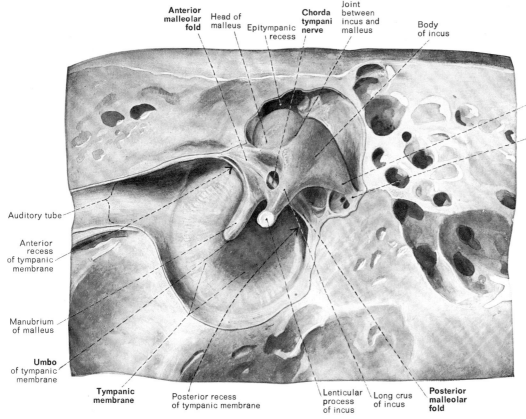

Anterior malleolar fold · Head of malleus · Epitympanic recess · **Chorda tympani nerve** · Joint between incus and malleus · Body of incus

Short crus of incus

Posterior ligament of incus

Auditory tube

Anterior recess of tympanic membrane

Manubrium of malleus

Umbo of tympanic membrane

Tympanic membrane · Posterior recess of tympanic membrane · Lenticular process of incus · Long crus of incus · **Posterior malleolar fold**

Fig. 584: Lateral Wall of the Right Tympanic Cavity (Viewed from the Medial Aspect)

NOTE: 1) the tympanic cavity is lined completely with a mucous membrane which attaches onto the surfaces of all the structures of the middle ear. This tympanic mucosa is continuous with that lining the mastoid air cells posteriorly and the auditory tube anteriorly.

2) reflections of the tympanic mucous membrane from the anterior and posterior malleolar folds. These are also reflected around the chorda tympani nerve as it curves along the medial side of the manubrium of the malleus.

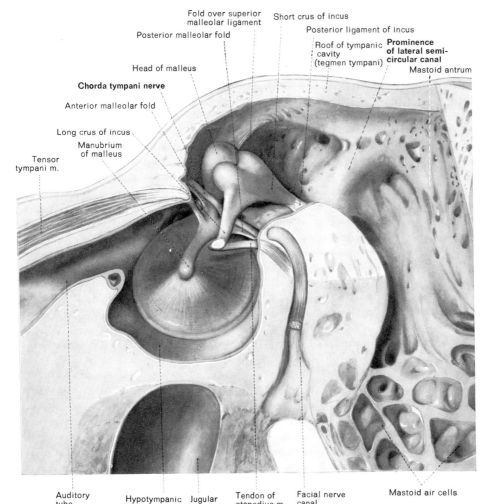

Fold over superior malleolar ligament · Short crus of incus

Posterior malleolar fold · Posterior ligament of incus

Head of malleus · Roof of tympanic cavity (tegmen tympani) · **Prominence of lateral semicircular canal**

Chorda tympani nerve · Mastoid antrum

Anterior malleolar fold

Long crus of incus

Manubrium of malleus

Tensor tympani m.

Auditory tube · Hypotympanic recess · Jugular fossa · Tendon of stapedius m. · Facial nerve canal · Mastoid air cells

Fig. 585: The Muscles, Chorda Tympani Nerve, and Ossicles of the Right Middle Ear

NOTE: 1) the tendon of the tensor tympani muscle inserting on the manubrium of the malleus and the short tendon of the stapedius as it inserts onto the neck of the stapes close to its articulation with the incus. The tensor tympani draws the manubrium medially thereby making the tympanic membrane taut. It is innervated by the mandibular division of the trigeminal nerve.

2) the stapedius is the smallest of the skeletal muscles in the body and it is supplied by the facial nerve. It pulls the head of the stapes posteriorly thereby tilting the base of the stapes in the vestibular window.

3) the direct communication between the nasopharynx, tympanic cavity and mastoid air cells has important clinical meaning, since oro-respiratory tract infections reach the middle ear readily by way of the auditory tube.

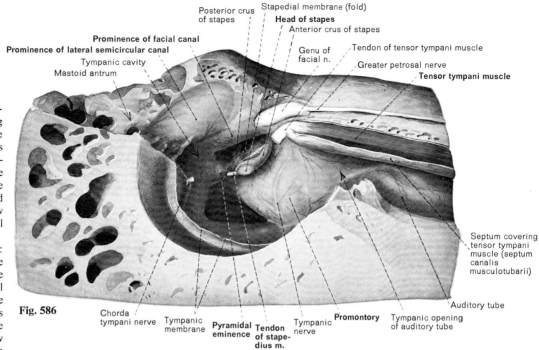

Fig. 586: Medial Wall of the Right Tympanic Cavity (Viewed from Lateral Aspect)

NOTE: 1) the tympanic membrane has been removed along with the bony roof of the tympanic cavity. The malleus and incus have also been removed and the tendon of the tensor tympani severed. Observe the stapes with its base directed toward the vestibular window and the stapedius muscle still attached to its neck.

2) several bony markings: a) the prominence containing the lateral semicircular canal, b) the curved prominence of the facial canal with its facial nerve, c) the rounded promontory, which is the thin bony covering over the cochlea and d) the hollow pyramidal eminence from which arises the stapedius muscle.

Fig. 586 labels: Posterior crus of stapes; Stapedial membrane (fold); Head of stapes; Anterior crus of stapes; Prominence of facial canal; Prominence of lateral semicircular canal; Genu of facial n.; Tendon of tensor tympani muscle; Tympanic cavity; Greater petrosal nerve; Mastoid antrum; Tensor tympani muscle; Septum covering tensor tympani muscle (septum canalis musculotubarii); Auditory tube; Chorda tympani nerve; Tympanic membrane; Pyramidal eminence; Tendon of stapedius m.; Tympanic nerve; Promontory; Tympanic opening of auditory tube

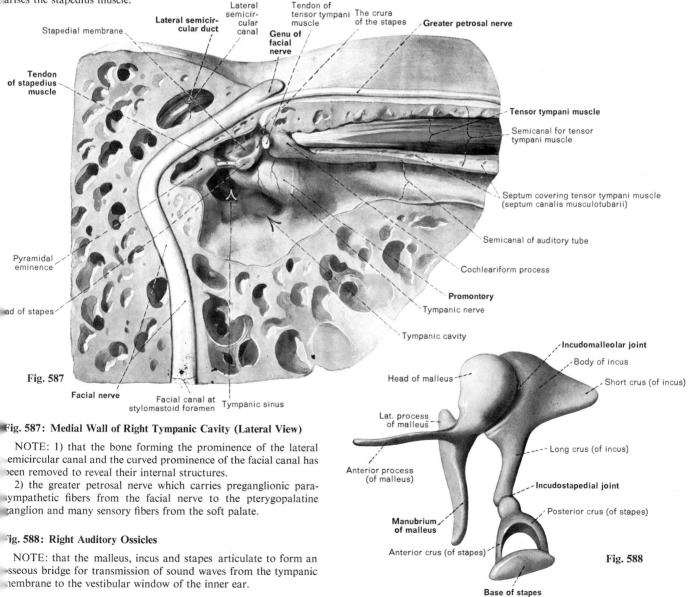

Fig. 587 labels: Stapedial membrane; Lateral semicircular duct; Lateral semicircular canal; Tendon of tensor tympani muscle; The crura of the stapes; Genu of facial nerve; Greater petrosal nerve; Tendon of stapedius muscle; Tensor tympani muscle; Semicanal for tensor tympani muscle; Septum covering tensor tympani muscle (septum canalis musculotubarii); Semicanal of auditory tube; Cochleariform process; Pyramidal eminence; Promontory; Tympanic nerve; Head of stapes; Tympanic cavity; Facial nerve; Facial canal at stylomastoid foramen; Tympanic sinus

Fig. 587: Medial Wall of Right Tympanic Cavity (Lateral View)

NOTE: 1) that the bone forming the prominence of the lateral semicircular canal and the curved prominence of the facial canal has been removed to reveal their internal structures.

2) the greater petrosal nerve which carries preganglionic parasympathetic fibers from the facial nerve to the pterygopalatine ganglion and many sensory fibers from the soft palate.

Fig. 588: Right Auditory Ossicles

NOTE: that the malleus, incus and stapes articulate to form an osseous bridge for transmission of sound waves from the tympanic membrane to the vestibular window of the inner ear.

Fig. 588 labels: Incudomalleolar joint; Body of incus; Short crus (of incus); Head of malleus; Long crus (of incus); Lat. process of malleus; Incudostapedial joint; Posterior crus (of stapes); Anterior process (of malleus); Manubrium of malleus; Anterior crus (of stapes); Base of stapes

Fig. 589: Medial Wall of the Right Tympanic Cavity Showing the Stapedius Muscle (Lateral View)

NOTE: 1) the lateral aspect of the pyramidal eminence was removed in order to demonstrate the stapedius muscle. Its tendon emerges through the apex of the eminence and inserts on the neck of the stapes. This muscle measures about 4 mm. in length and its action on the base of the stapes (pulling it laterally) protects the inner ear from damage caused by loud sounds.

2) the tympanic branch of the glossopharyngeal nerve (IX) coursing along the promontory. This nerve is sensory to the mucous membrane of the middle ear and is also known as the nerve of Jacobson. Its fibers are joined by sympathetic fibers and by branches from the facial nerve to form the tympanic plexus.

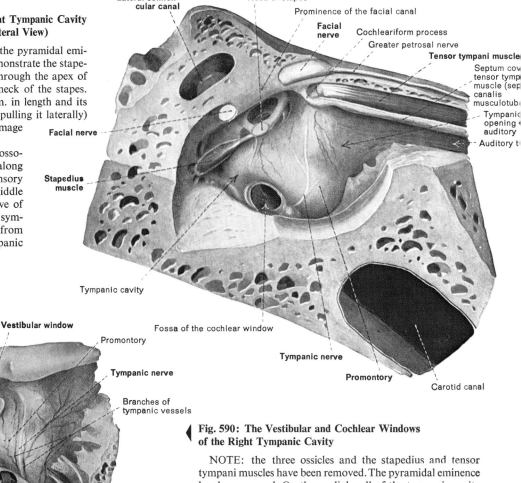

Lateral semicircular canal — Head of stapes — Prominence of the facial canal — **Facial nerve** — Cochleariform process — Greater petrosal nerve — **Tensor tympani muscle** — Septum cov tensor tymp muscle (sep canalis musculotub — Tympanic opening auditory — Auditory t

Facial nerve

Stapedius muscle

Tympanic cavity

Fossa of the cochlear window

Tympanic nerve

Promontory

Carotid canal

Prominence of facial canal — **Vestibular window** — Promontory

Fossa of vestibular window

Subiculum of promontory

Tympanic nerve

Facial nerve

Branches of tympanic vessels

Pyramidal eminence

Tympanic sinus

Bony separation between tympanic cavity and carotid canal

Fossa of cochlear window — **Secondary tympanic membrane**

Fig. 590: The Vestibular and Cochlear Windows of the Right Tympanic Cavity

NOTE: the three ossicles and the stapedius and tensor tympani muscles have been removed. The pyramidal eminence has been opened. On the medial wall of the tympanic cavity observe the oval vestibular window and the round cochlear window which communicate with the internal ear. Coursing along the surface of the promontory can be seen the tympanic vessels and nerve.

Fig. 591: The Right Membranous Labyrinth Partially Exposed within the Temporal Bone

NOTE: 1) the membranous labyrinth is in blue while the roots of the vestibulocochlear nerve are in yellow. The membranous labyrinth lies within the bony labyrinth and generally conforms to it in shape. Between them is found the perilymphatic fluid.

2) within the bony cochlea lie the coils of the cochlear duct. The bony labyrinth consists of the cochlea and the semicircular canals interconnected by the vestibule. In the lateral wall of the vestibule is situated the vestibular window where the stapes has access to the perilymph.

3) the basal end of the cochlear duct communicates with the saccule through the ductus reuniens. The saccule communicates with the utricle and the semicircular canals through the utriculosaccular duct.

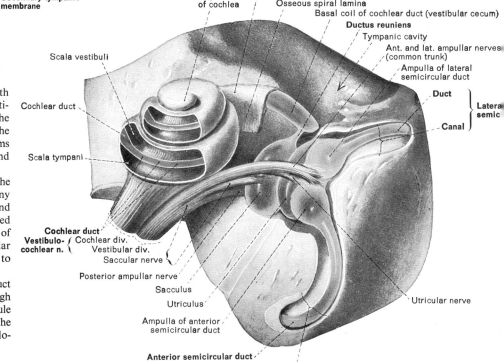

Basal coil of cochlea — Cupula of cochlea — Osseous spiral lamina — Basal coil of cochlear duct (vestibular cecum) — **Ductus reuniens** — Tympanic cavity — Ant. and lat. ampullar nerves (common trunk) — Ampulla of lateral semicircular duct — **Duct** — **Canal** — Latera semic

Scala vestibuli

Cochlear duct

Scala tympani

Cochlear duct — **Vestibulo-cochlear n.** — Cochlear div. — Vestibular div. — Saccular nerve

Posterior ampullar nerve

Sacculus

Utriculus

Ampulla of anterior semicircular duct

Anterior semicircular duct

Utricular nerve

Anterior semicircular canal

Fig. 592: The Bony Labyrinth Projected onto the Base of the Cranial Cavity

NOTE: that the location of the bony labyrinth in the temporal bone has been projected onto the inner surface of the base of the skull. A line has been drawn through the plane of the anterior semicircular canal posteriorly to the midsagittal plane to indicate the angle of location of that particular canal (about 55° away from the horizontal right angle of 90°).

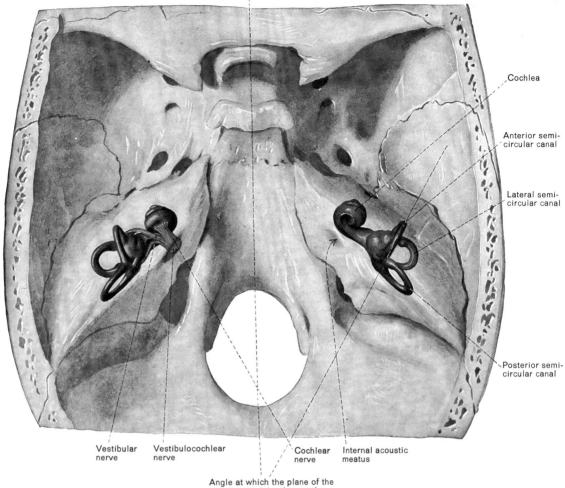

Cochlea

Anterior semicircular canal

Lateral semicircular canal

Posterior semicircular canal

Vestibular nerve

Vestibulocochlear nerve

Cochlear nerve

Internal acoustic meatus

Angle at which the plane of the anterior semicircular canal crosses the midsagittal plane

Fig. 593: The Right Membranous Labyrinth (Medial View)

NOTE: that the right membranous labyrinth and the branches of the vestibulocochlear nerve have been isolated from the bony labyrinth and shown somewhat diagrammatically. Observe the ampullae of the three semicircular ducts, the sacculus, the utriculus and the cochlear duct. The sites of connection of the endolymphatic duct to the utriculus and sacculus is also indicated.

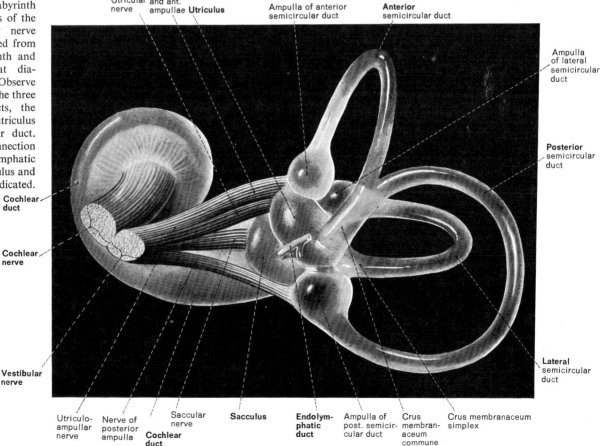

Nerve of lat. and ant. ampullae

Utricular nerve

Utriculus

Ampulla of anterior semicircular duct

Anterior semicircular duct

Ampulla of lateral semicircular duct

Posterior semicircular duct

Cochlear duct

Cochlear nerve

Vestibular nerve

Utriculo-ampullar nerve

Nerve of posterior ampulla

Saccular nerve

Cochlear duct

Sacculus

Endolymphatic duct

Ampulla of post. semicircular duct

Crus membranaceum commune

Crus membranaceum simplex

Lateral semicircular duct

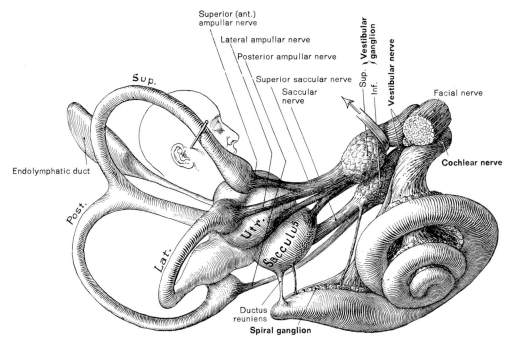

Fig. 594: The Right Membranous Labyrinth Viewed from the Lateral Aspect (Drawing by Max Brödel, 1934)

NOTE: 1) nerve branches from each of the ampullae of the semicircular ducts and from the utriculus and sacculus join to form the vestibular division of the vestibulocochlear nerve. The ganglion containing the sensory nerve cell bodies for this division is the vestibular (Scarpa's) ganglion and it has two parts, superior and inferior.

2) the cochlear division of the vestibulocochlear nerve serves the cochlear duct. Its ganglion, the spiral ganglion, is long and coiled. Observe the close relationship between the facial nerve and the vestibulocochlear nerve within the internal acoustic meatus. (Note that the superior semicircular duct is synonymous with the anterior semicircular duct.)

Fig. 595: Diagram of the Membranous Labyrinth Showing the Stapes

NOTE: 1) the bony structures are shown as cross hatched while the perilymphatic spaces are diagrammed as white. The membranous labyrinthine duct system (endolymphatic spaces) which contains the receptors is shown as black.

2) the stapes at the vestibular window. The cochlear window, shown close by, in life is covered by the second tympanic membrane.

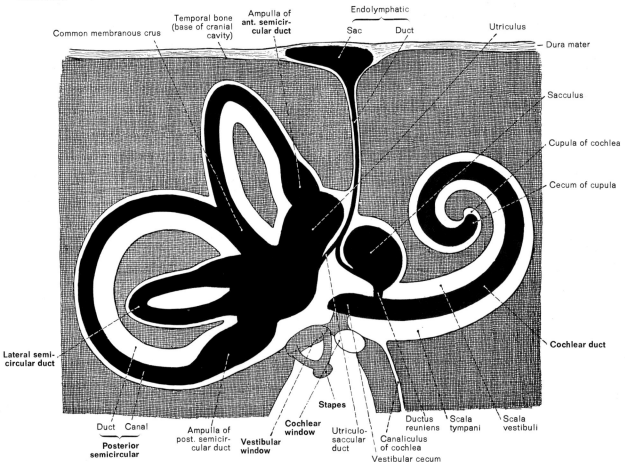

Index

Numbers in light-face type refer to figures in this *Atlas*. Numbers in **bold-face** type refer to pages in the 29th American Edition of *Gray's Anatomy* where additional relevant information concerning these structures may be obtained.

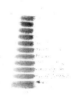

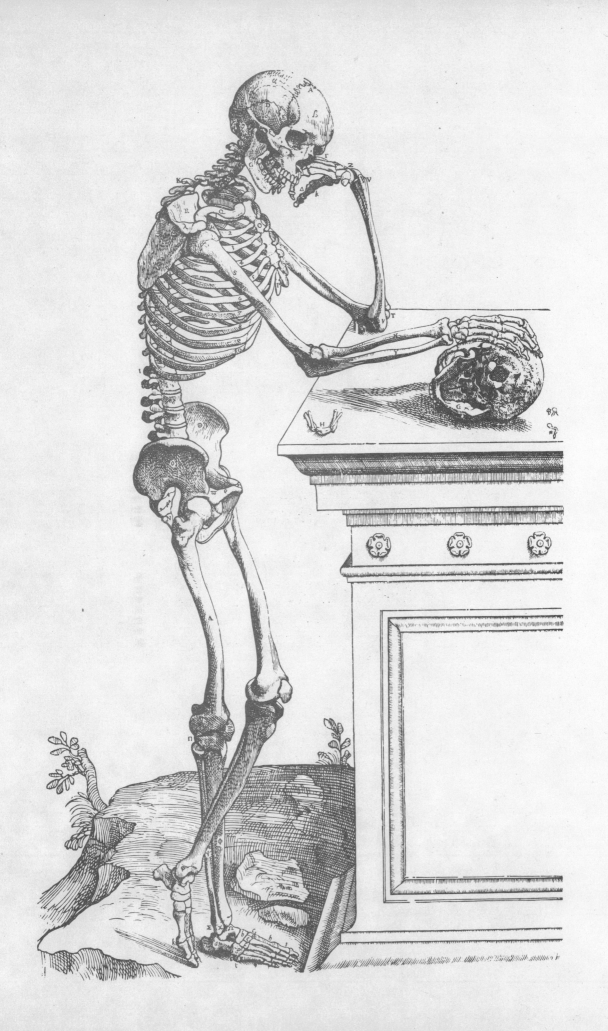